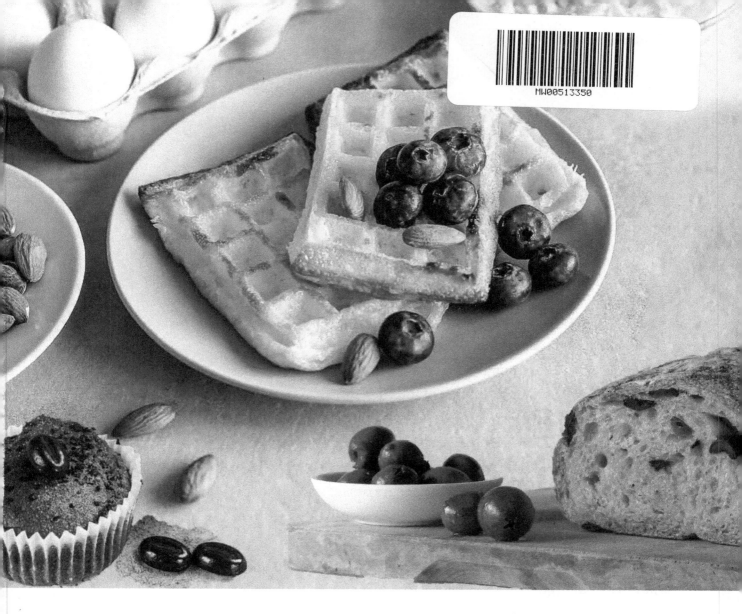

KETO DIET COOKBOOK FOR CARB LOVERS

3 BOOKS IN 1

ENJOY KETOGENIC WEIGHT-LOSS WITHOUT CARB CRAVINGS | EASY RECIPES FOR TRUE TO FLAVOR LOW-CARB FOOD | INCLUDES CHAFFLES, SNACKS & DESSERTS AND USING THE BREAD MACHINE

Amanda White

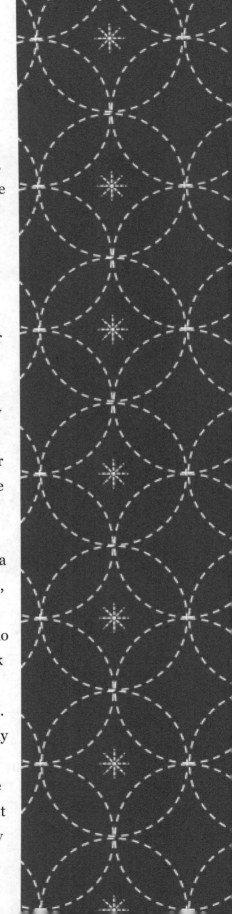

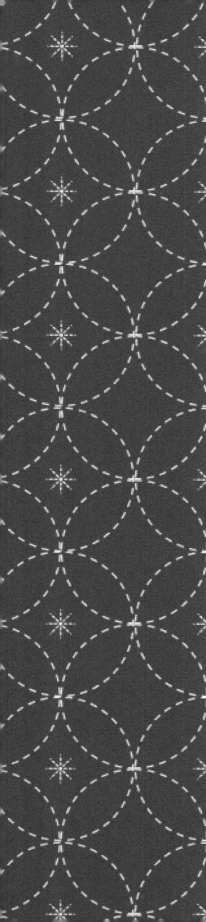

TABLE OF CONTENTS:

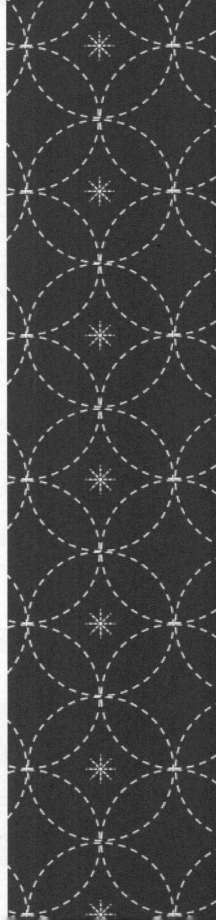

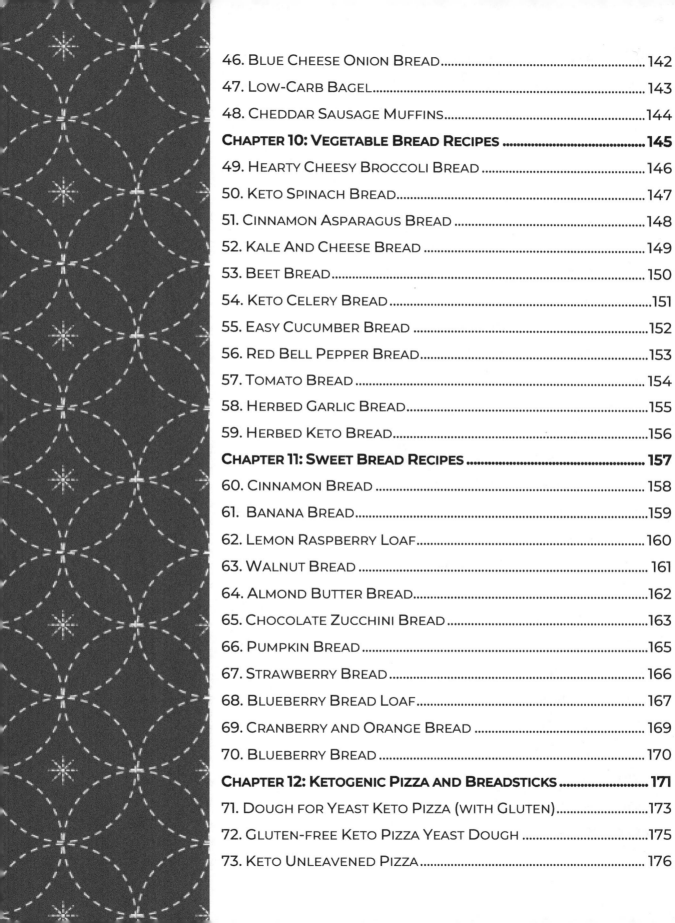

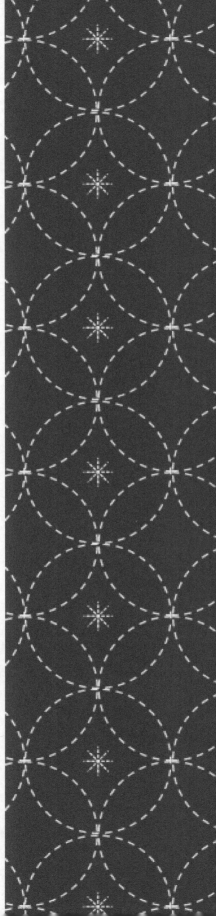

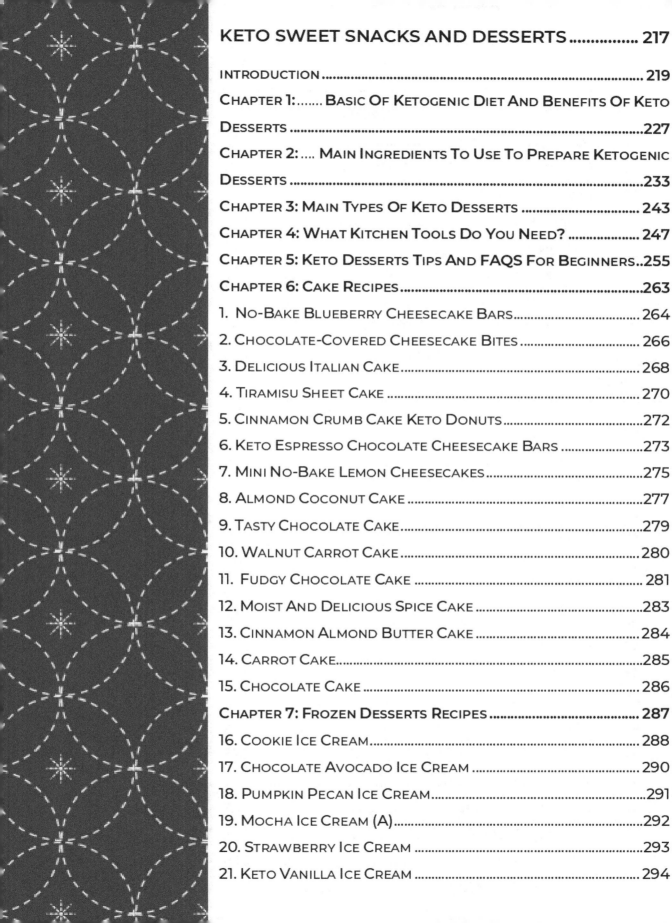

KETO SWEET SNACKS AND DESSERTS 217

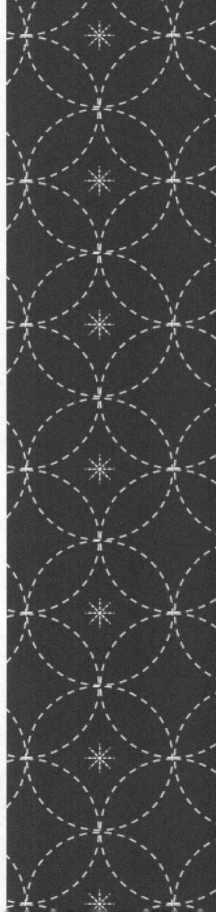

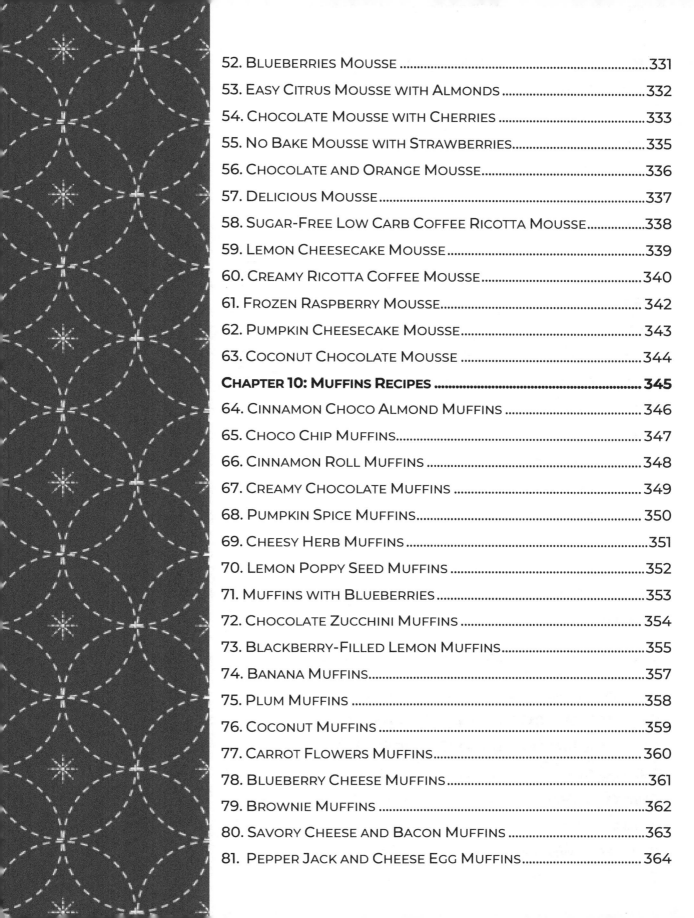

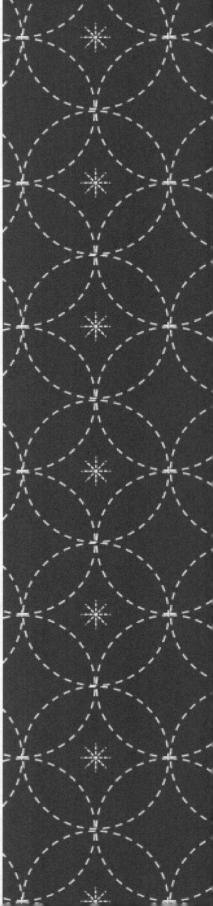

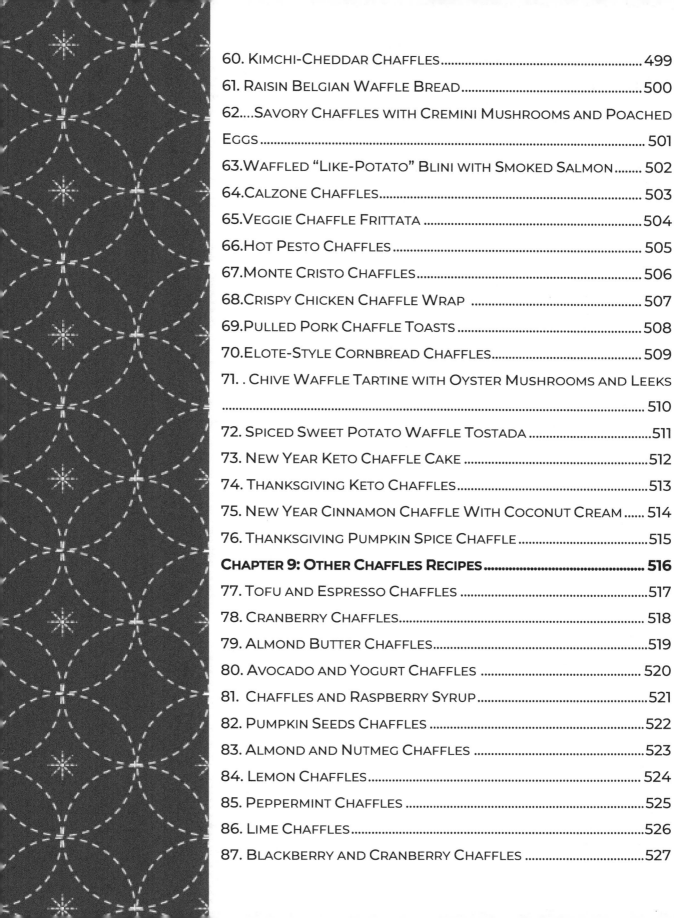

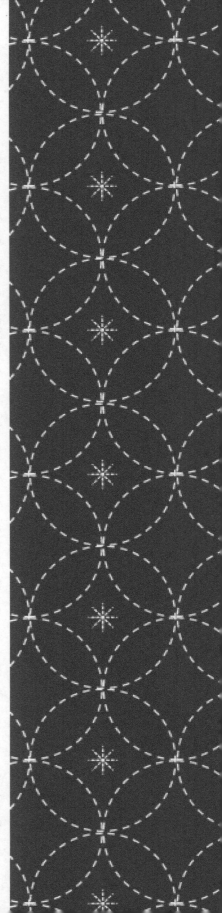

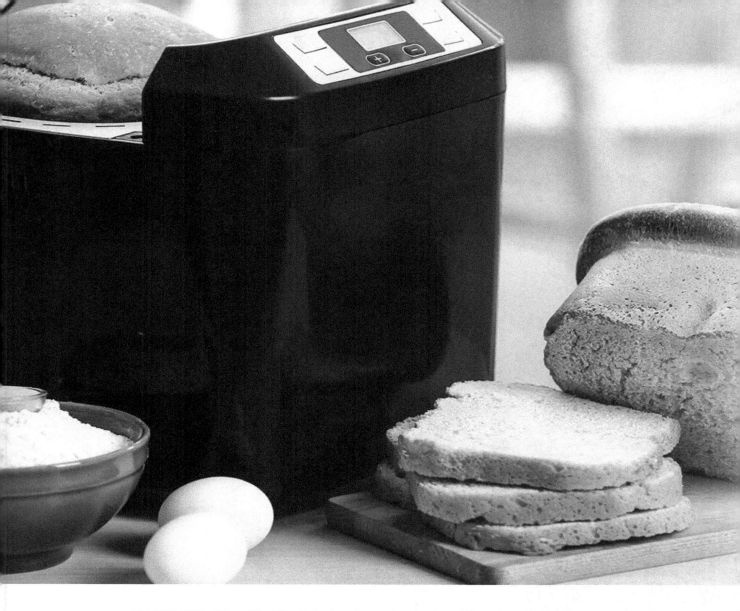

KETO BREAD MACHINE

THE ULTIMATE STEP-BY-STEP COOKBOOK WITH 101 QUICK AND EASY KETOGENIC BAKING RECIPES FOR COOKING DELICIOUS LOW-CARB AND GLUTEN-FREE HOMEMADE LOAVES IN YOUR BREAD MAKER

Amanda White

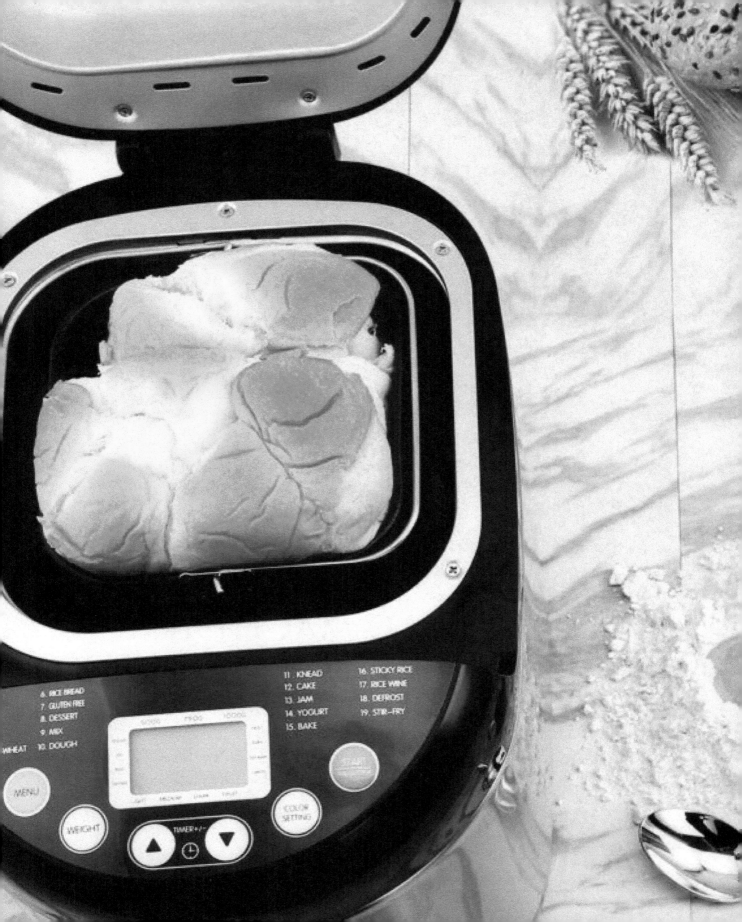

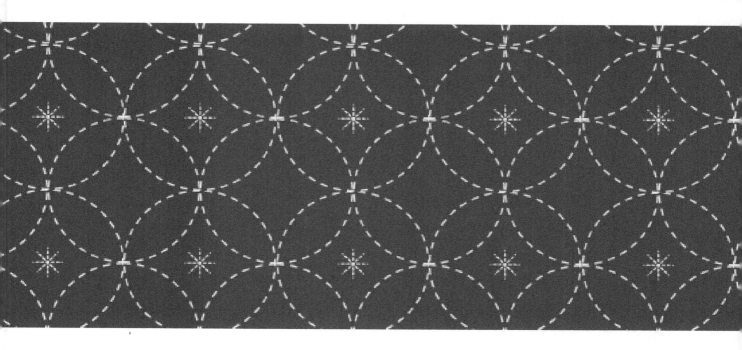

INTRODUCTION

Bread machine, also known as bread maker, a type of appliance that turns ingredients into baked bread. It comes with a bread pan at the bottom, which looks like paddles in a pizza oven. The bread machine is often controlled by a display panel.

The first bread maker was founded in Japan in 1986 by Panasonic. The purpose of this machine was to train the head bakers to knead bread. As it was industrialized, more companies started creating their own version of the bread machine. Some added a cooling fan at the bottom to allow the machine to cool off after use. Not too long after, it became famous in the United States, Europe, and Australia.

The bread machine is an all-in-one appliance. It takes the guesswork out of making bread by mixing, kneading, proving, and baking the dough. Usually, the bread machine takes a few hours to make a loaf.

Once done, the pan is removed from the bread-maker, which leaves a small hole on the rod where the paddle is attached. Do not be put off by the odd shape of the bread from the machine. It is normal to produce vertical, square, or cylindrical loaves, which is very different from commercialized loaves.

The bread machine is considerably smaller in size than the standard oven. And the usage is defined by the capacity of the bread machine itself. In most cases, the bread machine can accommodate up to 1.5 pounds or 700 grams of dough. There are also bread machines that can accommodate up to 900 grams of dough.

The typical bread maker comes with a built-in timer to control the start and end of the bread-making process. Most machines have a delayed start option, and this allows the bread to start baking even when you are asleep or at work, meaning you'll be greeted by a fresh loaf.

Homemade bread tends to go stale faster than commercial bread as it does not contain any preservatives. There is a natural way to preserve your bread, and it includes using a natural leaven and a pre-ferment in the bread machine. The reason behind this is that it contains a form of lactobacilli. The yeast is responsible for the flavor and the rising of the dough. The lactic acid is responsible for the preservation of the bread.

Before You Start!

Always remember to check the Directions on your bread machine. It varies across different models and types. So, before you start baking, make sure you know how to program your bread machine for the best quality bread. Your bread machine should come with a timing chart for the different types of bread.

There are bread machines that have their own weighing scale to ensure a proportionate amount of bread inside the machine. Check the capacity of your bread machine.

Basics About Ketogenic Diet and Bread

After this brief introduction where we have explained what a bread machine is, it is necessary to remember that in this cookbook, we are not going to bake classic bread made with cereal flours but, as you can understand from the title, the recipes will concern the preparation of bread that respects the rules of the ketogenic diet. In the first chapter, I'll explain in detail what the ketogenic diet is, but below I'll give you some quick tips to understand the subject of this cookbook. Probably you already know that the ketogenic diet is one of the most effective forms of weight loss. It helps you burn more fat using a diet that is high-fat and low-carbohydrates. The term "keto" originates from the "ketones" produced by the body when you are in ketosis. When you are in ketosis, your body has nothing to burn for fuel, so in place of the normal carbohydrates you consume, your body begins to burn your own excess body fat. When you keep yourself in ketosis long enough, you become "Fat Adapted", which means your body will automatically burn the excess fat.

Now you're probably wondering, "What is this ketogenic bread?" "How can I make it?"

As a staple food, bread is part of your daily meal plan, even if you are in ketosis. However, flour and sugar, as its main ingredient, make bread one of your number one enemy if you are in a keto diet. This does not mean though that you cannot have bread in your keto diet meal plan. As we'll see in chapter two, you can still eat any kind of bread by substituting flour with keto-friendly alternatives like almond flour and coconut flour.

All bread recipes are prepared with the bread machine and baked in the bread maker or, in some limited cases, in the normal kitchen oven.

But before you begin, you need to consider a few things. The ketogenic diet is not for everyone. If you are taking medications, consult your doctor first before engaging in this diet to avoid any complications.

Things to Keep in Mind as You Use the Recipes

You are probably going to come across a number of ingredients you haven't heard of before. Rest assured that these can be easily found in most local grocery stores. Some of these ingredients include:

Alternative keto-friendly flours, Psyllium Husk or Psyllium Husk Powder, Xanthan Gum, Inulin and others (see Chapter 2).

Sugar substitutes

As we've seen, sugar is not a food that is included in the keto diet. So, it is necessary to find low carb alternatives to replace the sweet taste of normal sugar. Some examples of substitutes that you can use are erythritol, stevia, sucralose, xylitol, and monk fruit sweetener. You will see this ingredient used in many recipes to give it some sweetness. It is also proven to help lower sugar levels in the body, making it a healthy alternative to traditional processed sugar. See Chapter 1 for best information on low-carb sweeteners.

Chapter 1: Everything You Need to Know About Ketogenic Diet

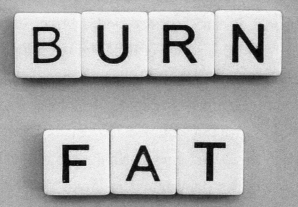

Thanks to the increasing demand for healthy diets and lifestyles, the ketogenic diet has taken center stage. Also known as a low-carb, high-fat meal plan, the keto diet restricts the intake of carbohydrates while promoting healthy fats. Usually, confectioneries and baked goods, snacks, and desserts contain the most carbs since they're predominantly made of sugars and flour. They're also the types of foods that people typically break their diets to eat.

Therefore, this cookbook is full of keto versions of snacks, desserts, and other treats that would normally be forbidden on the low-carb diet. Along with the recipes, you'll also get the ultimate ketogenic guidelines that explain basic information on ketogenic-friendly flours and sweeteners.

The Ketogenic Diet: Basic Concepts

After years of research and experimentation, scientists and nutritionists worked together to come up with an efficient formula that would not only treat mental illnesses like Alzheimer's and Parkinson's disease but also had a broad impact on general human health. This diet plan created miraculous effects like reducing obesity and controlling insulin in diabetic patients. It eventually came to be known as the ketogenic diet.

The word "keto" comes from the process of ketosis—a physical reaction in the body that this diet produces when appropriately followed. Ketosis is a metabolic process that uses stored fats for energy when there isn't enough glucose in the body to use. This makes it ideal for losing weight while also debunking the myth that fats in food are linked to weight gain. With this diet, the human body can harness more energy from food while producing ketones (a product of ketosis) that detoxify the blood and mind.

In order for any of this to work properly, you have to cut your carb intake using ketogenic carb recommendations. The main carb restriction states that your intake per meal should be no more than 13 grams of carbs. It also requires you to go to embrace high-fat foods instead. Combine this with regular exercise, and you can see the weight loss results you desire. To reduce carbohydrates in your diet, you'll need to remove or limit high-carb ingredients like all grains, lentils, legumes, potatoes, yams, yellow squash, sugars, honey, high-carb fruits, syrups, and the like. You can either avoid them or replace them with low-carb alternatives.

If a person successfully follows the ketogenic diet for about three to four weeks, they can witness marked changes in their physical and mental health. An obese person can lose about two to three pounds in this time period, and a diabetic patient can experience stable insulin levels. People with mental ailments can feel better control over their nerves and emotions, too. Following this diet and lifestyle over a long period of time can even decrease your risk of cancer and complicated cardiac diseases. Cholesterol levels can also be maintained following the ketogenic diet.

What to Eat and What Not to Eat on a Ketogenic Diet

Eating foods high in fat and low in carbs may sound simple, but it is more difficult to practically implement this idea if you are not familiar with the basics of nutrients. To help you, here is some brief insight regarding all the foods that are restricted and allowed on the ketogenic diet.

First, here are keto-friendly foods to add to your menu:

All dairy and plant fats are ideal for the ketogenic diet. This includes all forms of plants, oils, butter, ghee, cream, and cheese.

All dairy products except milk are suitable for a ketogenic diet. Since milk contains high traces of carbohydrates, it is restricted. When milk is processed to produce yogurt, cream cheese, cream, and other cheeses, the carbs are broken down, making them keto-friendly.

All vegetables low in carbs are allowed on the ketogenic diet, including all greens, above-ground vegetables, onions, garlic, ginger, and similar vegetables.

While most fruits should be limited or avoided, all berries and similar fruits are keto-friendly.

All sugar-free chocolates, sauces, and syrups are safe to use on a ketogenic diet. Ketogenic sugar substitutes are allowed.

Nut-based milk like almond milk, coconut milk, hemp milk, soy milk, etc. are also low-carb and, thus, safe to use.

While knowing what you can eat is great, knowing what not to eat on the ketogenic diet should be your major focus. First, get into the habit of reading labels and nutrition facts for every food you buy to make yourself comfortable with looking for carbs in food. You can't expect to control your carb intake without reading labels. Then, follow this list of high-carb ingredients while grocery shopping and keep them out of your kitchen.

All grains, legumes, lentils, and beans are rich in carbohydrates, so avoid them in any form. Rice, wheat, barley, oats, chickpeas, kidney beans, corn, sorghum, etc. are all a part of this category, too.

Potatoes, yams, beets, yellow squash, and similar vegetables are considered starchy vegetables and are high in carbs and should be avoided.

Apples, bananas, peaches, pears, melons, watermelons, mangoes, pineapples, and similar fruits are all carb-rich and are not allowed on the ketogenic diet.

Any amount of animal milk is restricted. Replace that with nut-based milk.

Flours from grains and lentils like wheat flour, all-purpose flours, and chickpea flour should be avoided and replaced with nut-based gluten-free flours.

White sugars, brown sugars, sugary syrups and beverages, maple syrups, honey, and dates are all forbidden on a ketogenic diet. Replace them with ketogenic sweeteners to add sweetness.

All processed foods with traces of carbohydrates need to be avoided.

Types of Gluten-Free Ketogenic Flours

Flours are an essential component of all baked desserts, bread, and confectioneries, so they can't be altogether avoided. Since grain- and lentil-based flours are not suitable for the ketogenic diet, look to other gluten-free options to produce the same products with a lower carb content. We will treat in more detail about these alternative flours in Chapter 2.

Low-carb Sweeteners

Sweeteners play an essential part in building the right balance of flavor in baked desserts. It's not just cakes or cookies that need sweeteners. Almost all desserts from custard to mousses, fat bombs, and ice creams need an excellent sweetener. Since sugar is not an option on a ketogenic diet, you should rely on other low-carb substitutes that are specially manufactured for such a diet. Those substitutes mainly include:

Stevia

Stevia is the strongest of all and tastes 200 times sweeter than ordinary white sugar. It should be used in minimal amounts. It is available in a range of varieties, including powdered and liquid form. Be extra careful while adding this intense sweetener to your recipes or use it as a blend with erythritol. One cup of sugar can be replaced with a teaspoon of stevia powder to get the same sweetness. Stevia is completely natural and comes from the stevia plant, so it doesn't have any adverse effects on your health. It has zero impact on blood sugar and is a great source of magnesium, zinc, potassium, vitamin B3.

Erythritol

Erythritol, a sugar alcohol produced naturally in fruits and from fermentation, is an exceptional natural and healthy low-carb sweetener that has bulking properties, which make it perfect for baking. Erythritol is a sweetener that leaves no aftertaste, and it is also easy on the stomach. Erythritol and erythritol blends can be used in keto snacks and desserts. Since erythritol has a sweetness level close to that of ordinary sugar, it is more commonly used for ketogenic desserts. As you'll see in the chart below, its conversion is simpler than stevia, too. Another plus point for erythritol is that it contains an extremely low amount of Calories. Where one gram of sugar has around four Calories, the same amount of erythritol contains only 0.24 Calories. Erythritol is available in a powdered form and can be used easily in baking.

Xylitol

Xylitol is also a naturally occurring sugar alcohol that can be used to sweeten ketogenic desserts. This is probably due to the taste and texture of this natural sweetener. It comes from plants like fruits and vegetables. Xylitol contains anti-bacterial properties that protect the mouth from bacteria that cause tooth decay. Due to its health benefits and curing powers, it is also added to medicines and mints to keep the gums and breath fresh. It is not only low in carbohydrates, but it contains few Calories and ranks very low on the glycemic index.

However, use Xylitol is small quantities to avoid gastrointestinal discomfort. Remind also to keep this product away from dogs because it is toxic to dogs.

Sorbitol

Another sugar alcohol, sorbitol, is found in several fruits, and it is also present in corn syrup. It is also known as a nutritive sweetener since it can provide as many as 2.6 kcals per gram. Like xylitol, it is also great for sweets, candies, mints, gummies, and bites. It has other medicinal properties that make it good for older people. Whether it's keto or any other diet, the use of this sweetener is always good for your health. It is 60 percent the sweetness of sugar, so 1 cup of sugar can be replaced with 1 ¼ cups of sorbitol.

Miscellaneous Sweeteners

In recent years, with the diffusion of low carbohydrate diets, a considerable number of sweetening blends have appeared on the market with the aim of replacing classic sugar. Below are some of the best known that we will use in the recipes of this cookbook:

Swerve

Swerve is a blend of oligosaccharides and erythritol; it is a natural and healthy low carb sweetener that has zero impact on blood sugar. Swerve is another ketogenic sweetener not only used in baking, but also for ice creams, mousses, fat bombs, and other desserts. Swerve is available in all forms, including powder, granulated, white, and even brown, making it perfect for adding texture to different baked items. It can also be added into tea or coffee with no aftertaste and can also be used to cook. Swerve can be used to replace sugar in any recipe, as the same amounts of sugar and swerve have equal sweetness.

Natvia

Natvia, a blend of stevia and erythritol, is also a natural sweetener. Natvia eliminates the intense aftertaste of stevia, yet retaining its sweetness and combining it with the bulking properties of erythritol to make a perfect healthy low carb sweetener suitable for baking.

Monk Fruit

Monk fruit sweetener is another good option to sweeten your ketogenic desserts and to give them pleasant taste and texture.

Conversion Chart

Below is a handy conversion table to make the replacement between white sugar and low carb sweeteners in an easy way:

SUGAR	1 TSP	1 TBSP	1/4 CUP	1/3 CUP	1/2 CUP	1 CUP
Erythritol	1 1/4 tsp	1 Tbsp + 1 tsp	1/3 cup	1/3 cup + 2 Tbsp	2/3 cup	1 1/3 cup
Xylitol	1 tsp	1 Tbsp	1/4 cup	1/3 cup	1/2 cup	1 cup
Swerve	1 tsp	1 Tbsp	1/4 cup	1/3 cup	1/2 cup	1 cup
Stevia	-	-	3/16 tsp	1/4 tsp	3/8 tsp	3/4 tsp
Liquid Stevia	3/8 tsp	3/8 tsp	1 1/2 tsp	2 tsp	3 tsp	2 Tbsp
Sukrin	1 tsp	1 Tbsp	1/4 cup	1/3 cup	1/2 cup	1 cup

Sugar Alcohols Glycemic Index

They are considered dietary fibers due to their chemical composition.

The glycemic index of a food is used to determine if it's suitable for the ketogenic diet. Since sugar has the highest glycemic value 60, all other sweeteners are compared to this value to calculate their glycemic values. Here is a list of commonly used sugar alcohols along with their glycemic values:

Sugar Alcohols	Glycemic Index
Xylitol	12
Glycerol	5
Sorbitol	4
Lactitol	3
Isomalt	2
Mannitol	2
Erythritol	1

Benefits of Ketogenic Diet

The Keto diet is famous not only because you are able to lose weight fast but also because it has many other benefits. Changing your eating habits will positively affect your body. Not only will you look good, but your body will feel good, too! You will start noticing changes in your body within the first week or two of being on this diet. Eliminating the toxins, you were used to ingesting will make a difference. The list below is not comprehensive by any means but will give you a good idea of what benefits that the Keto diet has to offer aside from the sought-out weight loss that the Keto diet is known for. Almost everyone will see significant improvements from the diet, whether it be from the list below or from other things that have not been mentioned. Since we are all different, and our bodies all react differently, you may experience things that others may or will not experience.

The following list is what I have thought to be profound benefits that the Keto diet has to offer.

Nonalcoholic Fatty Liver Disease

Nonalcoholic fatty liver disease is a disease when your liver stores too much in its cells. The fat cells that the liver stores are not related to actual fat but to carbs. The livers transform the carbs into triglycerides and store them as fat. This disease affects people of all ages who are at risk of being overweight or obese, have high blood pressure, have type 2 diabetes, to name a few. This disease could potentially have no sign or symptom, but some people have reported fatigue and pain in their upper right abdomen, spider-like blood vessels, jaundice (the yellowing of the skin) and edema (swelling of the legs). Since the possible warning signs are linked to other ailments, there are often other tests that your doctor may have you take, such as blood and imaging test.

Potential complications from this disease are the liver swelling. This swelling can cause scarring, which could potentially lead to liver or even liver failure. There are no medications to help this condition as of yet, but the Keto diet has helped countless people remove the carbs that their diets once had, therefore, lowering the triglycerides. The fat cells do not build up, but instead, the liver uses it as energy. In some cases, people who have had scarring on their livers show a significant improvement because the body is essentially going through a rejuvenation process that will lead to a healthy you!

High Blood Sugar

We have sugar in our blood. The correct amounts are vital because sugar causes our body's cells and organs to obtain the energy we need to survive. If your body receives too much sugar, instead of having an abundance of energy, you start to feel unwell. Your body cannot break down as much of the overflow of sugar, and this is why you start feeling the symptoms of high blood sugar. You feel drowsy, tired, have blurred vision, headaches, you have a hard time concentrating, tend to be thirsty, having to urinate quite often, to name a few. These are short-term complications for having high blood sugar. Long-term complications can possibly include a heart attack or stroke, kidney failure and nerve problems. There are many causes of having high blood pressure. Your medical professional is able to diagnose long-term issues with high blood pressure as type 1 or 2 diabetes and, in some cases, gestational diabetes. Diabetes is caused when your body is unable to make insulin, or there is not enough insulin to break down any sugar produced by carbs.

Gestational diabetes only occurs in women who are pregnant. Being on the Keto diet will help you be able to manage your diabetes by eliminating the carbs that are not able to be broken down by the insulin. You may also be able to reduce the medications you are prescribed. The lack of carbs in your system will make it easier for your body's functions.

Improved Digestion

Many of us have a problem with our digestive systems. From diarrhea, IBS (irritable bowel syndrome), constipation, and heartburn. We have all had at least three of these once in our lives. Constipation usually occurs when you are not eating enough fiber or not drinking enough water, among other things. On the opposite end, there is diarrhea. This can be caused by multiple things as well as consuming artificial sweeteners, or certain additives. Acid reflux or heartburn is caused by stomach fluids backing up into your esophagus. Different types of foods can cause this back up, especially if they are fatty or fried foods. Being overweight also has a high risk of heartburn. IBS or irritable bowel syndrome affects your large intestine. The symptoms for it are bloating, gas, cramping. Diarrhea or constipation. The triggers of IBS include but aren't limited to certain fatty foods, i.e., deep-fried and carbonated drinks. Removing all the fired, greasy and carbonated drinks from your diet will help you improve your digestion. Everyone can benefit from the Keto diet because we all have experienced digestive problems at one time or another. The Keto diet helps you stay on track to avoid all these foods and stick to the healthy ones that will not cause all the above-stated issues.

Lowering Triglycerides

Triglycerides, as stated before, are a type of fat found in your body. If you have high triglycerides, you are at risk for your arteries to harden, which dramatically increases your risk of a stroke, heart attack or heart disease. Your medical professional has probably checked your levels at one point with a "lipid panel". This is how they diagnosis this. If you focus on what you eat and exercise, you will have a better chance of lowering them. Avoiding sugar and refined carbs can increase these levels. In addition, eating foods with Trans fats or hydrogenated oils or fats can increase levels as well. Focusing on healthier fats such as red meat and fish will help combat high levels. If you are prescribed medications for high triglycerides, the medication and an improvement in your diet should help reduce those dangerous high levels.

Depression

Depression is categorized as a mood disorder that causes a constant feeling of sadness. It also causes people to lose interest in things they once loved. This mood disorder is a constant in your life, and you cannot one day wake up and be a happier you. Some symptoms of depression include hopelessness, anger, and frustration, being tired all the time, having no energy, trouble thinking, and anxiety feeling of guilt and sleep disturbances. There are still studies conducted on what exactly causes depression, but so far, research has shown that what can lead to depression may be brain chemistry and how neurotransmitters react with other chemicals that should create mood stability.

Some other studies have shown that it might be an inherited trait. A blood relative might have passed down a gene with this particular trait that lacks the function to balance out your moods. Your body needs to be able to convert glutamate (a transmitter that your body has to get "messages" to the brain; you're welcome! I didn't know what this was either!) Into GABA (this is the body's main neurotransmitter). You need the right balance of both to have your brain function normally. When you are on a high carb diet, your brain isn't able to convert enough glutamate to GABA. This means that your body is suffering from neurotoxicity. Having your body goes into Ketosis, it seems to encourage the balance of both glutamate and GABA, which alleviates the symptoms of depression.

Acne

Acne, as many of us know, is a skin condition that starts from adolescence during puberty and sometimes follows us into our adult life. The root cause of acne is when a pore in your skin becomes clogged, bacteria, excess of the androgens hormone, or excess oil production. There are different types of acne, which include whiteheads, blackheads, and pimples (zits). They can appear on your face, forehead, chest upper back, and shoulders. We know how slightly they can be and sometimes painful! There are many myths surrounded by what affects acne, such as the makeup you wear, hygiene and eating greasy foods. One of the actual triggers that can lead to acne is your diet.

Eating too many carbohydrate-rich foods. Eating all these carbs can alter your stomach bacteria because you are adding excess sugar to your bloodstream, which can cause inflammation of the skin, among other things. If you reduce your intake of these carbs, you reduce the risk of inflamed skin. You can also consume more fatty fish that are rich in omega-3, eat the lowest carb-filled vegetables and limit your dairy intake to maximize the benefit.

Heart Health

Keto can also benefit your heart health! Losing weight and can help you lessen the risk of heart disease. This is two for the price of one! Cardiovascular disease is actually an umbrella term that incorporates various issues that affect your health regarding blood vessels or heart problems. This disease is when your heart is damaged by the buildup of plaque in the heart's major blood vessels. The buildup limits the blood flow to the heart, and this will limit the flow of oxygen as well. Your doctor will typically run a lab test in order to diagnosis you. This disease is very common and affects approximately 3 million people across the United States. CAD can end up weakening the heart muscles, which in turn can cause heart failure. Heart failure is when your heart cannot pump the blood the rest of your body needs. CAD can also cause heart arrhythmias. Heart arrhythmias are changes in the way your heartbeats. Instead of having a steady beat, it is either beating too fast, too slow or irregularly. By reducing the intake of carbs, you can try and reduce or not add any more of the buildup of the fatty deposits that are associated with the CAD.

Brain Health

Epilepsy is a central nervous system disorder that causes brain activity to become abnormal. There are different types of symptoms, including twitching in the arms or possibly legs, as well as staring out into nothingness for a short period of time with a blank stare. Once you have a seizure, your seizures typically tend to stay the same, and nothing will change drastically. There are many causes of this disorder. A few are head trauma, brain conditions such as tumors or strokes, and injuries to the brain before birth, such as lack of oxygen and developmental disorders.

Your medical will evaluate your symptoms and order a neurological exam, which includes testing motor skills and mental focus as well as blood exams, EEGs, CT scans, MRI, PETs, to name a few. Several studies have shown that the Keto diet has been linked to patients who have seen a reduction in the number of seizure episodes they have. Having the body go into the ketosis stage helps in altering your brain's metabolism to reduce the risk of having seizures. Many experts use the Keto diet as an aid to reduce seizures. Patients are still medicated but are still on the Keto diet to bring out the best outcome for the patient. Studies are being conducted for more brain conditions in hopes of either finding a cure or helping patients live a better life.

Migraines

Migraines are caused when nerve cells are overactive ad send out the incorrect signals to the nerves that are connected to your head and face. Sending these signals causes the chemical to be released and cause the blood vessels in the lining of your brain to swell. This is what causes the unbearable pain you experience when you have a migraine. There are a few triggers for migraines like changes in the weather, changes in your sleeping habits, skipping meals, caffeine, stress, and food. When you suffer from migraines, you typically experience different "stages" before the actual onset of the migraine. Stage 1 is the prodromal stage. The second stage is called the Aura stage. Stage 3 is the Attack stage. The last stage is called the postdrome stage. In the first stage, you experience either high energy or being extremely depressed.

You can also experience cravings, the need to urinate quite often and sleepiness. In the second stage, you start noticing changes in your vision, and you may feel like you are on "pins and needles" and also may have difficulties with speaking or writing. In the third stage, the actual migraine begins. In this stage, you may have a migraine for, hopefully, just a few hours, or it can last for several days. You are sensitive to light, you feel throbbing, and it may only affect one side of your face or, in some cases, your whole face. Some people even have said they experience nausea and vomiting. In the last stage and when the migraine is over, you feel exhausted and sometimes confused.

A study done around 2009 showed that people who were on the Keto diet showed reduced signs of migraines. The researchers were first trying to have the patients lose weight to see if that would help them overall. The patients who were doing the Keto diet were the patients that had experienced the greatest reduction of migraines. They also had their non-overweight patients that suffer from migraines get on the Keto diet as well, and they too had reduced amounts of migraines. Because of the low carbs in the Keto diet, researchers have found that it reduces the migraine, causing inflammation of the blood vessels in the lining of your brain.

Muscle Mass and Performance

While you are on the Keto diet, you can increase your muscle mass as well. Carbs are not necessary to build the lean muscles some people are looking to create. In order to build muscle, you need to eat enough proteins, eating the calories in healthy fats and you need to weight train. You might gain muscle mass quicker if you are eating carbs, but you need to remember that in eating carbs, you will be eating the unhealthy fats that make you gain weight. If you are looking to maintain the lean muscles that you worked hard for, it is easier to maintain them on the Keto diet because you are losing fat and not your muscle mass. Studies have also shown that the Keto diet doesn't decrease your performance. Your body is just using a different way to energize itself. When you start the Keto diet, you will see a little slowdown in your performance, but this is expected because your body is going through a change that will take time to get adapted to. Once your body has now become accustomed to the way it is now converting fats into ketones, it will go back to where it once was performance-wise. You need to remember, though, to make sure that you are eating enough protein, calories, and training correctly, which are vital. The Keto diet will hurt your body's performance, nor will it hinder you from gaining or maintaining muscle mass. The benefits listed here are just the tip of the iceberg when it comes to all the health benefits that the Keto diet has to offer. Usually, enhanced weight loss is what people think of when they hear "Keto diet." Most are not aware of the vast benefits that are associated with the diet.

A quick non-in depth assessment of other benefits include helping to manage your appetite. It is a way to maintain your weight because your body is always burning your fat; it can help aid in the treatment of metabolic syndrome. It also aids in fighting different diseases, which can include Parkinson's, TBI (Traumatic Brain Injury), and Alzheimer's, to name just a few. Researchers are also starting to look into how the Keto diet may help with the possible removal of sugar consumption and replace it in hopes of killing off the cancer cells.

You will also feel more energized. Who doesn't want to feel this way!? Since your cutting the dreaded carbs, you will not be getting the effects of the sugar rushes that your body was used to, and you will always have that steady source of energy and not the sporadic one that we all wish would last for days. You will see a significant change in your overall mood and memory. Since you are eliminating ingredients that are not natural, your body will only be processing foods that it should be, therefore not sending out unhealthy toxins that affect your mood and memory. Wouldn't it be nice to remember where you placed your keys instead of looking for them for about ten minutes before you realize they are in your hands? No? Was that just me?

The Keto diet will also help with recovering faster from exercise. Deciding to add that extra five or ten pounds to your training regimen and dreading the next few days because of the achy and sore muscles will be a thing of the past. You will be able to recover faster because your body will not be as inflamed because of the reduction of carbs.

CHAPTER 2: MAIN INGREDIENTS TO USE TO PREPARE KETOGENIC BREAD

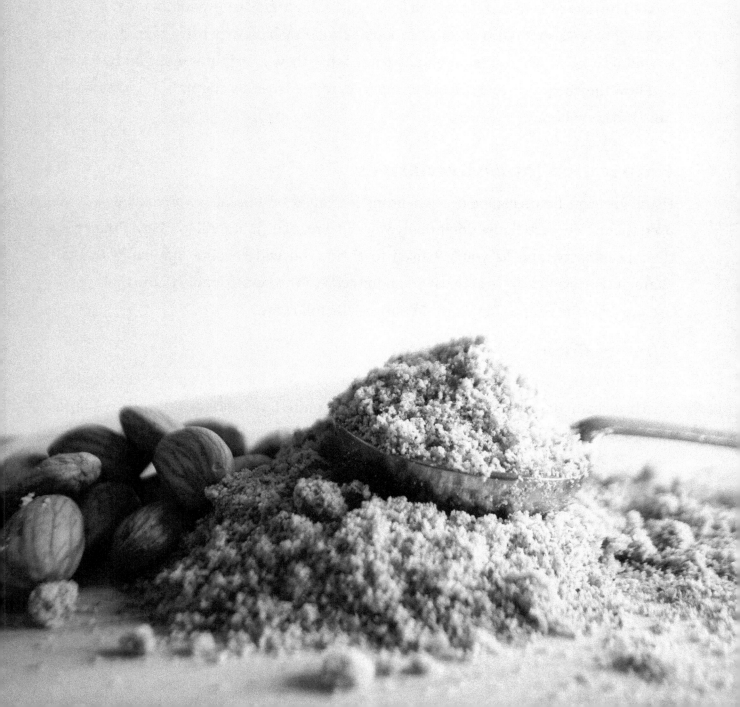

Enjoying the best flavors and textures of our baked bread ought to be more than having something to fold around a burger, satisfy your hungry appetite, or satisfying your cravings with excessive empty calories. I'm sure you must have heard about completely abstaining from bread if you want to live the Keto lifestyle, well I am happy to let you know that keto bread can now be an exciting addition to your daily nutritional goals. This is because, unlike your regular bread, keto bread is made with unique ingredients that uphold the law of keto dieting, which is low carbs, high-fat diet predominantly.

Even though we shall be spending our hard-earned cash on expensive ingredients, it is essential to know where they originate from, what they contribute to our body system, and how they help us. Here are the primary ingredients, and a couple of minors used in Keto bread making.

Ketogenic Flour Alternatives

Using low carb flours can be overwhelming for you at first because you may never have used them. Low carb flours don't really work like regular flours. All low carb flours have their peculiarity, and as you get used to them, you will become familiar with their characteristics and how best to use them in recipes. The keto-friendly flours that we will use most for the recipes in this cookbook are the following:

Almond flour

This flour comes from almonds finely ground into a powder and is used for baking low-carb bread and desserts. It is rich in minerals, vitamins, and also provides more calories than other nuts. Almond flours are made by blanching almonds to remove the skins and then grinding them until a fine floury-consistency is reached. ¼ cup or about 28g almond flour contains 160 Calories and 3g net carbs. Store almond flour in a well-lidded container and keep refrigerated after opening. The rules you need to follow are given below:

- Use only dried or fresh almonds.
- Grind a small number of almonds at a time.

- Don't grind a portion for over thirty seconds.
- Slightly shake the blender or grinder as you go.

Most almond flour brands are more coarsely ground, which influences the final texture in baked products. In thick or brisk-type bread, this doesn't generally make a difference. However, when we're trying to achieve more tender loaf— white bread, Challah, French-style—the appearance and taste response are important. Search for brands that show they are finely ground.

They are pricier, but you will be more joyful with the finished product.

Almond Meal

Almond meal, also known as ground almonds, has the same amount of macros as the almond flour and contains the same amounts of minerals and vitamins. The difference between almond meal and almond flour is the absence of blanching. The almonds are ground with their skin-on until a slightly rough consistency is reached. It can be used in many baking recipes as an alternative to almond flour. Almond meal can be likened to the consistency of cornmeal. But almond meal is not the same as almond flour. Meal is coarser and not ideal for every bread, dessert, or confectionery. Instead, it's only used when you need a crumbly texture for a recipe. Keep this differentiation in your mind when choosing ingredients; don't substitute one for the other.

The almond meal should also be stored in a well-lidded container and refrigerated after opening.

Coconut Flour

Coconut flour is another low-carb flour that is very high in fiber and protein and, as the name indicates, comes from the dehydrated white flesh of a coconut. It is so finely ground that it turns into flour and gives a nice texture and taste to recipes. The texture of coconut flour is not exactly like wheat flour; it is denser and can soak up more moisture than wheat flour. Due to this, extra water or liquid needs to be added to give coconut flour the same texture batters or doughs. The ability to absorb more moisture is one of the characteristics of coconut flour. This flour can also make lots of clumps in a batter; use a good beater or whisk your mixtures well with a fork to break up any clumps.

As a beginner, do not do without the extra moisture, butter, or eggs you find in recipes. 2 tbsp or 18 g coconut flour contains 45 Calories and 2 net carbs.

Store coconut flour in a well-lidded container or sealed bag and keep it in a dark pantry out of direct sunlight.

Advantages of coconut flour are given below:

- Coconut flour is rich in protein, fiber, and iron.
- The protein content in the coconut flour is comparable or higher than in whole-grain wheat.
- The coconut flour does not have the distinctive exotic taste like coconut butter, cream, and milk.

Disadvantages of coconut flour:

- The high-fiber content can cause a problem for some types of bread.

Secrets of cooking with coconut flour:

- Always sift the flour before using it.
- Mix dough more thoroughly than with usual flour.
- Watch the baking time.

White Bean Flour

It has a gentle, smooth nutty flavor and braces our shortlist of useable flours in keto bread making. It contains a one of a kind fiber called resistant starch, which implies that unlike refined carbohydrates that basically melts and blends into our circulatory systems, it goes through the small intestine, for the most part, as undigested fiber. It enhances digestive health by promoting the development of useful microorganisms and manages blood glucose levels because the energy is discharged later in the large intestine, averting sharp spikes and diminishes between meals. Other significant by-products of this flour's digestive process are chemical compounds called "short-chain unsaturated fatty acids," which help counteract colon disease by preventing the absorption of cancer-causing agents (carcinogens). When compared with other flours, it contains the most starches. However, its advantages are more.

Ground Flaxseed

Flaxseeds are a rich source of healthy fats, vitamins, minerals, and antioxidants, making them quite beneficial for digestion and heart health. Flaxseed flour and meal can both be used in the ketogenic diet.

Flaxseed bread, muffins, and cookie recipes are in this book to give you a simple idea on how to use this super nourishing seed flour or meal. Processed flaxseed flour is available at most grocery stores.

Flax Meal

Flaxseed or ground flax is very nourishing and a great source of Vitamin B1, Copper, and Omega – 3. Like an almond meal, flaxseed meal is coarser than the ground flaxseed so take that into account when following recipes. Ground flaxseeds are a good alternative for eggs in some baking recipes. Substitute a mixture of 3 tbsp. of water and 1 tbsp. ground flax meal for 1 egg and let sit until moisture is absorbed. This alternative only works for recipes that are not heavily egg-based. 2 tbsp. or 14 g of ground flax meal contains 70 Calories and 1 g Net Carb. To prevent staleness, store flax meal in a well-lidded mason jar and refrigerate or freeze before and after you open it.

Pumpkin seed/Sunflower seed meal

These flours can conveniently replace almond meal or almond flour in any recipe. You can use a food processor or coffee grinder to make your own homemade pumpkin seed or sunflower meals. Pumpkin and sunflower seeds meal can be stored in a cool, dark pantry for up to 4 months.

How to replace gluten?

No gluten-free flour, or any blend thereof, can copy the flexibility, gas–holding and binding characteristics of gluten. It does superb, magical things, allowing ease of kneading and stretching, creating superbly chewy, fluffy, and airy bread. Unfortunately, all the ketogenic flours we have seen are gluten-free. This can be appreciated by those who have a gluten intolerance, but its absence is felt when baking baked goods. So what are our other options to replace it?

Egg whites have been a major help; however, something more is needed to achieve the desired texture and suppleness we're searching for.

We have three essential gluten—substitution choices: xanthan gum, psyllium and oat fibers; there's also ground seeds like chia and flaxseeds that become gelatinous when water is added.

Xanthan Gum

Before we move onto the fun part of baking, you must learn that xanthan gum is going to be your new best friend. You may not realize this, but many of the gluten-free flour alternatives lack a binding agent. A binding agent is helpful to hold your food together, much like gluten does when used in baking and cooking. The moment you remove gluten, all mixtures will typically crumble and fall apart. Xanthan gum is made from lactose, sucrose, and glucose that have been fermented from a specific bacterium. When this is added to liquid, it creates a gum and is used with gluten-free baking. As a general guide, you will be using one teaspoon of xanthan gum for one cup of gluten-free flour that you use. For some mixes, this gum is already added, so when you are baking, you will always want to check the ingredient label. It should be noted that xanthan gum can be expensive, but it will last you a long time.

If you have an allergy to xanthan gum, you can find ways around it. Instead, you can try using psyllium husks, ground flaxseeds, or ground chia seeds. Psyllium can be sold in full husks or powder. As you bake more, you will soon find what works for you and what doesn't!

Psyllium Husk Powder

This commonly known husk is obtained from the seeds of Plantago ovata. Basically, it is an excellent soluble fiber supplement. Available in both powder and husk form, this supplement is also good for the ketogenic diet. Unflavored psyllium husks are sold both whole and as a ground powder. Powdered psyllium makes for dense bread. Psyllium seed husk helps to produce a bread-like texture, as it replaces gluten to a certain extent. The husk is highly absorbent, so although the bread will not have the same airy texture as gluten-rich bread, its inclusion produces a moisture loaf. There is no carbohydrate content since the husk is pure fiber.

The powder is suitable to use in several ketogenic breads, desserts, and confectioneries as it has a light and airy touch that gives food a fluffy and soft texture.

Oat fiber

Oat fiber is a powdered fiber. It is pure fiber, not a flour; it is obtained by grinding the skin and shell of oatmeal grains. It should not be confused with oatmeal, which is derived from the grain itself (separated from the peel) and, due to its high carbs content, is not suitable for preparing ketogenic foods.

Practically oat fibers consist only of ground husks and are generally not used as the main ingredient for baking. The product obtained by grinding the hull is made up of over 90% insoluble fibers and is practically free of carbohydrates and calories.

This type of fiber is known to absorb water easily (up to 7 times its weight). This allows it to bind easily to fat and retain moisture, making bakery products more workable. They are, therefore, ideal in addition to the other alternative flours mentioned in this chapter to improve the consistency of the dough.

Oat fibers also help intestinal regularity and are gluten-free.

Protein Source Ingredients

Natural Whey Protein Powder

This obviously cannot be described as flour for any reason; however, to make keto bread, it is an incredible substitution. Whey is the fluid that is left after the main phases of cheese production and then processed into a concentrated powder. It is viewed as total protein and contains every one of the nine essential amino acids. Studies have proven that, in addition to improving muscle quality (which helps the muscle to burn more calories), these essential amino acids help avert cardiovascular diseases, diabetes, and age-related bone loss. And there's more—from anti-cancer properties to improving food reaction in kids with asthma. Even though It must be enhanced with our other flours, it breaks down rapidly to help make delectable, healthy, nutrient-rich baked products.

You can find 100% natural unflavored whey protein from health food portions at online stores, and they are likely to be more affordable than the various brands sold in the grocery stores. It is important to search for products without any additives and also consider the brands and costs while shopping.

Egg Whites

Having lots of egg whites in a recipe are genuinely economical and simple to plan. I get them in two different ways; in powder form in a 36-ounce canister that equals 255 egg whites and; in the fluid form, which can be bought with discounts at stores like Costco or 1-quart containers in nearby staple goods. I have seen wide varieties in cost, so be sure to compare before buying. Since they are pasteurized, they won't whip so well as new whites, however adding a small quantity of cream of tartar will make excellent, fluffy steeps similarly as high as using fresh egg whites.

Egg whites are essentially 90% water and 10% proteins, which are long chains of amino acids. When we beat air into the whites, these chains become denatured, which implies they unwind and stretch into shapes that trap air, making light textures in what we bake. There is a school of thought that heating/cooking protein—which includes protein powders like whey—decimates the nutritional worth because our bodies can't assimilate "denatured" foods. This is false. If that were the case, we would need to eat everything raw, right?! Eggs, meat, all that we cook and prepare are denatured when warmed. The food leaves the stove changed in appearance, yet the protein isn't denatured; rather than being folded into tight molecular balls, the protein chains become long strands.

Cooked or raw, our bodies retain the same essential amino acids. Understanding what denaturing truly is, enables us to appreciate many healthy foods, unhindered by senseless arguments.

Ingredients for Leavening and Baking

Yeast

I buy ACTIVE dry yeast in economical 2-pound bundles and store it in a zip–lock bag in the freezer. It just takes two or three minutes for one tablespoon of yeast powder to warm to room temperature. I measure it straight from the freezer, (speedily returning it), regularly adding it to the bowl of dry ingredients without proofing (allowing it to break down and activate it into a froth before adding to the batter).

Yeast production today is very reliable. Proofing is only useful if it is past the expiry date, and you have to test whether it is still good and can be useful. It will activate when it interacts with the fluid fixings in the blending procedure. There is just one rise with low–carb bread. This is my hypothesis, though, however, since yeast has so little to eat—essentially only a tablespoon of Honey—I don't need it to generate the entirety of its energy in a different dish; I need its work to begin inside the batter. I tried this, one loaf with sealed yeast included and the other with the yeast entering the batter dry; the subsequent loaf rose higher. All brand name names of yeast sold in North America are without gluten except for brewer's yeast utilized in lager production.

Honey

Don't be scared to hear about honey or sugar in a ketogenic cookbook; I'm not crazy. Honey is important to give food to the yeast and activate it since the flours used in keto diet don't contain sugars to eat or starches to convert into glucose. For the same reason, you can use ordinary sugar, if you like. Obviously, just one tablespoon is used for the whole formula and separated into 8, 12, or 16 servings, and our portion is quite small. It should also be remembered that practically all this tablespoon will be used as food by the yeast and will be converted into alcohol and carbon dioxide. So there will be any sugar left in your ketogenic bread. According to the American Diabetes Association, consuming white sugar increases blood glucose levels somewhat quicker than Honey, which has a glycemic run somewhere in the range of 31 and 78 relying upon the variety.

Locust honey, for example, has a glycemic index (GI) of 32; clover honey has 69. You can investigate this further on online sites like the Glycemic Index Database. Local raw nectar additionally seems to help regular sensitivities since the honey bees gather region dust, which helps construct your invulnerability.

If you absolutely do not want to use that spoonful of sugar or honey, you can replace it with Inulin (see below).

Inulin

This ingredient you will find in most recipes that include yeast. In traditional bread recipes that use yeast, you need to have sugar to feed the yeast, which is what helps your bread double in size. Inulin is a naturally occurring substance that feeds yeast the same way sugar does in recipes.

Diastatic Malt Powder

Diastatic Malt Powder has, for some time, been a hidden secret of professional bakers. Albeit just one teaspoon is added to every one of the following recipes, it critically enhances the flavor and produces an appetizing home-baked bread aroma. It is listed as a discretionary element for gluten-free diets since it is produced from sprouted grains (for example, barley) that have been dried and ground. Luckily gluten-free varieties of malt and malt substitutes are additionally being created and are accessible on a limited basis. "Diastatic" alludes to the enzymes that are present as the grain newly sprouts, which convert starches into sugars and advances yeast growth.

I have not been able to decide whether these enzymes separate the resistant starches found in white bean flour; I just know the taste and texture are obviously better, and the bread remains fresh for a more extended period. It usually comes in a 1-pound pack that is generally cheap because only one teaspoon is utilized per portion. Note: Do not mistake this for non–diastatic, which is basically a sugar without any enzymes.

Oils and Fats

Oils rich in saturated fats, for example, corn oil and vegetable oil, are not allowed. Instead, select oils that are high in omega-3s, for example, olive, coconut, and avocado oil.

Oil And Butter Alternatives

Coconut Oil

There is a wide range of health benefits obtained from coconut oil. It's beneficial for your heart, your assimilation, and your resistant framework, and is additionally valuable in assisting with weight reduction. It has a light, however particular coconut flavor.

Almond Butter

Almonds top the chart of the "world's most beneficial foods" list on the earth. Almond butter gives a pleasant nutty flavor, which can be likened to peanut spread in your dishes.

Cashew Butter

Rich in a few distinct nutrients, cashew butter is additionally high in protein and is a great substitute for butter or nutty spread in a recipe. It does, obviously, have an aftertaste like cashews.

Macadamia Butter

Macadamia nuts are a rich source of dietary fiber and monounsaturated fats. The butter is sweet and velvety and lessens bad cholesterol in the body while increasing good cholesterol. Macadamia butter is a good substitution for the regular butter and has a sweet, nutty flavor.

Milk Alternatives

Almond Milk

Pressed from almond seeds, almond milk is high in protein and low in bad fats. It's a perfect, tasty swap for dairy and has a scarcely recognizable and very mellow flavor.

Coconut Milk

Pressed from the meat of the coconut, coconut milk keeps up stable glucose and advances cardiovascular, bone, muscle, and nerve wellbeing. It gives a rich, sweet coconut flavor to your dishes.

Other Ingredients

Meats and Proteins

Your meats need to come from grass-fed, organically produced livestock, free-range poultry, or wild-caught fish and assorted types of seafood. Wild game is excellent, as well, in case you're so interested. Meats, for example, venison, are very low in bad fats while high in good fats and lean protein, so don't hesitate to get some for yourself!

Fruits and Vegetables

If it is remotely possible, shop at your nearby ranchers' market for fresh organic fruits and veggies. Since the Paleo diet is dependent upon your inventiveness to finish a hot, new, delicious supper without the aid of flours, fats, and other no-no's, you will need to gain proficiency with various approaches to get ready healthy dishes within the shorts time. In addition, if you're offering a wide assortment of foods that your family knows and cherishes, you won't be under such a great amount of pressure to cook a simple dish that everyone will eat and really appreciate. Tomatoes are great for any serving of mixed greens and make a tasty base for soups and sauces. They're loaded with nutrients and have a great number of uses that you ought to have some close by consistently. Different meals ought to incorporate carrots, peppers, cauliflower, and celery.

For fruits, choose ones that are high in vitamins and generally low in sugar, for example, stone fruits and berries. Berries are likewise great sources of antioxidants, phytonutrients, and minerals. Apples are healthy organic snacks, as are peaches, oranges, and bananas. The dark tip of the banana that you take out is highly rich in Vitamin K, so do your body a huge favor and eat it!

Seasonings

Your success with making the change to the caveman diet (Paper diet) is, to a great extent, reliant on how delightful your food is. Thus, you're going to need to fuse different herbs and flavors to make your dishes heavenly. Here are a few that you ought to consistently have close by:

- All spice
- Dark pepper
- Basil
- Cayenne pepper
- Cinnamon
- Cloves
- Squashed red pepper
- Curry powder
- Dry mustard
- Garlic (fresh and powdered)
- Mustard seed
- Oregano
- Paprika
- Parsley
- Rosemary
- Thyme

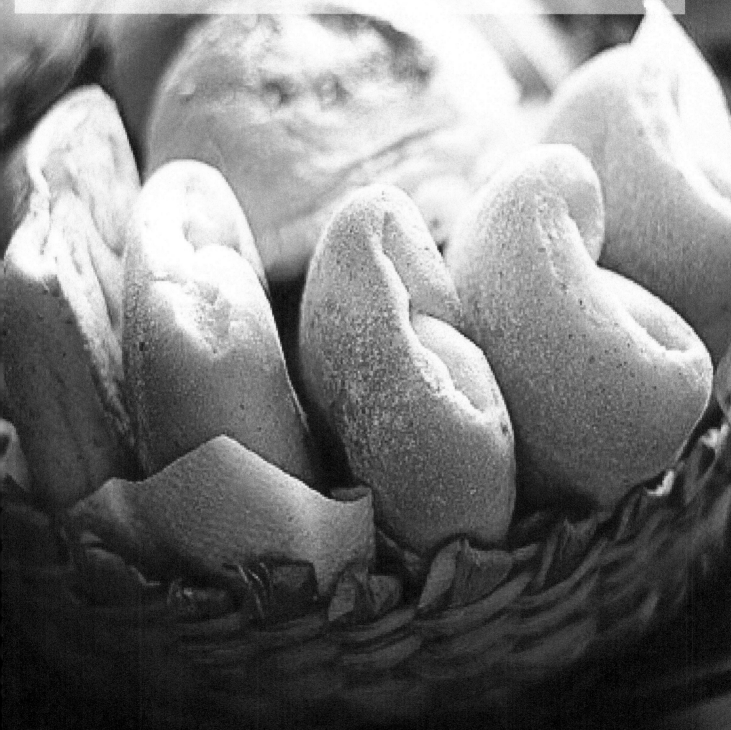

CHAPTER 3: BRIEF GENERAL EXPLANATION OF MAIN TYPES OF KETO BREAD

A staple food is a food regularly eaten in quantities that make it a predominantly standard diet for some people. Some common staple foods include meat, eggs, fish, cheese, root vegetables or tubers like potatoes and cassava, starchy tubers, and cereals from which bread is made.

Different Types of Bread

There are many types of bread, but only three categories to which they can be classified. The first is bread that rises high and has to be baked in pans like bread loaves and muffins; the second are breads with medium volume like baguettes, rye bread, and other French bread; and the last are those that hardly rise or more known as flatbread like naan bread, tortilla bread, pizza bread, and crackers.

Some of the most popular breads that people normally eat for breakfast, lunch or dinner include:

Loaves

These are rounded or oblong mass of dough baked in rectangular pans. Loaves come in white bread, multi-grain, brown bread, Ezekiel bread and many others. The loaves are the most common type of bread.

Bagels

Bagel is a type of bread resembling a doughnut, but unlike regular bread, bagels are prepared by boiling first in water before baking.

Pizza

Pizza is a round flatbread topped by tomato sauce, cheese and some added meat and vegetables. The pizza is of Italian origin. Pizza can also be prepared using a loaf bread. Muffins. Muffins are prepared and baked like cakes, but muffins are a type of bread and not cake. Muffins are usually eaten for breakfast and can be sweet or savory.

Breadsticks

Breadstick is a dry bread that resembles thin-sized pencils in form and normally used as a dipping stick. Breadstick originated from Turin, Italy, and is usually served as an appetizer.

Crackers

Cracker is a type of bread made from wheat flour and water and comes in many forms like rye and multi-grain.

CHAPTER 4: WHAT IS A BREAD MACHINE?

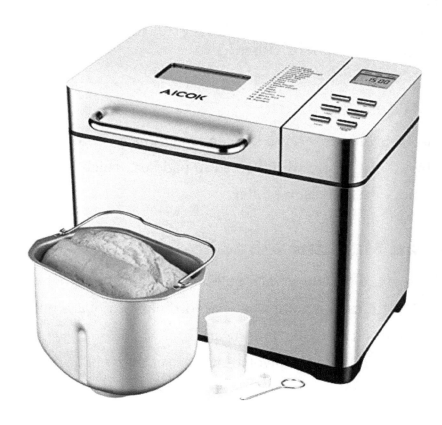

Bread is a baked food that can be set up from various kinds of batter. The mixture is ordinarily made of flour and water. Bread is prepared in several shapes, sizes, types, and surfaces. Extents and kinds of flour and different fixings shift, as do techniques for arrangement. Since the commencement, bread has been one of the most fundamental nourishments, as it is likewise one of the most established counterfeit nourishments. Truth be told, individuals were making bread since the beginning of horticulture.

Individuals in all societies serve bread in different structures with any dinner of the day. It tends to be eaten as a piece of the supper or as a different bite.

How Do You Cook Bread?

Bread is typically arranged from wheat flour mixture, which is made with yeast and permitted to rise. Normally, individuals heat bread in the stove. In any case, an ever-increasing number of individuals go to the extraordinary bread machines to prepare crispbread at home.

What Is A Bread Machine?

A bread machine, or bread maker, is a kitchen apparatus for heating bread. The gadget comprises of a bread dish or tin with worked in paddles, which is situated in the focal point of a little unique multi-reason broiler.

How Is Bread Machine Made?

This machine is essentially a conservative electric appliance that holds a solitary, huge bread tin inside. The tin itself is somewhat extraordinary – it has a hub at the base that is associated with an electric engine underneath.

A little metal oar is appended to the pivot at the base of the tin. The oar is answerable for manipulating the mixture. A waterproof seal secures the hub itself. We should investigate every one of the bread machine parts in detail:

- The top over the bread producer comes either with the survey window or without it
- The control board is likewise situated on the highest point of the bread machine with the end goal of comfort
- In the focal point of the top, there is a steam vent that depletes the steam during the heating procedure. A portion of the bread creators likewise have an air vent on the gadget for air to come inside the tin for the mixture to rise

How Does Bread Machine Work?

To begin with, you put the plying paddle inside the tin. At the point when the tin is out of the machine, you can gauge the fixings and burden them into the tin.

A while later, you simply need to put the skillet inside the stove (machine), pick the program you wish by means of the electronic board, and close the top. Here the bread producer enchantment dominates!

One of the main things the bread machine will do is working the batter – you will hear the sounds. On the off chance that your bread creator accompanies the preview window, you can watch the entire procedure of preparing, which is very interesting.

After the massaging stage, everything will go calm for quite a while – the rising stage comes. The machine allows the mixture to dough and rise. At that point, there will be another round of manipulating and a period of demonstrating.

At long last, the bread producer' broiler will turn on, and you will see the steam coming up through the steam vent. Although the typical bread making process is programmed, most machines accompany formula books that give you various intriguing propelled bread plans.

The best thing about using a bread-making machine is it gets the hard cycle of bread making easy. You can use the bread-making machine in complete cycle, especially for loaf bread, or you can just do the dough cycle if you are baking bread that needs to bake in an oven.

To use the bread-making machine, here are some steps to guide you:

Familiarize yourself with the parts and buttons of your bread-making machine.

Your bread-making machine has three essential parts, and without it, you will not be able to cook your bread. The first part is the machine itself, the second is the bread bucket, and the third is the kneading blade. The bread bucket and kneading blade are removable and replaceable. You can check with the manufacturer for parts to replace it if it's missing.

Learn how to operate your bread-making machine. Removing and placing the bread bucket back in is important. Practice snapping the bread bucket on and off the machine until you are comfortable doing it. This is important because you don't want the bucket moving once the ingredients are in place.

Know your bread bucket capacity.

This is an important step before you start using the machine. If you load an incorrect measurement, you are going to have a big mess on your hand. To check your bread bucket capacity:

- Use a liquid measuring cup and fill it with water.
- Pour the water on the bread bucket until it's full. Count how many cups of water you poured on the bread bucket.
- The number of cups of water will determine the size of your loaf bread
  - Less than 10 cups =1-pound loaf
  - 10 cups =1 to 1 ½ pounds loaf
  - 12 cups=1 or 1 ½ to 2 pounds loaf
  - 14 cups or more=1 or ½ to 2 or 2 ½ pounds loaf

Learn the basic buttons and settings of your bread-making machine.

Here are some tips you can do to familiarize yourself with the machine:

- Read all the button labels. The buttons indicate the cycle in which your machine will mix, knead, and bake the bread.
- Basic buttons include START/STOP, CRUST COLOR, TIMER/ARROW, SELECT (BASIC, SWEET, WHOLE WHEAT, FRENCH, GLUTEN FREE, QUICK/RAPID, QUICK BREAD, JAM, DOUGH.)
- The SELECT button allows you to choose the cycle you want in which you want to cook your loaf. It also includes DOUGH cycle for oven-cooked breads.

Using the Delay button.

When you select a cycle, the machine sets a preset timer to bake the bread. For example, if you select BASIC, time will be set by 3 hours. However, you want your bread cooked at a specific time, say, you want it in the afternoon, but it's only 7:00 in the morning. Your bread cooks for 3 hours, which means it will be done by 10:00 am, but you want it done by 12. You can use the up and down arrow key to set the delay timer. Between 7 am and 12 noon, there is a difference of 5 hours, so you want your timer to be set at 5. Press the arrow keys up to add 2 hours in your timer so that your bread will cook in 5 hours instead of 3 hours. Delay button does not work if you are using the DOUGH cycle.

Order of adding the ingredients

This only matters if you are using the delay timer. It is important to ensure that your yeast will not touch any liquid so as not to activate it early. Early activation of the yeast could make your bread rise too much. If you plan to start the cycle immediately, you can add the ingredients in any order. However, adding the ingredients in order will discipline you to do it every time and make you less likely to forget it when necessary. To add the ingredients, do it in the following order:

- First, place all the liquid ingredients in the bread bucket.
- Add the sugar and the salt.
- Add the flour to cover and seal in the liquid ingredients.
- Add all the other remaining dry ingredients.
- Lastly, add the yeast. The yeast should not touch any liquid until the cooking cycle starts. When adding the yeast, make a small well using your finger to place the yeast to ensure proper timing of yeast activation.

Using the Dough Cycle

You cannot cook all breads using the bread-making machine, but you can use the machine to make the bread-making process easier. All bread goes under the dough cycle. If your bread needs to be oven-cooked, you can still use the bread-making machine by selecting the DOUGH cycle to mix and knead your flour into a dough. To start the Dough cycle:

- Add all your bread recipe ingredients in your bread bucket.
- Select the DOUGH cycle. This usually takes between 40 to 90 minutes.
- Press the START button.
- After the cycle is complete, let your dough rest in the bread-making machine for 5 to 40 minutes.
- Take out the dough and start cutting into your desire shape.

Some machines have Pasta Dough or Cookie Dough cycle, which you can use for muffin recipes. However, if all you have is basic dough setting, you can use it for muffin recipe, but you need to stop the machine before the rising cycle begins.

How to Use a Bread Machine?

Independent of which bread machine you pick, the preparing procedure is basically the equivalent all over the place. You load fixings to the tin. At that point, place the bread container in the machine and pick the vital program.

The average heating process takes anyplace somewhere in the range of 2 and 5 hours, contingent upon the model. Toward the finish of the heating procedure, it is prescribed to put a portion on a wire rack to chill off before eating it.

Other than the principle fixings, you can include some other additional items you need, including raisins, nuts, chocolate chips, and so forth.

While bread heating procedure may appear to be exceptionally crude and straightforward, there are a few indications that will make you a star at bread preparing with a bread machine:

Check and adhere to the guidelines/manual. With some bread creators, the dry fixings ought to be included first, with others, the wet fixings go in first.

In addition, when perusing bread preparing plans, remember that not the entirety of the bread creators is made equivalent – some item 1 pound portions, others make 1, 5, and 2 pound portions. A portion of the bread machine models is equipped for heating 3-pound portions.

It is significant not to surpass the limit of the bread machine container.

In the event that the formula calls for milk, it isn't prescribed to utilize a deferred blend cycle.

Set the machine for 'Pizza Dough' program following the manual of your bread creator. After your mixture is prepared, you can move it to a gently floured surface for additional handling.

Benefits of a Bread Machine

While utilizing a bread machine for some may seem like a pointless advance, others don't envision the existence without newly home-heated bread. In any case, how about we go to the realities – underneath, we indicated the advantages of owning a bread machine.

As a matter of first importance, you can appreciate the crisply prepared handcrafted bread. Most bread creators additionally include a clockwork, which permits you to set the preparing cycle at a specific time. This capacity is extremely valuable when you need to have sweltering bread toward the beginning of the day for breakfast.

You can control what you eat. By preparing bread at home, you can really control what parts are coming into your portion. This choice is extremely valuable for individuals with sensitivities or for those, who attempt to control the admission of a fixings' portion.

It is simple. A few people believe that preparing bread at home is chaotic, and by and large, it is a hard procedure. In any case, preparing bread with a bread machine is a breeze. You simply pick the ideal choice and unwind - all the blending, rising, and heating process is going on within the bread producer, which additionally makes it a zero chaos process!

It sets aside you huge amounts of cash in the long haul. If you imagine that purchasing bread at a store is modest, you may be mixed up. In turns out that in the long haul, preparing bread at home will set aside your cash, particularly in the event that you have some dietary limitations.

Bread machines can create different sorts of bread: whole wheat bread, sans gluten bread, rye bread, and several different kinds. They can likewise make pizza mixture, pasta batter, jam, and different heavenly dishes.

Incredible taste and quality, you have to acknowledge it – nothing beats the quality and taste of a crisp heap of bread. Since you are the person who is making bread, you can ensure that you utilize just the fixings that are new and of a high caliber. Homemade bread consistently beats locally acquired bread as far as taste and quality.

What Else Can you Do with a Bread Machine?

We have just referenced that bread creator utilizes are not just constrained to heating various kinds of bread. Here, we might want to investigate some inventive thoughts regarding how to utilize a bread machine.

You Can Create Your Own Fruit or Vegetable Butters

Bread machine is an extraordinary apparatus for making creamy fruit spread. He featured that the gradual warmth inside the bread machine builds up the sugars in the organic product.

It Is Possible to Make Delicious tomato Sauce in a Bread Maker

A bread machine is in the same class as a stewing pot. Be that as it may, it accepts that the unsettling part makes the bread machine ideal for a sauce.

Prepare a Casserole? Of Course!

Any dish you can envision can be made in a bread creator rather than a customary stove.

Bread Makers Can Bake Cakes

Similarly, likewise, with ideal portions of bread, bread making machines are incredible for heating cakes.

Bread Machine Setting Programs

Most bread machines offer a number of settings. While they may be called slightly different things the most common include:

Basic

This is the most commonly used settings. Often used for traditional white loaves. This setting is what will be used for many savory yeast recipes. This setting should not be used when making sweet bread, which can cause over proofing and will result in overflowing.

Whole Wheat

If you are making a bread that uses whole wheat flour, then this is the setting you will use. Whole wheat flour requires a longer bake time. If you use a wheat gluten ingredient, then you may be able to use the basic setting instead. Double check your user manual to understand which settings are best based on the ingredients you are using.

Gluten-Free

Most of the time, the flours used in these recipes act differently than the everyday all-purpose flour or even wheat flour. Many gluten-free recipes will vary slightly or significantly, but most ingredients should be set out and used at room temperature. Many of these breads, although gluten-free, will still require a rise time.

Sweet Bread

This setting is also used often. This setting is what will be used for most sweet bread recipes that include yeast.

French

This setting is what will be used for not just French bread, but different types of artisan breads. When using this setting, you will have a bread that comes out with a crispy crust like that of a French or Italian loaf.

Quick/Rapid

This setting may also be labeled either quick cycle or rapid time. These breads will bake quickly and have short rise times. If using a rapid rising yeast, you can sometimes use this setting. To use this setting correctly, consult the user manual of your specific machine to ensure proper use.

Quick Bread

This setting is used for most breads that require no rising times and can be baked immediately. Banana bread is one example of a recipe you would use this setting for. This setting can also be used to bake cakes in your bread machine as well.

Jam

Some bread machines will offer special settings such as jam. This setting allows you to make your own homemade jams.

Dough

This is another special setting that some bread machines may offer. The dough setting can be used to make the dough for different breads, pies crust, and even cookie dough.

Basic Steps to Make Bread

Bread is usually prepared from combining flour and water to form a dough and commonly cooked by baking. Bread has played a significant role in the history of human-made food throughout the world.

Below is a basic guide on how to make bread:

- Scaling refers to measuring of ingredients and the most important in the bread-making process. A slight change in the measurement can affect how your bread will turn out.

- Mix all ingredients you measure to prepare it for fermentation and development of gluten. The key to mixing is time and speed.

- Next is allowing the dough to rise or the fermentation process. During this time, the yeast converts the dough's natural sugars into carbon dioxide and ethanol. The carbon dioxide is what makes the dough rise.

- After fermentation, you need to release some of the trapped carbon dioxide in the gluten. This is the punching or degassing process. This process also helps gluten to relax, distribute nutrients, and equalize the temperature of the dough inside and out.

- Next process is cutting or dividing. Dividing the dough will help you easily manage the dough during the next stages. You can cut and weigh the dough into smaller sizes.

- The next step is shaping your dough to your desired type of bread. You can shape it into a loaf, a ball, or a long torpedo.

- Next is resting or benching. You set aside your pre-shaped dough to rest and make the gluten relax. Resting time varies from a few minutes or more.

- The next process is the final shaping and panning. After resting, you can knead the dough and get it into its final shape. You can shape it into a ball, baguette, torpedo, braid, or loaf before putting it in the baking pan.

- Most breads with yeast undergo two fermentation. The first one is bulk fermentation, and the second is during proofing. During proofing, the dough can rise to its baking size.
- After proofing, the bread is ready to go into the oven to bake.
- Once baked, the bread goes on cooling racks to cool down.
- Last step is storing and packing of the bread.

What Kinds Of Bread Machines Are There?

Lion's share of the bread-making machines will be somewhat extraordinary. This is because of the way that every variety of bread creator is intended to fill a specific need. Beneath, we will talk about the most widely recognized kinds of bread creators accessible on the advanced market.

Vertical

The greater part of the bread machines heat portions that are situated vertically, as the bread tin is molded right now. This sort of bread machine includes just one massaging paddle.

Even

There are likewise some bread producers that have two working oars inside the tin. These bread machines prepare level bread, much the same as the one you get from the pastry kitchen of the shop.

Small

Little bread producers are extraordinary for the restricted kitchen space or if you don't eat a ton of bread. These little kitchen assistants don't take a significant part of the counter space and produce simply enough bread for a couple or one individual.

Huge

Huge bread machines prove to be useful in enormous families – bread can vanish immediately when you have many individuals at the table. The large bread creators that produce 3 lb portions of bread are equipped for sustaining a major family.

Gluten-Free

With the incredible wealth of the bread creator models available, there are unquestionably those, which are intended to provide food the requirements of smart dieting individuals.

Much the same as that, a bread machine that has a gluten setting is perfect for preparing this sort of bread.

Choosing the Right Bread Machine

When selecting the ideal bread machine for your home, there are several factors to have in mind. These factors include:

a) The size of the bread machine pan. If you are many in your household, then a bigger bread pan is ideal for getting bread big enough to satisfy the whole group. If you are by yourself or there are only two of you, a smaller bread pan may be ideal.

b) Bread machines are different, and they come with several cycles, as well. These cycles are what determine how best the dough will be mixed and kneaded. Bread machines with fewer cycles are ideal, but it all depends on what your needs are.

c) Bread machines come in different qualities, which also dictate their prices as well. The best qualities are, of course, more expensive. Consider what your needs are and what you can afford before purchasing one.

d) Consider the timer on your machine. Some have the timer on the dough only, which lets you know when it is ready to be removed and baked in an oven. Some have it on the bake cycle when the bread is to be baked on the bread maker itself.

e) Different machines produce bread in different shapes as well. Consider the shape you want before making a purchase. It is important to note that each shape has its challenges; one example is that horizontal-shaped pans have a problem when kneading the dough. They are notorious for leaving flour in the pan's corners.

Producers

Presently, as we have talked about the key minutes about bread creators, ample opportunity has already passed to take a gander at the organizations that produce them. While there are many bread machine makers, existent all-inclusive, we will concentrate on the most dependable and famous bread machine producers.

Zojirushi

The Zojirushi Corporation is a Japanese organization that produces different home machines, one of Zojirushi's product offerings - bread creators. Bread machines from this maker are known for their predominant quality.

The organization maker machines in two sizes that are mirroring the clients' inclinations. The 2 – lb Bread machines are ideal for heating customarily molded 2-lb portion. The 1-lb bread machine will be a solid match for one individual or individuals who eat less bread.

Bread machines from Zojirushi are equipped for making top-notch bread, cakes, and various dishes. Zojirushi bread creators offer the accompanying cycles: entire wheat, cake, jam, custom made (the natively constructed cycle permits you to program the work, rise and prepare times for your inclinations), and mixture.

Panasonic

We wager you previously caught wind of Panasonic – the notorious brand behind various electronic gadgets. Panasonic Corporation is likewise recently known as Matsushita Electric Industrial Co., Ltd. The organization is a Japanese worldwide gadget maker.

Panasonic bread creators are at the highest point of the value bushel, yet the cost can be clarified by various astonishing highlights that are offered by these apparatuses.

Panasonic offers five bread creators models, with one of them highlighting a programmed yeast administering framework.

Breadman

The organization is an American brand of kitchen machines. Breadman bread producers offer the chance to prepare proficient style bread at home. The brand is known for its unrivaled quality and reliable client service.

Breville

Breville is an Australian little home apparatuses maker, which was set up in Melbourne in 1932. The organization is demonstrated to utilize top-notch materials for their items, and it turned out to be very well known in New Zealand and the US.

West Bend

The West Bend Company was known as a West Bend, Wisconsin organization in the period somewhere in the range of 1911 and 2001. The West Bend Company has been creating aluminum cookware and electrical apparatuses. In any case, it is likewise known for assembling stroke cycle motors, for example, detachable pontoon engines.

With the extraordinary experience despite its good faith, West Bend Company is equipped for conveying the top of the line item to the clients. The Small Kitchen Appliance Division of the West Bend is known as West Bend Housewares.

How to Clean a Bread Maker?

There are a few straightforward advances you can follow to keep up your bread producer appropriately. Most importantly, you have to recall the accompanying guidelines for utilizing the bread machine:

- Clean your bread producer each time you use it;

- Never pour water or some other fluid straightforwardly into the bread creator, while cleaning. Just the bread tin is intended to have fluids inside;
- Make sure that the machine is unplugged and has cooled totally before playing out any upkeep or cleaning

Cleaning a Bread Machine

In the event that you need to draw out the life of your bread machine, it is important to deal with the apparatus all the time. To keep your bread creator in the ideal condition, you won't have to invest a lot of energy.

Stage One: Remove all the Crumbs & Residue from the Bread Tin

After you have unplugged the bread machine and it has totally chilled off, you can begin the cleaning procedure. Turn it as an afterthought over the sink, trash, or some other surface and delicately clear the pieces of remaining flour with some wipe or delicate brush.

If there is some mixture adhered to the dividers of the bread producer tin, leave it till it dries out – and afterward expel similarly as you did with the morsels. A similar procedure ought to be followed if there is some mixture of the warming component of the bread producer.

Remember that not the entirety of the removable pieces of your bread producer is dishwasher safe. Many bread machines have parts that can be washed in the dishwashing machine. In any case, it is in every case, better to double-check and read the manual to discover the similarity part.

Stage Two: Ensure Everything Is Dry Before Using Bread Maker Again

After you wrapped up the pieces of your bread machine, ensure that every one of them is totally dry before assembling them back. There's nothing more to it! It is that straightforward - three simple strides to keeping your bread machine consistently in incredible condition.

As a little something extra, we have arranged some more tips about cleaning and support of bread creators.

On the off chance that any fluid contacted the inward surface of the bread machine, utilize a microfiber fabric to absorb the dampness. Make a point to rehash a similar procedure until there is no wet left on the warming component.

It is critical to take great consideration of the warming component of your bread machine, as this is one of the most major pieces of the apparatus. Keep the warming component clean and don't let any earth/pieces go onto it – this represents a danger of fire. To clean the warming component, utilize a delicate fabric, and expel the earth tenderly.

CHAPTER 5: WHAT KITCHEN TOOLS DO YOU NEED?

In addition to the bread machine, which is obviously the indispensable device for preparing recipes that you will find in the next chapters, there are other tools that can make your job easier.

You probably already have many of them in your kitchen. Here are some of the most important:

Kitchen scale

Every kitchen should have a scale. It is a very important tool in baking, which is a must-have. It is practically not possible to prepare some types of foods without having a kitchen scale. For baking, a scale is necessary. It is recommended to make accurate measurements when preparing bread. This is because using a cup to measure may be wrong many times. A digital scale is recommended, as it is very accurate.

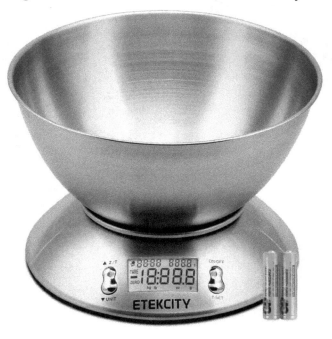

Bowls

I love using the large metal mixing bowl that I found at a restaurant supply store, but any bowl will do. Make sure you have a variety of sizes so you can measure out different quantities of ingredients. Whenever I shop at thrift stores, I like finding small bowls for a few cents here and there to add to my collection. Having little bowls for ingredients in smaller amounts, like salt, yeast, chopped herbs, and so on, is nice, but it's not absolutely necessary—any vessel will do.

Dough Scraper

I recommend getting metal and a plastic dough scraper. They cost just a few dollars at kitchen stores, at restaurant supply stores, or on Amazon, and they are so useful. A metal scraper is helpful for cutting and scraping dough off your work area, and a plastic scraper is flexible enough to help scrape the dough out of the bowl after rinsing.

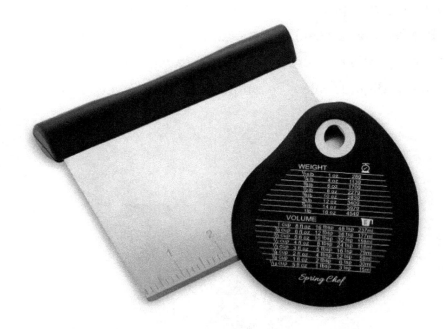

Pastry brush

Pastry brush or basting brush looks like a paintbrush. It is made of plastic fiber or nylon. It is used for spreading butter, oil, or glaze on food.

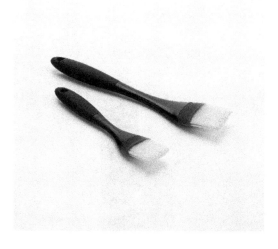

Blender

It is an essential kitchen appliance used for emulsifying, puree, or mix food.

Mixer

Every person needs a Mixer in their kitchen. It is a very handy kitchen tool, and it does the heaviest work – kneading the dough.

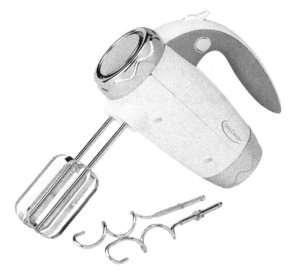

Food processor

A food processor is good for kneading and mixing doughs, pureeing, grating cheese, or shredding and grinding items.

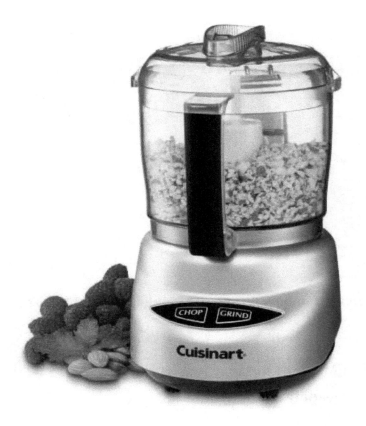

Oven

Usually, it is essential for baking, but in this recipe book, we will only use it in some recipes because the star will be the bread machine.

Cheese grater

Use a stainless-steel cheese grater to get your cheese perfectly grated.

Razor Blade or Lame

A razor blade is the best tool for slashing the top of a loaf of bread. A lame is a tool that holds the razor blade safely and has a nice handle, which makes it even easier to make precision slashes.

Rimmed Baking Sheet

This is an item you likely have in your kitchen already, and if not, it's a worthwhile investment. I usually use a 12-by-18-inch or a 16-by-24-inch baking sheet, which can be found at restaurant supply stores and online.

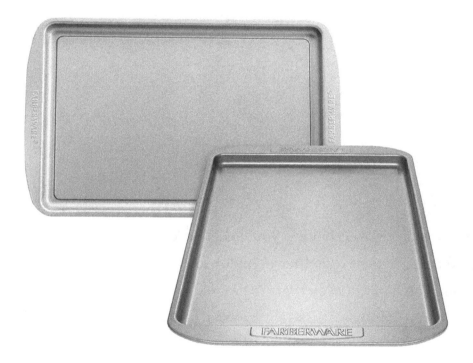

Banneton or Proofing Basket

For the final proof, the dough needs to be placed in a basket that will allow air to circulate. You can buy baskets specifically for this called bannetons, which are made of cane. If you aren't ready to invest in a couple of bannetons just yet, a round or oval basket from a thrift store can be lined with a floured kitchen towel for a more affordable option. When I first started out, I had a ragtag collection of round and oval-shaped baskets, and they worked just fine.

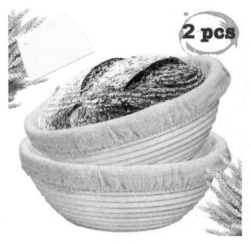

Thermometer

To achieve consistency in your baking, you'll need to know the temperature of your water and the ingredients. Buy a probe thermometer to check temperatures of ingredients. I also recommend you have an oven thermometer to be sure the temperature of your oven is accurate. You can purchase these for around $20 on Amazon and in most grocery stores.

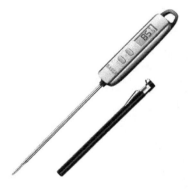

Finally, here is a small list with other useful tools that you will certainly have in the kitchen and that do not need any particular explanation:

- Kitchen towels
- Nonstick cooking spray
- Spoon
- Teaspoon
- Tablespoon
- Scissors
- Plastic wrap

Chapter 6:   Tips and FAQs For Bread Machine Beginners

Baking Tips

Do not get frustrated if a dish does not turn out perfectly as you are baking with new ingredients, which are usually fussy and will take some practice. However, read through these tips carefully to gain the knowledge that you will require to have your Keto breads turn out to be a success!

Temperature is everything

You want to use eggs, cream cheese, sour cream, milk and any other cooled items set at room temperature. This is due to cold items not mixing particularly well into the almond and coconut flours, which are used in Keto and if they are not brought down to room temperature, then your bread will not properly rise.

A trick for the eggs, in particular, is to use a bowl of warm water to immerse the eggs for the duration of 4 minutes. This will quickly bring them to room temperature, which is a nice trick in case you forgot to pull them out of the fridge.

Make sure that you measure your ingredients properly

This will lead to consistent results for all the Keto recipes that you find. The correct method in measuring is to spoon the ingredient into the cup rather than scooping it out of the bag directly. This will create perfect results every time as you will not over pack the ingredients using this method. You can also ensure that all the ingredients are the correct increments if you purchase a simple kitchen or baking scale.

Ensure the yeast is properly proofed

Not every recipe includes active dry yeast. However, for the ones that do, there is a specific process to follow as outlined in those particular recipes. It includes combining the yeast with honey for the yeast to feed upon. Do not worry about the sugar content as the honey is for the yeast to feed upon, creating the carbon dioxide required for the bread to rise. The sugar will be cooked off during the process and will not be present in the final result.

Once combined, you will blend water, which is the specific temperature of 105° - 110°, which can be checked with a kitchen thermometer, or it will be slightly warm to the touch. You will know that this process was successful by the mixture becoming bubbly after waiting for a period of 7 minutes.

If there are no bubbles, simply repeat the process with the correct temperature water. You will not waste a whole dish because this occurs at the beginning of the recipe.

Temperature is important during the rising process

You want to keep your rising bread in an environment where the temperature is not going to vary much and will be undisturbed during the rising time. You want to have the area to be slightly warm and humid, but not hot as this will stop the rising process. It is suggested to keep the covered tray on top of the stove, which is preheating.

Always Sift Your Coconut Flour:

Not sifting your coconut flour will result in a grainy bread full of coconut flour clumps...yuck! To sift your coconut flour, simply use a mesh strainer, and add the coconut flour. Sift over a large container or bowl.

Keep away from xylitol

When using any yeast in your recipes, you want to make sure that xylitol is not an additive in your ingredients as it rapidly decreases the rising of the dough and will cause them to become flat. You will find that Monk Fruit and Erythritol do not contain xylitol and may be used as a substitute for sweeteners that have this additive included.

Loaf pan size is important

There are a wide variety of baking pans out there. I have made it easy by including the particular pan that is required for each recipe. However, if you do not have that specific size, always opt to go with a pan that is the next size up rather than downsizing. This will ensure that the dough will not rise too far, causing the bread to burst over the pan.
The measurements for pans are calculated from the top of the pan and does not include the pan itself.

Pure ingredients are everything

Especially when dealing with the different varieties of cheese, you want to make sure there are no preservatives or additives. Also, opt for the skim or whole milk types as these will have less water to weep during the baking process.

When baking powder is being used, it is a priority to ensure that it is as fresh as possible. Since there is no gluten present, it needs to be of the best quality to make the rising process work properly.

Not sure if your baking powder is still active? Do a small test by combining it with boiling water. If bubbles occur immediately, then your baking powder will make your bread properly rise.

A perfect way to grease any pan

If you want to make sure that you do not run into the problem of your Keto breads sticking to the pan, this fail-proof trick will take the headache out of baking. Dissolve 2 tbps. of coconut oil in a saucepan and then apply to your pan with a pastry brush. Set in the freezer for a minimum of 20 minutes as the oil hardens. Pull out of the freezer before filling with your dough.

Separating the eggs is a necessary step

It may seem like a pain at the time, but there is a reason that you will find the eggs are separated. This simple measure also helps the Keto breads to rise. When incorporating the whipped eggs into the batter, do not over mix. This is due to you counteracting the airiness that has been created by whipping the eggs, and your breads will not rise properly.

Tips for Saving Time

The keto diet doesn't have to be either complicated or difficult. Although more and more keto-friendly products and food items are being made available these days, it's always better to cook your meals and bake goods at home. Though it might seem odd at the beginning, once you get the hang of things, this process will become faster, easier, and more enjoyable. Here are some time-saving tips for you:

Make riced cauliflower in bulk then use airtight containers to freeze it. That way, you can simply take the amount you need when your recipe calls for it.

For recipes that call for boiled low-carb food items, use an instant pot. This allows you to cook ingredients in bulk faster.

Stock up on parchment paper as you can use this to line your baking sheets, pans, and other similar items before placing them in the oven.

Use your freshly-baked bread loaves to make delicious sweet or savory sandwiches. Then store these in the refrigerator for meals on-the-go.

When planning which recipes to bake, check the ingredients to see if they share common items. This makes shopping a lot easier, especially if you want to make meal prepping part of your keto journey.

Tips for Saving Money

Apart from saving time, there are also things you can do in order to save money while following the keto diet. Starting a new diet is always challenging, no matter what type of diet you choose to follow. Most of the time, you won't even know where to start. Although you've already learned all that you can about the diet, actually taking the first step towards starting it can be very intimidating.

If you want to stick with your keto journey, then you must make sure that you don't break the bank just because of it. Otherwise, you might end up deciding that the diet isn't working for you since you're losing money on it. This doesn't have to be the case! To help you out, here are some clever money-saving tips you can try:

Create things from scratch

Whether you're baking pastries or cooking dishes, it's important to learn how to create things from scratch. Although it's easier and more convenient to purchase ready-made, prepackaged keto food products, doing so will surely make you lose a lot of money. If you want to stick with your budget, learning how to make homemade meals from scratch is of the essence.

Purchase fresh, whole ingredients

Buying ingredients that are fresh and whole allows you to whip up healthy meals and snacks that fit right into your keto diet. In fact, a proper keto diet should be built around these types of ingredients so you can get high-quality sources of macros and the rest of the nutrients. Also, fresh and whole ingredients are a lot cheaper, which means that you can save a lot of money.

Buy local produce, which is in season

Do research on which foods and food items are available each season. Purchasing local produce that is in season allows you to get the ingredients you need at an affordable price. As long as you know which ingredients are in season in your locale, you can start planning your meals and recipes easily and more effectively.

Buy ingredients in bulk

Speaking of saving money on ingredients, buying in bulk also allows you to save some money. Go around your locale and check out all the food shops, supermarkets, farmer's markets, and convenience stores. That way, you can determine which places offer the freshest ingredients, which ones have the best prices, and which places offer bulk or wholesale products.

Bake (and cook) in bulk

Of course, if you buy in bulk, it's a good idea to use these ingredients in bulk too. This is where meal prepping comes in. Once a week, set aside some time to plan your meals, shop for all of the ingredients and bake/cook all of your meals for the whole week. This is an excellent way to save money and ensure that you don't feel tempted to buy takeout or ready-made foods, which are less healthy and more expensive.

Maintaining a Low-Carb Diet

Although starting the low-carb keto diet may help you lose weight, there are some things for you to consider. First of all, if you really want to shed those unwanted pounds and enjoy all of the health benefits the keto diet has to offer, you must follow it properly.
Also, to stay on the safe side, you may want to consult with your doctor before you start this diet. This is especially true for people who are suffering from medical conditions or for those who have a complicated medical history. If you've already decided to go low-carb, here are some pointers for you:

Choose your carbs wisely

The main energy sources of the body come from simple and complex carbs. Simple carbs are naturally found in milk and fruits, but sweets such as candies also contain them. When choosing foods that contain carbs, opt for complex variety such as starchy veggies, lentils, beans, and legumes.

Opt for lean protein

Just because you're allowed to eat moderate amounts of protein while on the keto diet, this doesn't mean that you should eat all kinds of protein. If you want to lose weight and improve your health, then the best protein choices are eggs, beans, skinless turkey or chicken breast, and fish.

Make it a habit to read food labels

This allows you to choose the ingredients and food items that fit into your diet more effectively. When you read food labels, this gives you information about the food items you plan to purchase from stores.

Consume a lot of non-starchy veggies and fruits

Although these food items may contain simple carbs, that doesn't mean you should stop eating them. Fruits and veggies are the healthiest kinds of foods, so continue eating them as part of your diet to ensure your overall health.

Plan your meals

Meal planning can be your friend when you're following the keto diet. This involves planning your meals for a specific amount of time (like for one week), shopping for ingredients, then setting one day each week to cook all of the meals you've planned. It's an excellent way to save time, money, and to stick with your diet.

Maintain open communication with your doctor

Finally, it's important to maintain open communication with your doctor, especially when you experience any changes because of the diet. Whether you're at the peak of your health or you're suffering from any kind of medical condition, keeping your doctor in the loop is essential.

Learn How to Check Nutritional Information

As mentioned, it's important to check food labels. In fact, you should make this a habit if you decide to start the keto diet. The good news is that all of the big food companies have introduced new nutrition labels, which makes it easier to learn the nutritional information of the foods you plan to buy. Here are some steps to follow when checking nutritional information:

Check the serving size

This information tells you how many calories and nutrients you would get for each serving of the food item. When you know this, you can compare this serving size with the amount you actually consume.

Check the caloric information

This information tells you the amount of energy you obtain for each serving.

Check the percent daily value

This information tells you the percentage of nutrients on a scale which, in turn, tells you if the food item contains minimal or high amounts of nutrients. A DV of 5% and below is considered little, and a DV of 15% and above is considered a lot.

Search for these nutrients

Look for calcium, fiber, iron, vitamin A, and vitamin C.

Conversely, try to avoid these

Cholesterol, fat, saturated fat, sodium, and trans fat.

The great thing about nutrition labels is these make it easier to compare products, they allow you to find out the nutritional value of food items, and they help you determine whether or not different food items are appropriate for your diet.

FAQs

What is the difference between a ketogenic diet and a low-carb diet?

A low carb diet is a general term used to describe any diet containing 130 to 150 grams on the total. However, ketogenic diets are a subset of this general diet plan. It further restricts the amount of carbohydrate to minimum levels and, at the same time, requires an increased intake of fat. Thus, a ketogenic diet plan is more specific than the low carbohydrate plan.

Do I need to count calories? Are calories of importance?

Keeping track of caloric intake is important as it directly relates to weight gain. Whether on a low carb diet or a high one, it is necessary to keep check of the calories.

How can a person track carb intake/ macro?

Whenever you follow a recipe, look for its contents and the nutritional value available with the recipe. If it is not available, look for online nutrition calculators, which enables you to calculate the nutritional value within a few minutes.

What is the time taken to get to ketosis?

If you are a person of discipline and routine, then it typically takes two to three days to start a keto routine. However, it is a gradual process and goes through different stages. Exercise helps boosts the speed of the process. For people with sedentary lifestyles, it can also take weeks.

Can I eat dairy?

This is perhaps the most frequently asked question by the people who are new to a keto diet. Not all dairy products are keto-friendly as raw dairy products are high in carbs. But those fermented or processed loses their carbohydrates and are good to use. These include butter, cheese and yogurt.

Can I eat peanuts?

Not all legumes are not keto-friendly, peanuts are one of them. There is a great misconception that peanuts can be taken on a keto diet, but it is clearly not true as they are low on carbs and high in fats. When taken in small amounts, they do not disrupt the balance of the ketogenic diet.

Is ketosis bad?

There is no proven evidence that could suggest that ketosis is dangerous. Many people confuse ketosis with ketoacidosis, the latter is a health problem which only occurs in patients with diabetes type 1. During ketoacidosis, the ketones level in the blood exceeds up to a critical value. Ketosis, on the other hand, is completely normal and doesn't pose any danger to a person's health.

Are the high-fat foods healthy? Does eating a lot of fat make people fat?

Most of us believe that high fats are unhealthy, but it is nothing but a myth. Fats can only be unhealthy if taken with a high amount of carbohydrates. However, when taken with low carbs or no carbs, these fats become a direct and active source of energy for the body. They easily break down and release essential compounds, including ketones.

Can I go off of the ketogenic diet plan and still keep the weight off?

Unfortunately, when you see-saw on any diet plan, you're going to gain the weight back. Some individuals don't understand that you're making a lifestyle change.

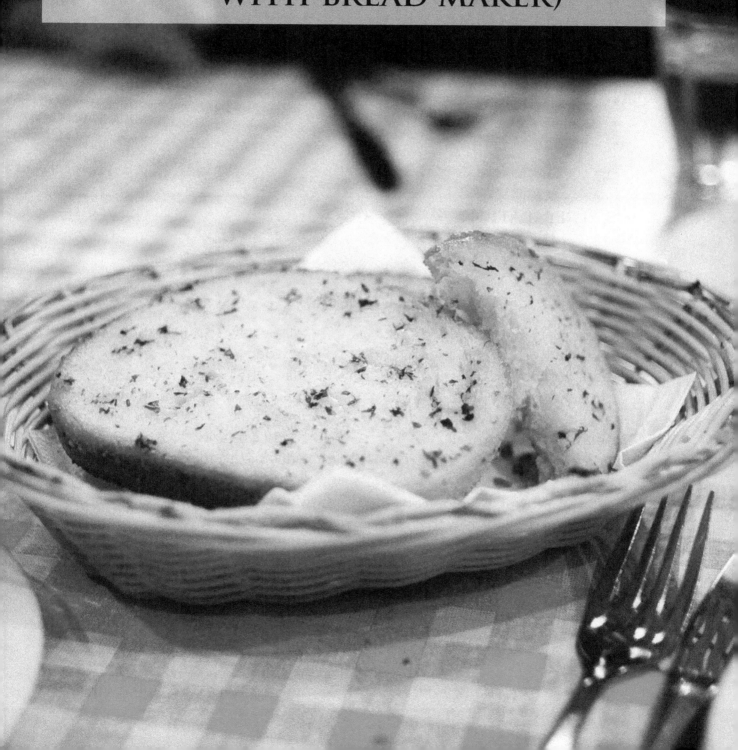

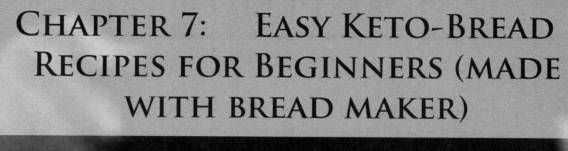

Chapter 7: Easy Keto-Bread Recipes for Beginners (made with bread maker)

1. BEST KETO BREAD

INGREDIENTS

- 1 ½ cup almond flour
- 6 drops liquid stevia
- 1 pinch Pink Himalayan salt
- ¼ tsp. cream of tartar
- 3 tsp. baking powder
- ¼ cup butter, melted
- 6 large eggs, separated

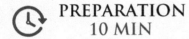 **PREPARATION**
10 MIN

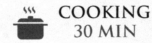 **COOKING**
30 MIN

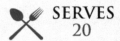 **SERVES**
20

DIRECTIONS

1. In a bowl, to the egg whites, add cream of tartar and beat until soft peaks are formed.
2. Into another bowl, combine stevia, salt, baking powder, almond flour, melted butter. Mix well.
3. Grease the machine loaf pan with ghee.
4. Following the instructions on your machine's manual, mix the dry ingredients into the wet ingredients and pour in the bread machine loaf pan, taking care to follow how to mix in the baking powder.
5. Place the bread pan in the machine, and select the basic bread setting, together with the bread size and crust type, if available, then press start once you have closed the lid of the machine.
6. When the bread is ready, using oven mitts, remove the bread pan from the machine.
7. Let it cool before slicing.
8. Cool, slice, and enjoy.

Nutrition: Calories 90, Fat 7 g, Carb 2 g, Protein 3 g

2. YEAST BREAD

INGREDIENTS

- 2 ¼ teaspoons dry yeast
- ½ teaspoon and 1 tablespoon erythritol sweetener, divided
- 1 1/8 cups warm water, at 100°F / 38°C
- 3 tablespoons avocado oil
- 1 cup / 100 grams almond flour
- ¼ cup / 35 grams oat fiber
- ¾ cup / 100 grams soy flour
- ½ cup / 65 grams ground flax meal
- 1 ½ teaspoons baking powder
- 1 teaspoon salt

 PREPARATION
10 MIN

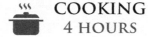 **COOKING**
4 HOURS

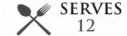 **SERVES**
12

DIRECTIONS

1. Gather all the ingredients for the bread and plug in the bread machine having the capacity of 2 pounds of bread recipe.
2. Pour water into the bread bucket, stir in ½ teaspoon sugar and yeast and let it rest for 10 minutes until emulsified.
3. Meanwhile, take a large bowl, place the remaining ingredients in it and stir until mixed.
4. Pour flour mixture over yeast mixture in the bread bucket, shut the lid, select the "basic/white" cycle or "low-carb" setting and then press the up/down arrow button to adjust baking time according to your bread machine; it will take 3 to 4 hours.
5. Then press the crust button to select light crust if available, and press the "start/stop" button to switch on the bread machine.
6. When the bread machine beeps, open the lid, then take out the bread basket and lift out the bread.
7. Let bread cool on a wire rack for 1 hour, then cut it into twelve slices and serve.

Nutrition: Calories 162, Fat 11.3 g, Protein 8.1 g, Carb 7 g, Fiber 2.8 g, Net Carb 4 g

3. CREAM CHEESE BREAD

INGREDIENTS

- ¼ cup / 60 grams butter, grass-fed, unsalted
- 1 cup and 3 tablespoons / 140 grams cream cheese, softened
- 4 egg yolks, pasteurized
- 1 teaspoon vanilla extract, unsweetened
- 1 teaspoon baking powder
- ¼ teaspoon of sea salt
- 2 tablespoons monk fruit powder
- ½ cup / 65 grams peanut flour

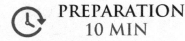 **PREPARATION** 10 MIN

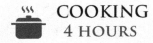 **COOKING** 4 HOURS

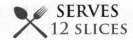 **SERVES** 12 SLICES

DIRECTIONS

1. Gather all the ingredients for the bread and plug in the bread machine having the capacity of 2 pounds of bread recipe.
2. Take a large bowl, place butter in it, beat in cream cheese until thoroughly combined and then beat in egg yolks, vanilla, baking powder, salt, and monk fruit powder until well combined.
3. Add egg mixture into the bread bucket, top with flour, shut the lid, select the "basic/white" cycle or "low-carb" setting and then press

the up/down arrow button to adjust baking time according to your bread machine; it will take 3 to 4 hours.

4. Then press the crust button to select light crust if available, and press the "start/stop" button to switch on the bread machine.
5. When the bread machine beeps, open the lid, then take out the bread basket and lift out the bread.
6. Let bread cool on a wire rack for 1 hour, then cut it into twelve slices and serve.

Nutrition: Calories 98, Fat 7.9 g, Protein 3.5 g, Carb 2.6 g, Fiber 0.4 g, Net Carb 2.2 g

4. LEMON POPPY SEED BREAD

INGREDIENTS

- 3 eggs, pasteurized
- 1 ½ tablespoons butter, grass-fed, unsalted, melted
- 1 ½ tablespoons lemon juice
- 1 lemon, zested
- 1 ½ cups / 150 grams almond flour
- ¼ cup / 50 grams erythritol sweetener
- ¼ teaspoon baking powder
- 1 tablespoon poppy seeds

 PREPARATION
10 MIN

 COOKING
4 HOURS

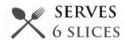 **SERVES**
6 SLICES

DIRECTIONS

1. Gather all the ingredients for the bread and plug in the bread machine having the capacity of 1 pound of bread recipe.
2. Take a large bowl, crack eggs in it and then beat in butter, lemon juice, and lemon zest until combined.
3. Take a separate large bowl, add flour in it and then stir in sweetener, baking powder, and poppy seeds until mixed.
4. Add egg mixture into the bread bucket, top with flour mixture, shut the lid, select the "basic/white"

cycle or "low-carb" setting and then press the up/down arrow button to adjust baking time according to your bread machine; it will take 3 to 4 hours.
5. Then press the crust button to select light crust if available, and press the "start/stop" button to switch on the bread machine.
6. When the bread machine beeps, open the lid, then take out the bread basket and lift out the bread.
7. Let bread cool on a wire rack for 1 hour, then cut it into six slices and serve.

Nutrition: Calories 201, Fat 17.5 g, Protein 8.2 g, Carb 5.8 g, Fiber 3 g, Net Carb 2.8 g

5. ALMOND MEAL BREAD

INGREDIENTS

- 4 eggs, pasteurized
- ¼ cup / 60 ml melted coconut oil
- 1 tablespoon apple cider vinegar
- 2 ¼ cups / 215 grams almond meal
- 1 teaspoon baking soda
- ¼ cup / 35 grams ground flaxseed meal

- 1 teaspoon onion powder
- 1 tablespoon minced garlic
- 1 teaspoon of sea salt
- 1 teaspoon chopped sage leaves
- 1 teaspoon fresh thyme
- 1 teaspoon chopped rosemary leaves

 PREPARATION
10 MIN

 COOKING
4 HOURS

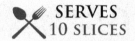 **SERVES**
10 SLICES

DIRECTIONS

1. Gather all the ingredients for the bread and plug in the bread machine having the capacity of 2 pounds of bread recipe.

2. Take a large bowl, crack eggs in it and then beat in coconut oil and vinegar until well blended.

3. Take a separate large bowl, place the almond meal in it, add remaining ingredients, and stir until well mixed.

4. Add egg mixture into the bread bucket, top with flour mixture, shut the lid, select the "basic/white" cycle or "low-carb" setting and then press the up/down arrow button to adjust baking time according to your bread machine; it will take 3 to 4 hours.

5. Then press the crust button to select light crust if available, and press the "start/stop" button to switch on the bread machine.

6. When the bread machine beeps, open the lid, then take out the bread basket and lift out the bread.

7. Let bread cool on a wire rack for 1 hour, then cut it into ten slices and serve.

Nutrition: Calories 104, Fat 8.8 g, Protein 4 g, Carb 2.1 g, Fiber 1.8 g, Net Carb 0.3 g

6. MACADAMIA NUT BREAD

INGREDIENTS

- 1 cup / 135 grams macadamia nuts
- 5 eggs, pasteurized
- ½ teaspoon apple cider vinegar
- ¼ cup / 30 grams coconut flour
- ½ teaspoon baking soda

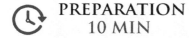 **PREPARATION**
10 MIN

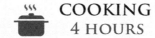 **COOKING**
4 HOURS

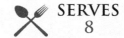 **SERVES**
8

DIRECTIONS

1. Gather all the ingredients for the bread and plug in the bread machine having the capacity of 1 pound of bread recipe.
2. Place nuts in a blender, pulse for 2 to 3 minutes until mixture reaches a consistency of butter, and then blend in eggs and vinegar until smooth.
3. Stir in flour and baking soda until well mixed.
4. Add the batter into the bread bucket, shut the lid, select the "basic/white" cycle or "low-carb" setting and then press the up/down arrow button to adjust baking time according to your bread machine; it will take 3 to 4 hours.
5. Then press the crust button to select light crust if available, and press the "start/stop" button to switch on the bread machine.
6. When the bread machine beeps, open the lid, then take out the bread basket and lift out the bread.
7. Let bread cool on a wire rack for 1 hour, then cut it into eight slices and serve.

Nutrition: Calories 155, Fat 14.3 g, Protein 5.6 g, Carb 3.9 g, Fiber 3 g, Net Carb 0.9 g

7. CAULIFLOWER AND GARLIC BREAD

INGREDIENTS

- 5 eggs, pasteurized, separated
- 2/3 cup / 85 grams coconut flour
- 1 ½ cup / 300 grams riced cauliflower
- 1 teaspoon minced garlic
- ½ teaspoon of sea salt
- ½ tablespoon chopped rosemary
- ½ tablespoon chopped parsley
- ¾ tablespoon baking powder
- 3 tablespoons melted butter, grass-fed, unsalted

 PREPARATION
10 MIN

 COOKING
4 HOUR

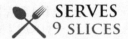 **SERVES**
9 SLICES

DIRECTIONS

1. Gather all the ingredients for the bread and plug in the bread machine having the capacity of 2 pounds of bread recipe.

2. Take a medium bowl, place cauliflower rice in it, cover with a plastic wrap, and then microwave for 3 to 4 minutes until steamed.

3. Then drain the cauliflower, wrap in cheesecloth and twist well to squeeze out moisture as much as possible, set aside until required.

4. Place egg whites in a large bowl and whisk by using an electric whisker until stiff peaks form.

5. Then transfer one-fourth of whipped egg whites into a food processor, add remaining ingredients except for cauliflower and pulse for 2 minutes until blended.

6. Add cauliflower rice, pulse for 2 minutes until well combined, and then pulse in remaining egg whites until just mixed.

7. Add batter into the bread bucket, shut the lid, select the "basic/white" cycle or "low-carb"

setting and then press the up/down arrow button to adjust baking time according to your bread machine; it will take 3 to 4 hours.

8. Then press the crust button to select light crust if available, and press the "start/stop" button to switch on the bread machine.

9. When the bread machine beeps, open the lid, then take out the bread basket and lift out the bread.

10. Let bread cool on a wire rack for 1 hour, then cut it into nine slices and serve.

Nutrition: Calories 108, Fat 8 g, Protein 6 g, Carb 8 g, Fiber 5 g, Net Carb 3 g

8. ROSEMARY BREAD

INGREDIENTS

- 6 eggs, pasteurized
- 8 tablespoons butter, grass-fed, unsalted, melted
- ½ cup /65 grams coconut flour
- 1 teaspoon baking powder
- ¼ teaspoon salt
- ½ teaspoon onion powder
- 1 teaspoon garlic powder
- 2 teaspoons dried rosemary

 PREPARATION 10 MIN

 COOKING 4 HOURS

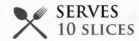 **SERVES** 10 SLICES

DIRECTIONS

1. Gather all the ingredients for the bread and plug in the bread machine having the capacity of 1 pound of bread recipe.
2. Take a large bowl, crack eggs in it, and then slowly beat in the melted butter until well combined.
3. Take a separate large bowl, place flour in it, and then stir in remaining ingredients until mixed.
4. Add egg mixture into the bread bucket, top with flour mixture, shut the lid, select the "basic/white" cycle or "low-carb" setting and then press the up/down arrow button to adjust baking time according to your bread machine; it will take 3 to 4 hours.
5. Then press the crust button to select light crust if available, and press the "start/stop" button to switch on the bread machine.
6. When the bread machine beeps, open the lid, then take out the bread basket and lift out the bread.
7. Let bread cool on a wire rack for 1 hour, then cut it into ten slices and serve.

Nutrition: Calories 147, Fat 12.5 g, Protein 4.6 g, Carb 3.5 g, Fiber 2 g, Net Carb 1.5 g

9. SESAME AND FLAX SEED BREAD

INGREDIENTS

- 3 eggs, pasteurized
- ½ cup / 100 grams cream cheese, softened
- 6 ½ tablespoons heavy whipping cream
- ¼ cup / 60 ml melted coconut oil
- ½ cup / 50 grams almond flour
- ¼ cup /35 grams flaxseed
- 6 ½ tablespoons coconut flour
- 2 2/3 tablespoons sesame seeds
- ½ teaspoon salt
- 1½ teaspoon baking powder
- 2 tablespoons ground psyllium husk powder
- ½ teaspoon ground caraway seeds

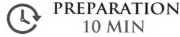 **PREPARATION** 10 MIN   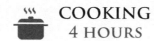 **COOKING** 4 HOURS   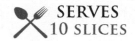 **SERVES** 10 SLICES

DIRECTIONS

1. Gather all the ingredients for the bread and plug in the bread machine having the capacity of 2 pounds of bread recipe.
2. Take a large bowl, crack eggs in it and then beat in cream cheese, whipping cream, and coconut oil until well blended.
3. Take a separate large bowl, place flours in it, and then stir in remaining ingredients until mixed.
4. Add egg mixture into the bread bucket, top with flour mixture, shut the lid, select the "basic/white" cycle or "low-carb" setting and then press the up/down arrow button to adjust baking time according to your bread machine; it will take 3 to 4 hours.
5. Then press the crust button to select light crust if available, and press the "start/stop" button to switch on the bread machine.
6. When the bread machine beeps, open the lid, then take out the bread basket and lift out the bread.
7. Let bread cool on a wire rack for 1 hour, then cut it into ten slices and serve.

Nutrition: Calories 230, Fat 21 g, Protein 6.3, Carb 6.2 g, Fiber 2 g, Net Carb 3.2 g

10. 3-SEED BREAD

INGREDIENTS

- 2 eggs, pasteurized
- ¼ cup / 50 grams butter melted
- 1 cup / 250 ml water warm, at 100°F / 38°C
- ¼ cup / 35 grams chia seeds
- ½ cup / 75 grams pumpkin seeds
- ½ cup / 75 grams psyllium husks
- ½ cup / 75 grams sunflower seeds
- ¼ cup / 25 grams coconut flour
- 1/4 teaspoon salt
- 1 teaspoon baking powder

 PREPARATION 10 MIN

 COOKING 4 HOURS

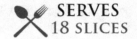 **SERVES** 18 SLICES

DIRECTIONS

1. Gather all the ingredients for the bread and plug in the bread machine having the capacity of 2 pounds of bread recipe.
2. Take a medium bowl, crack eggs in it and then beat in the butter until well blended.
3. Take a separate large bowl, place flour in it, and then stir in remaining ingredients except for water until mixed.
4. Pour water into the bread bucket, add egg mixture, top with flour mixture, shut the lid, select the "basic/white" cycle or "low-carb" setting and then press the up/down arrow button to adjust baking time according to your bread machine; it will take 3 to 4 hours.
5. Then press the crust button to select light crust if available, and press the "start/stop" button to switch on the bread machine.
6. When the bread machine beeps, open the lid, then take out the bread basket and lift out the bread.
7. Let bread cool on a wire rack for 1 hour, then cut and serve.

Nutrition: Calories 139, Fat 10 g, Protein 5 g, Carb 5.6 g, Fiber 3.6 g, Net Carb 2 g

11. BACON AND CHEDDAR BREAD

INGREDIENTS

- 2 eggs, pasteurized
- ¼ cup / 60 ml beer
- 2 tablespoons butter, grass-fed, unsalted, melted
- ¼ cup / 50 grams bacon, pasteurized, cooked, crumbled
- ½ cup / 120 grams shredded cheddar cheese
- ½ tablespoon coconut flour
- 1 cup / 100 grams almond flour
- ¼ teaspoon salt
- ½ tablespoon baking powder

 PREPARATION 10 MIN

 COOKING 4 HOURS

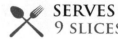 **SERVES** 9 SLICES

DIRECTIONS

1. Gather all the ingredients for the bread and plug in the bread machine having the capacity of 2 pounds of bread recipe.
2. Take a large bowl, crack eggs in it, beat in beer and butter until blended, and then fold in bacon and cheese until just mixed.
3. Take a separate large bowl, place flours in it, and then stir in salt and baking powder until mixed.
4. Add egg mixture into the bread bucket, top with flour mixture, shut the lid, select the "basic/white" cycle or "low-carb" setting and then press the up/down arrow button to adjust baking time according to your bread machine; it will take 3 to 4 hours.
5. Then press the crust button to select light crust if available, and press the "start/stop" button to switch on the bread machine.
6. When the bread machine beeps, open the lid, then take out the bread basket and lift out the bread.
7. Let bread cool on a wire rack for 1 hour, then cut it into nine slices and serve.

Nutrition: Calories 140, Fat 12 g, Protein 5 g, Carb 3 g, Fiber 1 g, Net Carb 2 g

12. OLIVE BREAD

INGREDIENTS

- 4 eggs, pasteurized
- 4 tablespoons avocado oil
- 1 tablespoon apple cider vinegar
- ½ cup / 65 grams coconut flour
- 1 tablespoon baking powder
- 2 tablespoons psyllium husk powder
- 1 ½ tablespoons dried rosemary
- 1/2 teaspoon salt
- 1/3 cup / 75 grams black olives, chopped
- ½ cup / 120 ml water

 PREPARATION
10 MIN

 COOKING
4 HOURS

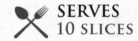 **SERVES**
10 SLICES

DIRECTIONS

1. Gather all the ingredients for the bread and plug in the bread machine having the capacity of 2 pounds of bread recipe.

2. Take a medium bowl, crack eggs in it, blend in oil until combined, stir in vinegar and fold in olives until mixed.

3. Take a separate medium bowl, place flour in it, and then stir in husk powder, baking powder, salt, and rosemary until mixed.

4. Add egg mixture into the bread bucket, top with flour mixture, shut the lid, select the "basic/white" cycle or "low-carb" setting and then press the up/down arrow button to adjust baking time according to your bread machine; it will take 3 to 4 hours.

5. Then press the crust button to select light crust if available, and press the "start/stop" button to switch on the bread machine.

6. When the bread machine beeps, open the lid, then take out the bread basket and lift out the bread.

7. Let bread cool on a wire rack for 1 hour, then cut it into ten slices and serve.

Nutrition: Calories 85, Fat 6.5 g, Protein 2 g, Carb 3.4 g, Fiber 2.5 g, Net Carb 1 g

13. JALAPENO CHEESE BREAD

INGREDIENTS

- 2 tablespoons Greek yogurt, full-fat
- 4 eggs, pasteurized
- 1/3 cup / 40 grams coconut flour
- ½ teaspoon of sea salt
- 2 tablespoons whole psyllium husks
- 1 teaspoon baking powder
- ¼ cup / 30 grams diced pickled jalapeños

- ¼ cup / 30 grams shredded cheddar cheese, divided

 PREPARATION 10 MIN

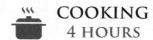 **COOKING** 4 HOURS

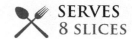 **SERVES** 8 SLICES

DIRECTIONS

1. Gather all the ingredients for the bread and plug in the bread machine having the capacity of 1 pound of bread recipe.
2. Take a large bowl, add yogurt and eggs in it and then beat until well combined.
3. Take a separate bowl, place flour in it, add remaining ingredients, and stir until mixed.
4. Add egg mixture into the bread bucket, top with flour mixture, shut the lid, select the "basic/white" cycle or "low-carb" setting and then press the up/down arrow button to adjust baking time according to your bread machine; it will take 3 to 4 hours.
5. Then press the crust button to select light crust if available, and press the "start/stop" button to switch on the bread machine.
6. When the bread machine beeps, open the lid, then take out the bread basket and lift out the bread.
7. Let bread cool on a wire rack for 1 hour, then cut it into eight slices and serve.

Nutrition: Calories 105, Fat 6.2 g, Protein 6.6 g, Carb 3.4 g, Fiber 1.7 g, Net Carb 1.7 g

14. BREAD DE SOUL

INGREDIENTS

- ¼ tsp. cream of tartar
- 2 ½ tsp. baking powder
- 1 tsp. xanthan gum
- 1/3 tsp. baking soda
- ½ tsp. salt
- 2/3 cup unflavored whey protein
- ¼ cup olive oil
- ¼ cup heavy whipping cream
- 2 drops of liquid sugar-free sweetener
- 4 eggs
- ¼ cup butter
- 12 oz. softened cream cheese

 PREPARATION 10 MIN　　 **COOKING** 45 MIN　　 **SERVES** 16

DIRECTIONS

1. Prepare bread machine loaf pan greasing it with cooking spray.
2. In a bowl, mix together the dry ingredients. Until well combined.
3. Into a separate bowl, microwave cream cheese and butter for 1 minute.
4. Remove and blend well with a hand mixer.
5. Add olive oil, eggs, heavy cream, and few drops of sweetener and blend well.
6. Following the instructions on your machine's manual, mix the dry ingredients into the wet ingredients and pour in the bread machine loaf pan, taking care to follow how to mix in the baking powder.
7. Place the bread pan in the machine, and select the basic bread setting, together with the bread size and crust type, if available, then press start once you have closed the lid of the machine.
8. When the bread is ready, using oven mitts, remove the bread pan from the machine.
9. Let it cool before slicing.
10. Cool, slice, and enjoy.

Nutrition: Calories 200, Fat 15.2 g, Carb 1.8 g, Protein 10 g

15. CHIA SEED BREAD

INGREDIENTS

- ½ tsp. xanthan gum
- ½ cup butter
- 2 tbsp. coconut oil
- 1 tbsp. baking powder
- 1 tbsp. sesame seeds
- 1 tbsp. chia seeds
- ½ tsp. salt
- ¼ cup sunflower seeds
- 2 cups almond flour
- 7 eggs

 PREPARATION 10 MIN   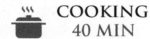 **COOKING** 40 MIN   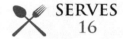 **SERVES** 16

DIRECTIONS

1. Preheat the oven to 350F.
2. Beat eggs in a bowl on high for 1 to 2 minutes.
3. Beat in the xanthan gum and combine coconut oil and melted butter into eggs, beating continuously.
4. Set aside the sesame seeds, but add the rest of the ingredients.
5. Prepare bread machine loaf pan greasing it with cooking spray and place the mixture in it. Top the mixture with sesame seeds.
6. Place the bread pan in the machine, and select the basic bread setting, together with the bread size and crust type, if available, then press start once you have closed the lid of the machine.
7. When the bread is ready, using oven mitts, remove the bread pan from the machine.
8. Let it cool before slicing.
9. Cool, slice, and enjoy.

Nutrition: Calories 405, Fat 37 g, Carb 4g, Protein 14 g

16. SPECIAL KETO BREAD

INGREDIENTS

- 2 tsp. baking powder
- ½ cup water
- 1 tbsp. poppy seeds
- 2 cups fine ground almond meal
- 5 large eggs
- ½ cup olive oil
- ½ tsp. fine Himalayan salt

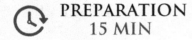
PREPARATION
15 MIN

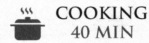
COOKING
40 MIN

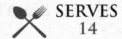
SERVES
14

DIRECTIONS

1. Prepare bread machine loaf pan greasing it with cooking spray.
2. In a bowl, mix together salt, almond meal, and baking powder until well combined.
3. Following the instructions on your machine's manual, mix the dry ingredients into the wet ingredients and pour in the bread machine loaf pan, taking care to follow how to mix in the baking powder.
4. Place the bread pan in the machine, and select the basic bread setting, together with the bread size, if available, then press start once you have closed the lid of the machine.
5. When the bread is ready, using oven mitts, remove the bread pan from the machine.
6. Let it cool for 30 minutes before slicing.
7. Enjoy.

Nutrition: Calories 227, Fat 21 g, Carb 4 g, Protein 7 g

17. KETO FLUFFY CLOUD BREAD

INGREDIENTS

- pinch salt
- ½ tbsp. ground psyllium husk powder
- ½ tbsp. baking powder
- ¼ tsp. cream of tarter
- 4 eggs, separated
- ½ cup, cream cheese

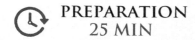 **PREPARATION**
25 MIN

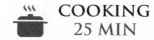 **COOKING**
25 MIN

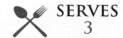 **SERVES**
3

DIRECTIONS

1. Preheat the oven to 300F and line a baking tray with parchment paper.
2. Whisk egg whites in a bowl until soft peaks are formed.
3. Mix egg yolks with cream cheese, salt, cream of tartar, psyllium husk powder, and baking powder in a bowl.
4. Fold in the egg whites carefully and transfer to the baking tray.
5. Place in the oven and bake for 25 minutes.
6. Remove from the oven and serve.

Nutrition: Calories 185, Fat 16.4 g, Carb 3.9 g, Protein 6.6 g

18. SPLENDID LOW-CARB BREAD

INGREDIENTS

- ½ tsp. herbs, such as basil, rosemary, or oregano
- ½ tsp. garlic or onion powder
- 1 tbsp. baking powder
- 5 tbsp. psyllium husk powder
- ½ cup almond flour
- ½ cup coconut flour
- ¼ tsp. salt
- 1 ½ cup egg whites

- 1 tbsp. oil or melted butter
- 1 tbsp. apple cider vinegar
- 1/3 to ¾ cup hot water

 PREPARATION 15 MIN   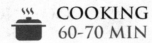 **COOKING** 60-70 MIN   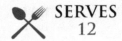 **SERVES** 12

DIRECTIONS

1. Prepare bread machine loaf pan greasing it with cooking spray.
2. In a bowl, mix together salt, psyllium husk powder, onion or garlic powder, coconut flour, almond flour, and baking powder. Until well combined.
3. Following the instructions on your machine's manual, mix the dry ingredients into the wet ingredients and pour in the bread machine loaf pan, taking care to follow how to mix in the baking powder.
4. Place the bread pan in the machine, and select the basic bread setting, together with the bread size, if available, then press start once you have closed the lid of the machine.
5. When the bread is ready, using oven mitts, remove the bread pan from the machine.
6. Cool and serve.

Nutrition: Calories 97, Fat 5.7 g, Carb 7.5 g, Protein 4.1 g

19. COCONUT FLOUR ALMOND BREAD

INGREDIENTS

- 2 tbsp. butter, melted
- 1 tbsp. coconut oil, melted
- 6 eggs
- 1 tsp. baking soda
- 2 tbsp. ground flaxseed
- 1 ½ tbsp. psyllium husk powder
- 5 tbsp. coconut flour
- 1 ½ cup almond flour

 PREPARATION 10 MIN   **COOKING** 30 MIN   **SERVES** 4

DIRECTIONS

1. Prepare bread machine loaf pan greasing it with cooking spray.
2. Mix the eggs in a bowl for a few minutes.
3. Add in the butter and coconut oil and mix once more for 1 minute.
4. Following the instructions on your machine's manual, add the almond flour, coconut flour, baking soda, psyllium husk, and ground flaxseed to the mixture and pour in the bread machine loaf pan.
5. Place the bread pan in the machine, and select the basic bread setting, together with the bread size, if available, then press start once you have closed the lid of the machine.
6. When the bread is ready, using oven mitts, remove the bread pan from the machine.
7. Cool and serve.

Nutrition: Calories 475, Fat 38 g, Carb 7 g, Protein 19 g

20. QUICK LOW-CARB BREAD LOAF

INGREDIENTS

- 2/3 cup coconut flour
- ½ cup butter, melted
- 3 tbsp. coconut oil, melted
- 1/3 cup almond flour
- ½ tsp. xanthan gum
- 1 tsp. baking powder
- 6 large eggs
- ½ tsp. salt

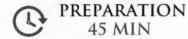 **PREPARATION**
45 MIN

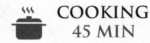 **COOKING**
45 MIN

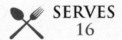 **SERVES**
16

DIRECTIONS

1. Prepare bread machine loaf pan greasing it with cooking spray.
2. Beat the eggs until creamy.
3. Add in the coconut flour and almond flour, mixing them for 1 minute. Next, add the xanthan gum, coconut oil, baking powder, butter, and salt and mix them until the dough turns thick.
4. Pour mixture in the bread machine loaf pan.
5. Place the bread pan in the machine, and select the basic bread setting, together with the bread size, if available, then press start once you have closed the lid of the machine.
6. When the bread is ready, using oven mitts, remove the bread pan from the machine.
7. Cool and serve.

Nutrition: Calories 174, Fat 15 g, Carb 5 g, Protein 5 g

21. KETO BAKERS BREAD

INGREDIENTS

- Pinch of salt
- 4 tbsp. light cream cheese softened
- ½ tsp. cream of tartar
- 4 eggs, yolks, and whites separated

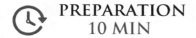 **PREPARATION**
10 MIN

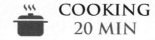 **COOKING**
20 MIN

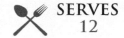 **SERVES**
12

DIRECTIONS

1. Heat 2 racks in the middle of the oven at 350F.
2. Line 2 baking pan with parchment paper, then grease with cooking spray.
3. Separate egg yolks from the whites and place them in separate mixing bowls.
4. Beat the egg whites and cream of tartar with a hand mixer until stiff, about 3 to 5 minutes. Do not over-beat.
5. Whisk the cream cheese, salt, and egg yolks until smooth.
6. Slowly fold the cheese mix into the whites until fluffy.
7. Spoon ¼ cup measure of the batter onto the baking sheets, 6 mounds on each sheet.
8. Bake in the oven for 20 to 22 minutes, alternating racks halfway through.
9. Cool and serve.

Nutrition: Calories 41, Fat 3.2 g, Carb 1 g, Protein 2.4 g

22. ALMOND FLOUR LEMON BREAD

INGREDIENTS

- 1 tsp. French herbs
- 1 tsp. lemon juice
- 1 tsp. salt
- 1 tsp. cream of tartar
- 1 tsp. baking powder
- ¼ cup melted butter
- 5 large eggs, divided
- ¼ cup coconut flour
- 1 ½ cup almond flour

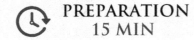 **PREPARATION** 15 MIN

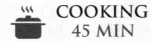 **COOKING** 45 MIN

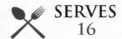 **SERVES** 16

DIRECTIONS

1. Prepare bread machine loaf pan greasing it with cooking spray.
2. Whip the whites and cream of tartar until soft peaks form.
3. In a bowl, combine salt, egg yolks, melted butter, and lemon juice. Mix well.
4. Add coconut flour, almond flour, herbs, and baking powder. Mix well.
5. To the dough, add 1/3 the egg whites and mix until well-combined.
6. Add the remaining egg whites mixture and slowly mix to incorporate everything. Do not over mix.
7. However, take a look to the manufacturer's instructions for mixing dry and wet ingredients.
8. Pour mixture in the bread machine loaf pan.
9. Place the bread pan in the machine, and select the basic bread setting, together with the bread size, if available, then press start once you have closed the lid of the machine.

Nutrition: Calories 115, Fat 9.9 g, Carb 3.3 g, Protein 5.2 g

23. SEED AND NUT BREAD

INGREDIENTS

- 3 eggs
- ¼ cup avocado oil
- 5 tsp. psyllium husk powder
- 1 tsp. apple cider vinegar
- ¾ tsp. salt
- 5 drops liquid stevia
- 1 ½ cups raw unsalted almonds
- ½ cup raw unsalted pepitas
- ½ cup raw unsalted sunflower seeds
- ½ cup flaxseeds

 PREPARATION
10 MIN

 COOKING
40 MIN

 SERVES
24

DIRECTIONS

1. Prepare bread machine loaf pan greasing it with cooking spray.
2. In a large bowl, whisk together the oil, eggs, psyllium husk powder, vinegar, salt, and liquid stevia.
3. Stir in the pepitas, almonds, sunflower seeds, and flaxseeds until well combined.
4. However, take a look to the manufacturer's instructions for mixing dry and wet ingredients.
5. Pour mixture in the bread machine loaf pan.
6. Place the bread pan in the machine, and select the basic bread setting, together with the bread size, if available, then press start once you have closed the lid of the machine.
7. When the bread is ready, using oven mitts, remove the bread pan from the machine.
8. Cool, slice, and serve.

Nutrition: Calories 131, Fat 12 g, Carb 4 g, Protein 5 g

24. DILL AND CHEDDAR BREAD

INGREDIENTS

- 4 eggs, pasteurized
- ¼ teaspoon cream of tartar
- 5 tablespoons butter, grass-fed, unsalted
- 2 cups / 470 grams grated cheddar cheese,
- 1 ½ cups / 150 grams almond flour
- 1 scoop of egg white protein
- 1/4 teaspoon salt

- 1 teaspoon garlic powder
- 4 teaspoons baking powder
- ¼ tablespoon dried dill weed

 PREPARATION
10 MIN

 COOKING
4 HOURS

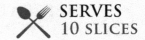 **SERVES**
10 SLICES

DIRECTIONS

1. Gather all the ingredients for the bread and plug in the bread machine having the capacity of 2 pounds of bread recipe.
2. Take a large bowl, crack eggs in it, beat until blended and then beat in cream of tartar, butter, and cheese until just mixed.
3. Take a separate large bowl, place flour in it, and then stir in egg white protein, salt, garlic powder, baking powder, and dill until mixed.
4. Add egg mixture into the bread bucket, top with flour mixture, shut

the lid, select the "basic/white" cycle or "low-carb" setting and then press the up/down arrow button to adjust baking time according to your bread machine; it will take 3 to 4 hours.
5. Then press the crust button to select light crust if available, and press the "start/stop" button to switch on the bread machine.
6. When the bread machine beeps, open the lid, then take out the bread basket and lift out the bread.
7. Let bread cool on a wire rack for 1 hour, then cut it and serve.

Nutrition: Calories 292, Fat 25.2 g, Protein 14.3 g, Carb 6.1 g, Fiber 2.6 g, Net Carb 3.5 g

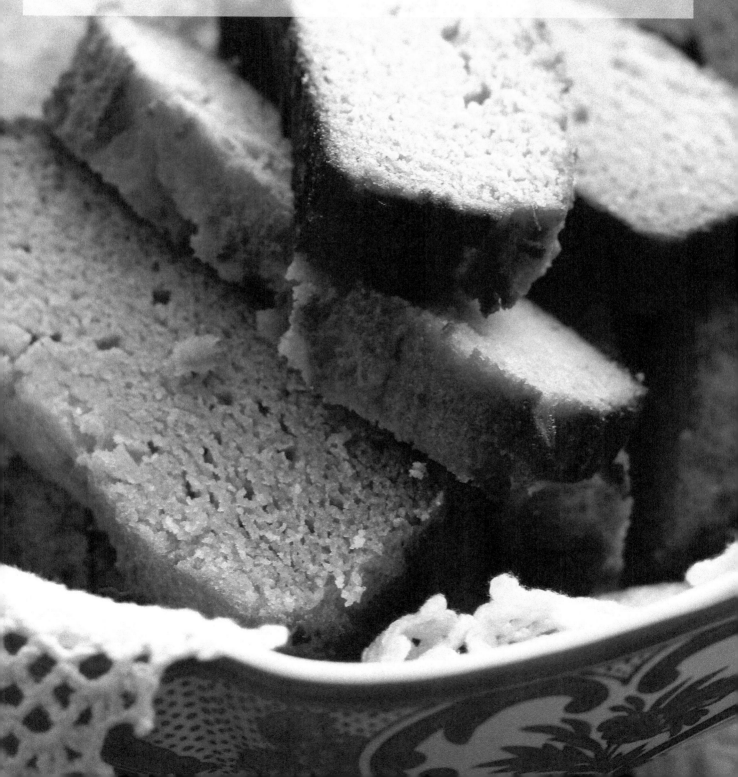

CHAPTER 8: GLUTEN FREE BREAD RECIPES

25. CLASSIC GLUTEN FREE BREAD

INGREDIENTS

- 1/2 cup butter, melted
- 3 tbsp coconut oil, melted
- 6 eggs
- 2/3 cup sesame seed flour
- 1/3 cup coconut flour
- 2 tsp baking powder
- 1 tsp psyllium husks
- 1/2 tsp xanthan gum
- 1/2 tsp salt

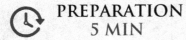 **PREPARATION**
5 MIN

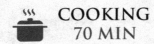 **COOKING**
70 MIN

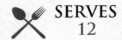 **SERVES**
12

DIRECTIONS

1. Pour in eggs, melted butter, and melted coconut oil into your bread machine pan.
2. Add the remaining Ingredients to the bread machine pan.
3. Set bread machine to gluten free.
4. When the bread is done, remove bread machine pan from the bread machine.
5. Let cool slightly before transferring to a cooling rack.
6. You can store your bread for up to 3 days.

Nutrition: Calories 146, Carbohydrates 1.2 g, Protein 3.5 g, Fat 14 g

26. GLUTEN FREE CHOCOLATE ZUCCHINI BREAD

INGREDIENTS

- 1 ½ cups coconut flour
- ¼ cup unsweetened cocoa powder
- ½ cup erythritol
- ½ tsp cinnamon
- 1 tsp baking soda
- 1 tsp baking powder
- ¼ tsp salt
- ¼ cup coconut oil, melted
- 4 eggs
- 1 tsp vanilla
- 2 cups zucchini, shredded

 PREPARATION 5 MIN   **COOKING** 80 MIN   **SERVES** 12

DIRECTIONS

1. Shred the zucchini and use paper towels to drain excess water, set aside.
2. Lightly beat eggs with coconut oil then add to bread machine pan.
3. Add the remaining Ingredients to the pan.
4. Set bread machine to gluten free.
5. When the bread is done, remove bread machine pan from the bread machine.
6. Let cool slightly before transferring to a cooling rack.
7. You can store your bread for up to 5 days.

Nutrition: Calories 185, Carbohydrates 6 g, Protein 5 g, Fat 17 g

27. NOT YOUR EVERYDAY BREAD

INGREDIENTS

- 2 tsp active dry yeast
- 2 tbsp inulin
- ½ cup warm water
- ¾ cup almond flour
- ¼ cup golden flaxseed, ground
- 2 tbsp whey protein isolate
- 2 tbsp psyllium husk finely ground
- 2 tsp xanthan gum
- 2 tsp baking powder
- 1 tsp salt
- ¼ tsp cream of tartar
- ¼ tsp ginger, ground
- 1 egg
- 3 egg whites
- 2 tbsp ghee
- 1 tbsp apple cider vinegar
- ¼ cup sour cream

 PREPARATION 5 MIN

 COOKING 30 MIN

 SERVES 12

DIRECTIONS

1. Pour wet Ingredients into bread machine pan.
2. Add dry Ingredients, with the yeast on top.
3. Set bread machine to basic bread setting.
4. When the bread is done, remove bread machine pan from the bread machine.
5. Let cool slightly before transferring to a cooling rack.
6. You can store your bread for up to 5 days.

Nutrition: Calories 175, Carbohydrates 6 g, Protein 5 g, Fat 14 g

28. BANANA CAKE LOAF

INGREDIENTS

- 1 ½ cups almond flour
- 1 tsp baking powder
- ½ cup butter
- 1 ½ cups erythritol
- 2 eggs
- 2 bananas, extra ripe, mashed
- 2 tsp whole almond milk

 PREPARATION
5 MIN

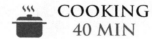 **COOKING**
40 MIN

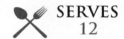 **SERVES**
12

DIRECTIONS

1. Mix butter, eggs, and almond milk together in a mixing bowl.
2. Mash bananas with a fork and add in the mashed bananas.
3. Mix all dry Ingredients together in a separate small bowl.
4. Slowly combine dry Ingredients with wet Ingredients.
5. Pour mixture into bread machine pan.
6. Set bread machine for bake.
7. When the cake is done remove from bread machine and transfer to a cooling rack.
8. Allow to cool completely before serving.
9. You can store your banana cake loaf bread for up to 5 days in the refrigerator.

Nutrition: Calories 168, Carbohydrates 7 g, Protein 5 g, Fat 14 g

29. ALMOND BUTTER BROWNIES

INGREDIENTS

- 1 cup almond butter
- 2 tbsp cocoa powder, unsweetened
- ½ cup erythritol
- ¼ cup dark chocolate chips, sugar-free
- 1 egg
- 3 tbsp almond milk, unsweetened

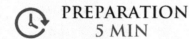 **PREPARATION**
5 MIN

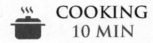 **COOKING**
10 MIN

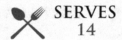 **SERVES**
14

DIRECTIONS

1. Beat egg and almond butter together in a mixing bowl.
2. Add in erythritol and cocoa powder.
3. If the mixture is too crumbly or dry, add in almond milk until you have a smooth consistency.
4. Fold in dark chocolate chips.
5. Pour mixture into bread machine pan.
6. Set bread machine to bake.
7. When done remove from bread machine and transfer to a cooling rack.
8. Cool completely before serving, you can store for up to 5 days in the refrigerator.

Nutrition: Calories 141, Carbohydrates 3 g, Protein 5 g, Fat 12 g

30. ALMOND BUTTER BREAD

INGREDIENTS

- 1 cup coconut almond butter, creamy
- 3 eggs
- ½ tsp baking soda
- 1 tbsp apple cider vinegar

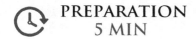
PREPARATION
5 MIN

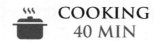
COOKING
40 MIN

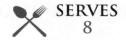
SERVES
8

DIRECTIONS

1. Combine all Ingredients in a food processor.
2. When the mixture is smooth transfer to bread machine baking pan.
3. Set bread machine to bake.
4. When done baking, remove from the pan from your bread machine.
5. Allow to cool completely before slicing.
6. You can store for up to 5 days in the refrigerator.

Nutrition: Calories 175, Carbohydrates 6 g, Protein 5 g, Fat 14 g

31. GLUTEN-FREE ALMOND BREAD

INGREDIENTS

- 2 cups almond flour, blanched
- ½ cup butter, melted
- 7 eggs
- 2 tbsp. avocado oil
- ½ tsp. xanthan gum
- ½ tsp. baking powder
- ½ tsp. salt

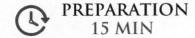 **PREPARATION** 15 MIN 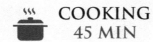 **COOKING** 45 MIN 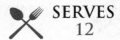 **SERVES** 12

DIRECTIONS

1. Prepare bread machine loaf pan greasing it with cooking spray.
2. In a bowl, mix together dry Ingredients until well combined.
3. In another bowl whisk eggs for 3 minutes or until they reach a creamy consistency.
4. Following the instructions on your machine's manual, mix the dry ingredients into the wet ingredients and pour in the bread machine loaf pan, taking care to follow how to mix in the baking powder.
5. Place the bread pan in the machine, and select the basic bread setting, or gluten-free program, if available, then press start once you have closed the lid of the machine.
6. When the bread is ready, using oven mitts, remove the bread pan from the machine.
7. Let it cool before slicing.
8. Cool, slice, and serve.

Nutrition: Calories 247, Fat 22.8 g, Carb 4.9 g, Protein 7.7 g

32. KETO ALMOND BREAD

INGREDIENTS

- ½ cups almond flour
- 2 tsp. baking powder
- 2 tbsp. butter, melted
- ¼ tsp. cream of tartar
- 6 eggs, whites and yolks separated
- Pinch of salt

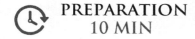
PREPARATION
10 MIN

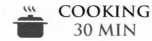
COOKING
30 MIN

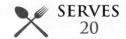
SERVES
20

DIRECTIONS

1. In a bowl, beat the cream of tartar and egg whites until soft peaks form.
2. Keep the mix on the side.
3. In a food processor, mix almond flour, salt, baking powder, egg yolks, and butter.
4. Add 1/3 cup egg whites to food processor and pulse until combined.
5. Add rest of the egg whites and mix until combined.
6. Pour mixture into bread machine pan.
7. Set bread Basic program and start.
8. When baking is complete remove from bread machine and transfer to a cooling rack.
9. When it is cool, slice, and serve.

Nutrition: Calories 271, Fat 22 g, Carb 6 g, Protein 5 g

33. CARROT CAKE

INGREDIENTS

- ½ cup erythritol
- ½ cup butter
- ½ tbsp vanilla extract
- 1 ¾ cups almond flour
- 1 ½ tsp baking powder
- 1 ½ tsp cinnamon
- ¼ tsp sea salt
- 1 ½ cup carrots, grated
- 1 cup pecans, chopped

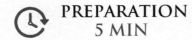 **PREPARATION**
5 MIN

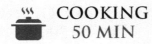 **COOKING**
50 MIN

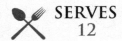 **SERVES**
12

DIRECTIONS

1. Grate carrots and place in a food processor.
2. Add in the rest of the Ingredients, except the pecans, and process until well-incorporated.
3. Fold in pecans.
4. Pour mixture into bread machine pan.
5. Set bread machine to bake.
6. When baking is complete remove from bread machine and transfer to a cooling rack.
7. Allow to cool completely before slicing. (you can also top with a sugar-free cream cheese frosting, see recipe below).
8. You can store for up to 5 days in the refrigerator.

Nutrition: Calories 350, Carbohydrates 8 g, Protein 7 g, Fat 34 g

34. SEEDED LOAF

INGREDIENTS

- 7 eggs
- 1 cup almond flour
- ½ cup butter
- 2 tbsp olive oil
- 2 tbsp chia seeds
- 2 tbsp sesame seeds
- 1 tsp baking soda
- ½ tsp xanthan gum
- ¼ tsp salt

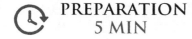 **PREPARATION** 5 MIN   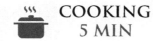 **COOKING** 5 MIN   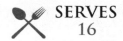 **SERVES** 16

DIRECTIONS

1. Add eggs and butter to the bread machine pan.
2. Top with all other Ingredients.
3. Set bread machine to the gluten free setting.
4. Once done remove from bread machine and transfer to a cooling rack.
5. This bread can be stored in the fridge for up to 5 days or 3 weeks in the freezer.

Nutrition: Calories 190, Carbohydrates 8 g, Fats 18 g, Protein 18 g

35. SIMPLE KETO BREAD

INGREDIENTS

- 3 cups almond flour
- 2 tbsp inulin
- 1 tbsp whole milk
- ½ tsp salt
- 2 tsp active yeast
- 1 ¼ cups warm water
- 1 tbsp olive oil

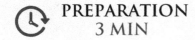 **PREPARATION**
3 MIN

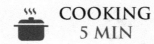 **COOKING**
5 MIN

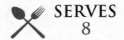 **SERVES**
8

DIRECTIONS

1. Use a small mixing bowl to combine all dry Ingredients, except for the yeast.
2. In the bread machine pan add all wet Ingredients.
3. Add all of your dry Ingredients, from the small mixing bowl, in the bread machine pan. Top with the yeast.
4. Set the bread machine to the basic bread setting.
5. When the bread is done, remove bread machine pan from the bread machine.
6. Let cool slightly before transferring to a cooling rack.
7. The bread can be stored for up to 5 days on the counter and for up to 3 months in the freezer.

Nutrition: Calories 85, Carbohydrates 4 g, Fats 7 g, Protein 3 g

36. CLASSIC KETO BREAD

INGREDIENTS

- 7 eggs
- ½ cup ghee
- 2 cups almond flour
- 1 tbsp baking powder
- ¼ tsp salt

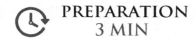

PREPARATION
3 MIN

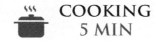

COOKING
5 MIN

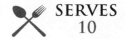

SERVES
10

DIRECTIONS

1. Pour eggs and ghee into bread machine pan.
2. Add remaining Ingredients.
3. Set bread machine to quick setting.
4. Allow bread machine to complete its cycle.
5. When the bread is done, remove bread machine pan from the bread machine.
6. Let cool slightly before transferring to a cooling rack.
7. The bread can be stored for up to 4 days on the counter and for up to 3 months in the freezer.

Nutrition: Calories 167, Carbohydrates 2 g, Fats 16 g, Protein 5 g

CHAPTER 9:   CHEESE BREAD RECIPES

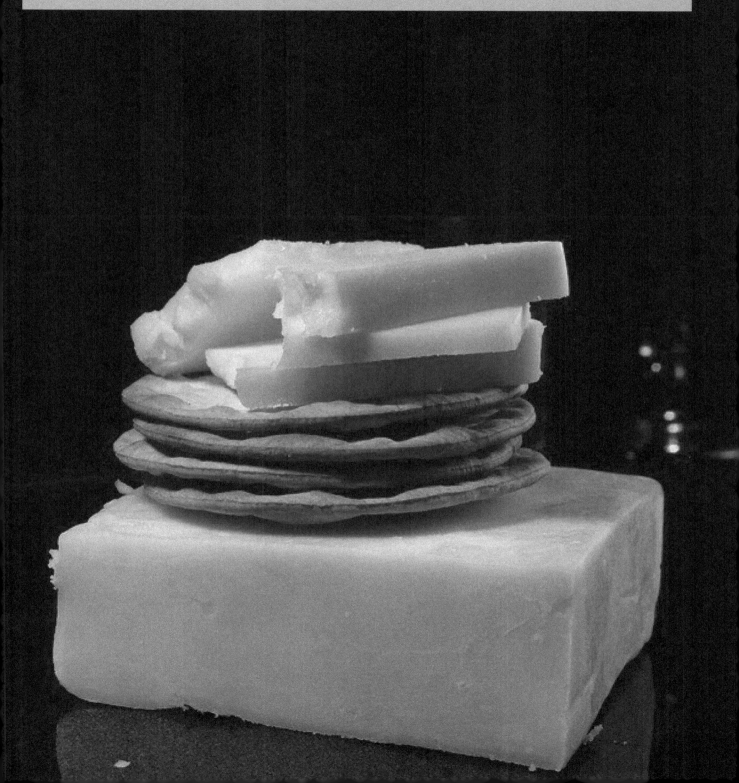

37. CHEESY GARLIC BREAD

INGREDIENTS

For Bread:
- ¾ cup mozzarella, shredded
- ½ cup almond flour
- Salt, to taste
- 1 egg

For topping:
- 2 tbsp melted butter
- ½ tsp parsley
- 1 tsp garlic clove, minced

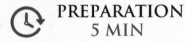 **PREPARATION**
5 MIN

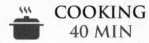 **COOKING**
40 MIN

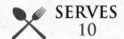 **SERVES**
10

DIRECTIONS

1. Mix together your topping Ingredients and set aside.
2. Pour the remaining wet Ingredients into the bread machine pan.
3. Add the dry Ingredients.
4. Set bread machine to the gluten free setting.
5. When the bread is done, remove bread machine pan from the bread machine.
6. Let cool slightly before transferring to a cooling rack.
7. Once on a cooling rack, drizzle with the topping mix.
8. You can store your bread for up to 7 days.

Nutrition: Calories 29, Carbohydrates 1 g, Protein 2 g, Fat 2 g

38. CHEESY GARLIC BREAD (VERS. 2)

INGREDIENTS

For the Bread:
- 5 eggs, pasteurized
- 2 cups / 200 grams almond flour
- ½ teaspoon xanthan gum
- 1 teaspoon garlic powder
- 1 teaspoon salt
- 1 teaspoon parsley
- 1 teaspoon Italian seasoning
- 1 teaspoon dried oregano
- 1 stick of butter, grass-fed, unsalted, melted

- 1 cup / 100 grams grated mozzarella cheese
- 2 tablespoons ricotta cheese
- 1 cup / 235 grams grated cheddar cheese
- 1/3 cup / 30 grams grated parmesan cheese

For the Topping:
- ½ stick of butter, grass-fed, unsalted, melted
- 1 teaspoon garlic powder

 PREPARATION 10 MIN

 COOKING 4 HOURS

 SERVES 16

DIRECTIONS

1. Gather all the ingredients for the bread and plug in the bread machine having the capacity of 2 pounds of bread recipe.
2. Take a large bowl, crack eggs in it and then whisk until blended.
3. Take a separate large bowl, place flour in it, and stir in xanthan gum and all the cheeses until well combined.
4. Take a medium bowl, place butter in it, add all the seasonings in it, and stir until mixed.
5. Add egg mixture into the bread bucket, top with seasoning mixture and flour mixture, shut the lid, select the "basic/white" cycle or "low-carb" setting and then press the up/down arrow button to adjust baking time according to your bread machine; it will take 3 to 4 hours.
6. Then press the crust button to select light crust if available, and press the "start/stop" button to switch on the bread machine.
7. When the bread machine beeps, open the lid, then take out the bread basket and lift out the bread.
8. Prepare the topping by mixing together melted butter and garlic

powder and brush the mixture on top of the bread.

9. Let bread cool on a wire rack for 1 hour, then cut it into sixteen slices and serve.

Nutrition: Calories 250, Fat 14.5 g, Protein 7.2 g, Carb 3 g, Fiber 1.6 g, Net Carb 1.4 g

39. CHEESE BLEND BREAD

INGREDIENTS

- 5 oz cream cheese
- 2 tsp baking powder
- ½ tsp himalayan salt
- ½ cup parmesan cheese, shredded
- 3 tbsp water
- 3 eggs
- ½ cup mozzarella cheese, shredded

 PREPARATION
5 MIN

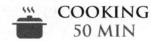 **COOKING**
50 MIN

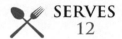 **SERVES**
12

DIRECTIONS

1. Place wet Ingredients into bread machine pan.
2. Add dry Ingredients.
3. Set the bread machine to the gluten free setting.
4. When the bread is done, remove bread machine pan from the bread machine.
5. Let cool slightly before transferring to a cooling rack.
6. You can store your bread for up to 5 days.

Nutrition: Calories 132, Carbohydrates 4 g, Protein 6 g, Fat 8 g

40. CHEESY VEG TORTILLAS

INGREDIENTS

- 1 ½ cups riced cauliflower
- 100g shredded cheddar cheese
- 2 free range eggs
- ½ teaspoon sea salt
- ¼ teaspoon garlic powder
- ¼ teaspoon onion powder

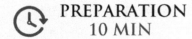 **PREPARATION** 10 MIN
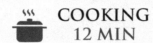 **COOKING** 12 MIN
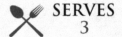 **SERVES** 3

DIRECTIONS

1. Preheat your oven to 400 degrees f. Line three baking sheets with parchment paper and set aside.
2. Combine all Ingredients in a food processor and puree until all the Ingredients come together into a smooth texture.
3. Pour mixture in bread machine pan.
4. Place the bread pan in the machine, and select the pasta or cookies setting.
5. Then press start once you have closed the lid of the machine.
6. Remove dough from bread machine when cycle is complete.
7. Use a 3-tablespoon cookie scoop to portion the mixture onto the baking sheets, leaving room for rolling them out.
8. Cover the mounds with a piece of parchment paper. Roll the mounds out into circles until they are about 4-to 4 1/2-inches across. Remove the wax paper.
9. Bake the tortillas for 12 minutes, until golden. Cool on the baking sheets for 3-5 minutes before peeling off the parchment paper.

Nutrition: Calories 160, Fat 11 g, Carb 4 g, Dietary Fiber 8 g, Protein 9 g, Cholesterol 100 mg, Sodium 419 mg

41. CHEESE & FRUIT STUFFED PANINI

INGREDIENTS

- Low carb flat bread (10 slices)
- 2 tbsp. Dijon mustard
- 2 tbsp. Mayonnaise
- 250g aged ham
- 120g brie thinly sliced
- 1 green apple very thinly sliced
- Oil or melted butter for brushing

 PREPARATION
10 MIN

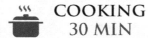 **COOKING**
30 MIN

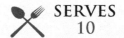 **SERVES**
10

DIRECTIONS

1. Start by preheating your panini maker.
2. Cut through the center of each slice of bread to get two very flat and thin slices.
3. Combine mustard and mayonnaise in a small bowl and spread one side of all the slices with the combo.
4. Form sandwiches with the cheese and ham.
5. Brush the outer parts of the sandwiches with the melted butter and put in the panini maker leaving it grill until golden.

Nutrition: Calories 288, Total Fat 12 g, Carb 15.5 g, Dietary Fiber 7.1 g, Protein 13.6 g, Cholesterol 217 mg, Sodium 329 mg

42. CHEESY LOW CARB BUTTER & GARLIC BREAD

INGREDIENTS

For Bread:
- 4 tablespoons melted butter
- 5 eggs
- 2 tablespoons ricotta cheese
- 1 cup mozzarella cheese
- 1 cup cheddar cheese
- 1/3 cup parmesan cheese
- 2 cups almond flour
- 1/2 teaspoon xanthan gum
- 1 teaspoon italian seasoning
- 1 teaspoon garlic powder
- 1 teaspoon oregano
- 1 teaspoon parsley
- 1 teaspoon salt

For garlic butter spread:
- 1 teaspoon garlic powder
- 2 tablespoons melted butter

 PREPARATION 5 MIN

 COOKING 15 MIN

 SERVES 16

DIRECTIONS

1. Prepare bread machine loaf pan greasing it with cooking spray.
2. In a bowl, mix together dry Ingredients until well combined.
3. In another bowl, whisk together wet Ingredients until well blended
4. Following the instructions on your machine's manual, mix the dry ingredients into the wet ingredients and pour in the bread machine loaf pan, taking care to follow how to mix in the baking powder.
5. Place the bread pan in the machine, and select the basic bread setting, together with the bread size and crust type, if available, then press start once you have closed the lid of the machine.
6. When the bread is ready, using oven mitts, remove the bread pan from the machine.
7. Let it cool before slicing.
8. In a small bowl, whisk together melted butter and garlic until well blended. Brush with garlic butter and serve.

Nutrition: Calories 240, Total Fat 14 g, Carb 4 g, Dietary Fiber 1.5 g, Sugars 1 g, Protein 7 g, Cholesterol 286 mg, Sodium 302 mg

43. GOAT CHEESE BREAD

INGREDIENTS

- 1 cup of almond blanched fine flour
- ½ cup of soy flour
- ¼ of salt
- 2 tsp. Of fresh thyme, crushed
- ½ cup of coconut milk, melted
- 1 tsp. Of pepper cayenne
- 2 Eggs
- 1 teaspoon Mustard of dijon
- 1 cup Crumbled fresh goat cheese
- 1 teaspoon baking powder
- 1/3 olive oil, extra virgin
- 1 teaspoon active dry yeast

 PREPARATION 5 MIN

 COOKING 15 MIN

 SERVES 10

DIRECTIONS

1. Get a mixing container and combine the almond flour, soy flour, fresh thyme, cayenne pepper, salt, crumbled fresh goat cheese, and baking powder.

2. Get another mixing container and combine extra virgin olive oil, eggs, coconut milk, and dijon mustard.

3. As per the instructions on the manual of your machine, pour the ingredients in the bread pan, taking care to follow how to mix in the yeast.

4. Place the bread pan in the machine, and select the basic bread setting, together with the bread size and crust type, if available, then press start once you have closed the lid of the machine.

5. When the bread is ready, using oven mitts, remove the bread pan from the machine. Use a stainless spatula to extract the bread from the pan and turn the pan upside down on a metallic rack where the bread will cool off before slicing it.

Nutrition: Calories 134, Fat 6.8 g, Carb 4.2 g, Protein 12.1 g

44. RICOTTA CHIVE BREAD

INGREDIENTS

- 1 cup lukewarm water
- 1/3 cup whole or part-skim ricotta cheese
- 1 ½ tsp salt
- 1 tablespoon granulated sugar (needed to activate yeast)
- 3 cups almond flour
- ½ cup chopped chives
- 2 ½ tsp instant yeast

 PREPARATION
5 MIN

 COOKING
3 HOURS

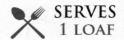 **SERVES**
1 LOAF

DIRECTIONS

1. Add ingredients to bread machine pan except dried fruit following order in your bread machine's manual instructions, taking care on how to mix in the yeast.

2. Place the bread pan in the machine, and select the basic bread setting, together with the bread size and light/medium crust type, if available, then press start once you have closed the lid of the machine.

3. When the bread is ready, using oven mitts, remove the bread pan from the machine.

4. Use a stainless spatula to extract the bread from the pan and turn the pan upside down on a metallic rack where the bread will cool off before slicing it.

NOTE: Top with spreads and greens for tea time snacks.

Nutrition: Calories 145, Fat 18 g, Sodium 207 mg, Carb 4 g, Fiber 1 g, Protein 8 g

45. MOZZARELLA HERBS BREAD

INGREDIENTS

- 1 cup grated cheese mozzarella
- ½ cup grated cheese parmesan
- ½ teaspoon salt
- 1 teaspoon baking powder
- 1 cup almond flour
- 1 cup coconut flour
- ½ cup warm water
- 1 teaspoon stevia
- ¼ teaspoon dried thyme
- 1 teaspoon grounded garlic
- 1 teaspoon dried basil
- 1 teaspoon olive oil extra virgin
- 2 teaspoons unsalted melted butter
- 1/3 cup unsweetened almond milk

 PREPARATION 5 MIN   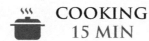 **COOKING** 15 MIN   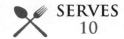 **SERVES** 10

DIRECTIONS

1. In a mixing container, mix the almond flour, baking powder, salt, parmesan cheese, mozzarella cheese, coconut flour, dried basil, dried thyme, garlic powder, and stevia powder.

2. Get another mixing container and mix warm water, unsweetened almond milk, melted unsalted butter, and extra virgin olive oil.

3. As per the instructions on the manual of your machine, pour the ingredients in the bread pan.

4. Place the bread pan in the machine, and select the basic bread setting, together with the bread size and crust type, if available, then press start once you have closed the lid of the machine.

5. When the bread is ready, using oven mitts, remove the bread pan from the machine. Use a stainless spatula to extract the bread from the pan and turn the pan upside down on a metallic rack where the bread will cool off before slicing it.

Nutrition: Calories 49, Fat 2 g, Carb 2 g, Protein 4 g

46. BLUE CHEESE ONION BREAD

INGREDIENTS

- ½ cup of blue cheese, crumbled
- 1 tsp. unsalted melted butter
- 1 tsp. fresh rosemary, chopped
- 1 ½ cup of almond fine flour
- 3 teaspoons olive oil extra virgin
- 1 teaspoon baking powder
- ½ cup warm water
- 1 yellow onion sliced and sautéed in butter until golden brown
- 2 garlic cloves, crushed
- 1 teaspoon Swerve sweetener
- 1 teaspoon salt

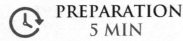 **PREPARATION** 5 MIN   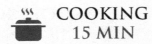 **COOKING** 15 MIN   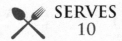 **SERVES** 10

DIRECTIONS

1. Prepare a mixing container, where you will combine the almond flour, swerve sweetener, baking powder, freshly chopped rosemary, crumbled blue cheese, sautéed sliced onion, salt, and crushed garlic.

2. Get another container, where you will combine the warm water, melted butter, and extra virgin olive oil.

3. As per the instructions on the manual of your machine, pour the ingredients in the bread pan.

4. Place the bread pan in the machine, and select the basic bread setting, together with the bread size and crust type, if available, then press start once you have closed the lid of the machine.

5. When the bread is ready, using oven mitts, remove the bread pan from the machine.

6. Use a stainless spatula to extract the bread from the pan, and turn the pan upside down on a metallic rack where the bread will cool off before slicing it.

7.

Nutrition: Calories 100, Fat 6 g, Carb 3 g, Protein 11 g

47. LOW-CARB BAGEL

INGREDIENTS

For Bagel:
- 1 cup Protein powder, unflavored
- 1/3 cup coconut flour
- 1 tsp. Baking powder
- ½ tsp. Sea salt
- ¼ cup ground flaxseed
- 1/3 cup sour cream
- 12 eggs

Seasoning topping:
- 1 tsp. Dried parsley
- 1 tsp. Dried oregano
- 1 tsp. Dried minced onion
- ½ tsp. Garlic powder
- ½ tsp. Dried basil
- ½ tsp. Sea salt

 PREPARATION 15 MIN

 COOKING 25 MIN

 SERVES 12

DIRECTIONS

1. In a mixer, blend sour cream and eggs until well combined.
2. Whisk together the flaxseed, salt, baking powder, Protein powder, and coconut flour in a bowl.
3. Whisk the topping seasoning together in a small bowl. Set aside.
4. Following the instructions on your machine's manual, mix the dry ingredients into the wet ingredients and pour in the bread pan, taking care to follow how to mix in the baking powder.
5. Place the bread pan in the machine, and select the basic bread setting, together with the bread size and crust type, if available, then press start once you have closed the lid of the machine.
6. When the bread is ready, using oven mitts, remove the bread pan from the machine.
7. Sprinkle pan with about 1 tsp. Topping seasoning and evenly pour batter into each.
8. Let the bread cool before slice it.
9. Sprinkle the top of each bagel evenly with the rest of the seasoning mixture.
10. Serve.

Nutrition: Calories 134, Fat 6.8 g, Carb 4.2 g, Protein 12.1 g

48. CHEDDAR SAUSAGE MUFFINS

INGREDIENTS

- 6 oz. Cooked sausage, grease drained, thinly sliced
- ¼ cup water
- 1 tbsp. baking powder
- ¼ cup heavy cream
- 1 cup shredded sharp white cheddar cheese
- 1 ½ cups almond flour
- ½ tsp. Italian seasoning
- ½ tsp. Sea salt
- 1 tbsp. Chopped fresh chives
- 2 minced large garlic cloves
- 1 large egg
- 4 oz. Softened cream cheese

 PREPARATION 15 MIN

 COOKING 25 MIN

 SERVES 8

DIRECTIONS

1. Using a hand mixer on low speed, whip the eggs and cream cheese in a bowl.
2. Add the garlic, chives, sea salt, Italian seasoning, then mix into the egg cheese mixture.
3. Add the water, almond flour, heavy cream, and cheddar cheese. Mix well.
4. Slowly mix in the sausage into the mixture using a spatula.
5. However, take a look to the manufacturer's instructions for mixing dry and wet ingredients.
6. Pour mixture in the bread machine loaf pan.
7. Place the bread pan in the machine, and select the dough cycle setting, or specific muffin program, if available.
8. Then press start once you have closed the lid of the machine.
9. Remove dough from bread machine when cycle is complete.
10. Preheat the oven to 350 F
11. Lightly grease muffin pan with cooking spray.
12. Drop a heap mold of dough into 8 wells on the muffin top pan.
13. Bake in the oven for 25 minutes.
14. Cool and serve.

Nutrition: Calories 321, Fat 28 g, Carb 3.5 g, Protein 13 g

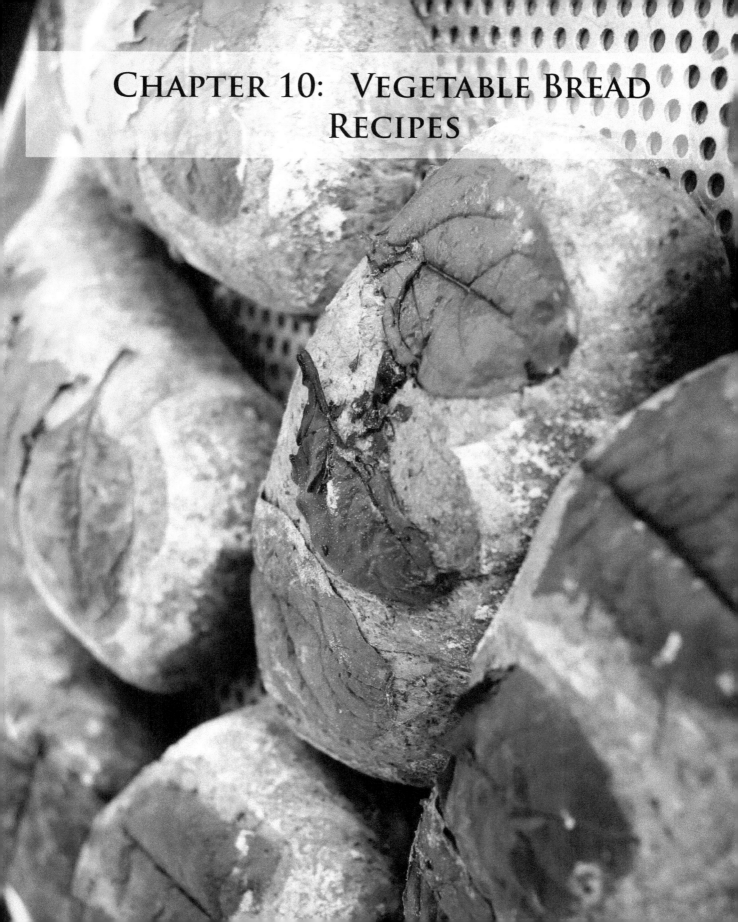

CHAPTER 10: VEGETABLE BREAD RECIPES

49. HEARTY CHEESY BROCCOLI BREAD

INGREDIENTS

- 5 eggs, whisked
- 2 teaspoons baking powder
- 1 cup cheddar, shredded
- 1 cup broccoli florets, separated
- 4 tablespoons coconut flour
- Cooking spray

 PREPARATION 10 MIN

 COOKING 30 MIN

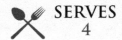 **SERVES** 4

DIRECTIONS

1. In a bowl, mix all the ingredients except the cooking spray and stir the batter really well.
2. Pour batter in the bread machine pan pre-greased with cooking spray.
3. Set the bread machine to the basic bread setting.
4. When the bread is done, remove bread machine pan from the bread machine.
5. Let cool slightly before transferring to a cooling rack.
6. Cool the bread down, slice and serve.

Nutrition: Calories 123, Fat 6 g, Fiber 1 g, Carbs 3 g, Protein 6 g

50. KETO SPINACH BREAD

INGREDIENTS

- ½ cup spinach, chopped
- 1 tablespoon olive oil
- 1 cup water
- 3 cups almond flour
- A pinch of salt and black pepper
- 1 tablespoon stevia
- 1 teaspoon baking powder
- 1 teaspoon baking soda
- ½ cup cheddar, shredded

 PREPARATION
10 MIN

 COOKING
30 MIN

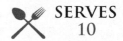 **SERVES**
10

DIRECTIONS

1. Use a small mixing bowl to combine the flour, with salt, pepper, stevia, baking powder, baking soda and the cheddar and stir well.
2. In the bread machine pan add all wet Ingredients.
3. Add all of your dry Ingredients, from the small mixing bowl, in the bread machine pan.
4. Set the bread machine to the basic bread setting.
5. When the bread is done, remove bread machine pan from the bread machine.
6. Let cool slightly before transferring to a cooling rack.
7. Slice and serve.

Nutrition: Calories 142, Fat 7 g, Fiber 3 g, Carbs 5 g, Protein 6 g

51. CINNAMON ASPARAGUS BREAD

INGREDIENTS

- 1 teaspoon stevia
- ¾ cup coconut oil, melted
- 1 and ½ cups almond flour
- 2 eggs, whisked
- A pinch of salt
- 1 teaspoon baking soda
- 1 teaspoon cinnamon powder
- 2 cups asparagus, chopped
- Cooking spray

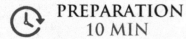 **PREPARATION** 10 MIN   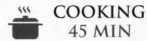 **COOKING** 45 MIN   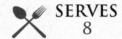 **SERVES** 8

DIRECTIONS

1. In a bowl, mix all the ingredients except the cooking spray and stir the batter really well.
2. Pour batter in the bread machine pan pre-greased with cooking spray.
3. Set the bread machine to the basic bread setting.
4. When the bread is done, remove bread machine pan from the bread machine.
5. Let cool slightly before transferring to a cooling rack.
6. Cool the bread down, slice and serve.

Nutrition: Calories 165, Fat 6 g, Fiber 3 g, Carbs 5 g, Protein 7 g

52. KALE AND CHEESE BREAD

INGREDIENTS

- 2 cups kale, chopped
- 1 cup warm water
- 1 teaspoon baking powder
- 1 teaspoon baking soda
- 2 tablespoons olive oil
- 2 teaspoons stevia
- 1 cup parmesan, grated
- 3 cups almond flour
- A pinch of salt
- 1 egg
- 2 tablespoons basil, chopped

 PREPARATION
10 MIN

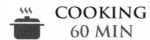 **COOKING**
60 MIN

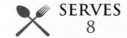 **SERVES**
8

DIRECTIONS

1. In a bowl, mix the flour, salt, parmesan, stevia, baking soda and baking powder and stir.
2. Pour batter in the bread machine pan pre-greased with cooking spray.
3. Add the rest of the ingredients gradually and following order in manufacturer's manual instructions
4. Set the bread machine to the basic bread setting.
5. When the bread is done, remove bread machine pan from the bread machine.
6. Let cool slightly before transferring to a cooling rack.
7. Cool the bread down, slice and serve.

Nutrition: Calories 231, Fat 7 g, Fiber 2 g, Carbs 5 g, Protein 7 g

53. BEET BREAD

INGREDIENTS

- 1 cup warm water
- 3 ½ cups almond flour
- 1 and ½ cups beet puree
- 2 tablespoons olive oil
- A pinch of salt
- 1 teaspoon stevia
- 1 teaspoon baking powder
- 1 teaspoon baking soda

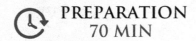 **PREPARATION 70 MIN**   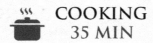 **COOKING 35 MIN**   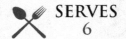 **SERVES 6**

DIRECTIONS

1. Add all ingredients gradually in the bread machine's pan, following the manufacturer's instructions for mixing dry and wet ingredients.
2. Set the bread machine to the basic bread setting.
3. When the bread is done, remove bread machine pan from the bread machine.
4. Let cool slightly before transferring to a cooling rack.
5. Cool the bread down, slice and serve.

Nutrition: Calories 200, Fat 8 g, Fiber 3 g, Carbs 5 g, Protein 6 g

54. KETO CELERY BREAD

INGREDIENTS

- ½ cup celery, chopped
- 3 cups almond flour
- 1 teaspoon baking powder
- 1 teaspoon baking soda
- A pinch of salt
- 2 tablespoons coconut oil, melted
- ½ cup celery puree

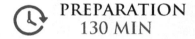
PREPARATION
130 MIN

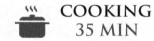
COOKING
35 MIN

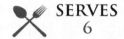
SERVES
6

DIRECTIONS

1. Add all ingredients gradually in the bread machine's pan, following the manufacturer's instructions for mixing dry and wet ingredients.
2. Set the bread machine to the basic bread setting.
3. When the bread is done, remove bread machine pan from the bread machine.
4. Let cool slightly before transferring to a cooling rack.
5. Cool the bread down, slice and serve.

Nutrition: Calories 162, Fat 6 g, Fiber 2 g, Carbs 6 g, Protein 4 g

55. EASY CUCUMBER BREAD

INGREDIENTS

- 1 cup erythritol
- 1 cup coconut oil, melted
- 1 cup almonds, chopped
- 1 teaspoon vanilla extract
- A pinch of salt
- A pinch of nutmeg, ground
- ½ teaspoon baking powder
- A pinch of cloves
- 3 eggs
- 1 teaspoon baking soda
- 1 tablespoon cinnamon powder
- 2 cups cucumber, peeled, deseeded and shredded
- 3 cups coconut flour
- Cooking spray

 PREPARATION
10 MIN

 COOKING
50 MIN

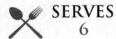 **SERVES**
6

DIRECTIONS

1. In a bowl, mix the flour with cucumber, cinnamon, baking soda, cloves, baking powder, nutmeg, salt, vanilla extract and the almonds and stir well.

2. Add the rest of the ingredients, stir well and transfer the dough in the bread machine loaf pan pre-greased with cooking spray.

3. However, take a look to the manufacturer's instructions for mixing dry and wet ingredients.

4. Place the bread pan in the machine, and select the basic bread setting, together with the bread size, if available, then press start once you have closed the lid of the machine.

5. When the bread is ready, using oven mitts, remove the bread pan from the machine.

6. Cool and serve.

Nutrition: Calories 243, Fat 12 g, Fiber 3 g, Carbs 6 g, Protein 7 g

56. RED BELL PEPPER BREAD

INGREDIENTS

- 1 ½ cups red bell peppers, chopped
- 1 teaspoon baking powder
- 1 teaspoon baking soda
- 2 tablespoons warm water
- 1 and ¼ cups parmesan, grated
- A pinch of salt
- 4 cups almond flour
- 2 tablespoons ghee, melted
- 1/3 cup almond milk
- 1 egg

 PREPARATION 10 MIN

 COOKING 30 MIN

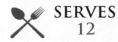 **SERVES** 12

DIRECTIONS

1. In a bowl, mix the flour with salt, parmesan, baking powder, baking soda and the bell peppers and stir well.
2. Add the rest of the ingredients, stir well and transfer the dough in the bread machine loaf pan pre-greased with cooking spray.
3. However, take a look to the manufacturer's instructions for mixing dry and wet ingredients.
4. Place the bread pan in the machine, and select the basic bread setting, together with the bread size, if available, then press start once you have closed the lid of the machine.
5. When the bread is ready, using oven mitts, remove the bread pan from the machine.
6. Cool and serve.

Nutrition: Calories 100, Fat 5 g, Fiber 1 g, Carbs 4 g, Protein 4 g

57. TOMATO BREAD

INGREDIENTS

- 6 cups almond flour
- ½ teaspoon basil, dried
- ¼ teaspoon rosemary, dried
- 1 teaspoon oregano, dried
- ½ teaspoon garlic powder
- 2 tablespoons olive oil
- 2 cups tomato juice
- ½ cup tomato sauce
- 1 teaspoon baking powder
- 1 teaspoon baking soda
- 3 tablespoons swerve

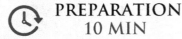 **PREPARATION**
10 MIN

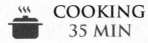 **COOKING**
35 MIN

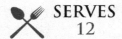 **SERVES**
12

DIRECTIONS

1. In a bowl, mix the flour with basil, rosemary, oregano and garlic and stir.
2. Add the rest of the ingredients, stir well and transfer the dough in the bread machine loaf pan pre-greased with cooking spray.
3. However, take a look to the manufacturer's instructions for mixing dry and wet ingredients.
4. Place the bread pan in the machine, and select the basic bread setting, together with the bread size, if available, then press start once you have closed the lid of the machine.
5. When the bread is ready, using oven mitts, remove the bread pan from the machine.
6. Cool down and serve.

Nutrition: Calories 102, Fat 5 g, Fiber 3 g, Carbs 7 g, Protein 4 g

58. HERBED GARLIC BREAD

INGREDIENTS

- ½ cup coconut flour
- 8 tbsp. melted butter, cooled
- tsp. baking powder
- 6 large eggs
- 1 tsp. garlic powder
- tsp. rosemary, dried
- ¼ tsp. salt
- ½ tsp. onion powder

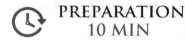 **PREPARATION** 10 MIN

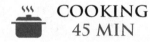 **COOKING** 45 MIN

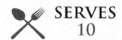 **SERVES** 10

DIRECTIONS

1. Prepare bread machine loaf pan greasing it with cooking spray.
2. In a bowl, add coconut flour, baking powder, onion, garlic, rosemary, and salt into a bowl. Combine and mix well.
3. Into another bowl, add eggs and beat until bubbly on top.
4. Add melted butter into the bowl with the eggs and beat until mixed.
5. Following the instructions on your machine's manual, mix the dry ingredients into the wet ingredients and pour in the bread machine loaf pan, taking care to follow how to mix in the baking powder.
6. Place the bread pan in the machine, and select the basic bread setting, together with the bread size and crust type, if available, then press start once you have closed the lid of the machine.
7. When the bread is ready, using oven mitts, remove the bread pan from the machine.
8. Let it cool before slicing.
9. Cool, slice, and enjoy.

Nutrition Facts per Serving: Calories 147, Fat 12.5 g, Carb 3.5 g, Protein 4.6 g

59. HERBED KETO BREAD

INGREDIENTS

- 3 cups coconut flour
- 1 teaspoon baking powder
- 1 teaspoon baking soda
- 2 teaspoons stevia
- 1 ½ cups warm water
- ½ teaspoon basil, dried
- 1 teaspoon oregano, dried
- ½ teaspoon thyme, dried
- ½ teaspoon marjoram, dried
- 2 tablespoons olive oil

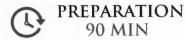 **PREPARATION** 90 MIN   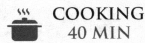 **COOKING** 40 MIN   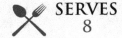 **SERVES** 8

DIRECTIONS

1. In a bowl, mix the flour with baking powder, baking soda, stevia, basil, oregano, thyme, and the marjoram and stir.
2. Add the rest of the ingredients, stir well and transfer the dough in the bread machine loaf pan pre-greased with cooking spray.
3. However, take a look to the manufacturer's instructions for mixing dry and wet ingredients.
4. Place the bread pan in the machine, and select the basic bread setting, together with the bread size, if available, then press start once you have closed the lid of the machine.
5. When the bread is ready, using oven mitts, remove the bread pan from the machine.
6. Cool the bread down before serving.

Nutrition: Calories 200, Fat 7 g, Fiber 3 g, Carbs 5 g, Protein 6 g

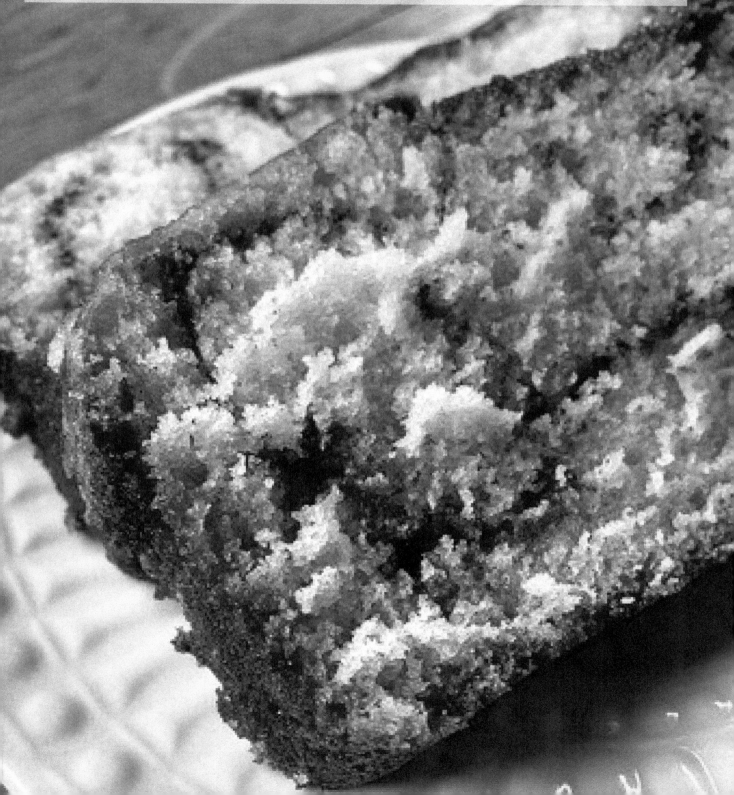

60. CINNAMON BREAD

INGREDIENTS

- 3 tablespoons sour cream
- 3 eggs, pasteurized
- 2 teaspoons vanilla extract, unsweetened
- ¼ cup / 60 grams melted butter, grass-fed, unsalted
- 2 cups / 200 grams almond flour
- 1/3 cup / 65 grams erythritol sweetener
- 2 tablespoons cinnamon
- 1 teaspoon baking soda
- 1 teaspoon baking powder

 PREPARATION
10 MIN

 COOKING
4 HOURS

 SERVES
10

DIRECTIONS

1. Gather all the ingredients for the bread and plug in the bread machine having the capacity of 2 pounds of bread recipe.
2. Take a large bowl, place sour cream in it and then beat in eggs, vanilla, and butter until combined.
3. Take a separate large bowl, place flour in it, and then stir in sweetener, cinnamon, baking powder, and soda until mixed.
4. Add egg mixture into the bread bucket, top with flour mixture, shut the lid, select the "basic/white" cycle setting and then press the up/down arrow button to adjust baking time according to your bread machine; it will take 3 to 4 hours.
5. Then press the crust button to select light crust if available, and press the "start/stop" button to switch on the bread machine.
6. When the bread machine beeps, open the lid, then take out the bread basket and lift out the bread.
7. Let bread cool on a wire rack for 1 hour, then cut it into ten slices and serve.

Nutrition: Cal 169, Fat 14.5 g, Protein 5.4 g, Carb 5.2, Fiber 2 g, Net Carb 2.2 g

61. BANANA BREAD

INGREDIENTS

- 2 eggs, pasteurized
- 1 teaspoon banana extract, unsweetened
- ¼ cup / 50 grams erythritol sweetener
- 3 tablespoons butter, grass-fed, unsalted, softened
- 2 tablespoons almond milk, unsweetened
- 1 cup / 100 grams almond flour
- 2 tablespoons coconut flour
- ¼ cup / 50 grams walnuts, chopped
- 1 teaspoons baking powder
- ¼ teaspoon xanthan gum
- ⅛ teaspoon of sea salt
- 1 teaspoon cinnamon

 PREPARATION 10 MIN

 COOKING 4 HOURS

 SERVES 12

DIRECTIONS

1. Gather all the ingredients for the bread and plug in the bread machine having the capacity of 2 pounds of bread recipe.
2. Take a large bowl, crack eggs in it and then beat in the banana extract, sweetener, butter, and milk until blended.
3. Take a separate large bowl, place flours in it, and then stir in remaining ingredients until mixed.
4. Add egg mixture into the bread bucket, top with flour mixture, shut the lid, select the "basic/white" cycle setting and then press the up/down arrow button to adjust baking time according to your bread machine; it will take 3 to 4 hours.
5. Then press the crust button to select light crust if available, and press the "start/stop" button to switch on the bread machine.
6. When the bread machine beeps, open the lid, then take out the bread basket and lift out the bread.
7. Let bread cool on a wire rack for 1 hour, then cut it into twelve slices and serve.

Nutrition: 240 Cal, 21 g Fat, 8.5 g Protein, 6.8 g Carb, 4.2 g Fiber, 2.6 g Net Carb

62. LEMON RASPBERRY LOAF

INGREDIENTS

- 2 eggs, pasteurized
- 4 tablespoons sour cream
- 1 teaspoon vanilla extract, unsweetened
- 1 teaspoon lemon extract, unsweetened
- 4 tablespoons butter, grass-fed, unsalted, melted
- ¼ cup / 50 grams erythritol sweetener
- 2 tablespoons lemon juice
- ½ cup / 100 grams raspberries preserves
- 2 cups / 200 grams almond flour
- 1 ½ teaspoons baking powder

 PREPARATION 10 MIN   **COOKING** 4 HOURS   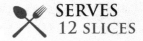 **SERVES** 12 SLICES

DIRECTIONS

1. Gather all the ingredients for the bread and plug in the bread machine having the capacity of 2 pounds of bread recipe.
2. Take a large bowl, place flour in it, and then stir in baking soda until mixed.
3. Take a separate large bowl, crack eggs in it, beat in sour cream, extracts, butter, sweetener, and lemon juice until blended and then stir in raspberry preserve until just combined.
4. Add egg mixture into the bread bucket, top with flour mixture, shut the lid, select the "basic/white" cycle setting and then press the up/down arrow button to adjust baking time according to your bread machine; it will take 3 to 4 hours.
5. Then press the crust button to select light crust if available, and press the "start/stop" button to switch on the bread machine.
6. When the bread machine beeps, open the lid, then take out the bread basket and lift out the bread.
7. Let bread cool on a wire rack for 1 hour, then cut it and serve.

Nutrition: Cal 171, Fat 14,3 g, Protein 4.6 g, Carb 5 g, Fiber 2.4 g, Net Carb 2.6 g

63. WALNUT BREAD

INGREDIENTS

- 4 eggs, pasteurized
- 2 tablespoons apple cider vinegar
- 4 tablespoons coconut oil
- ½ cup / 120 ml lukewarm water
- 1 cup / 200 grams walnuts chopped
- ½ cup / 65 grams coconut flour
- 1 tablespoon baking powder
- 2 tablespoons psyllium husk powder
- ½ teaspoon salt

 PREPARATION 10 MIN 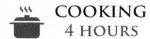 **COOKING** 4 HOURS 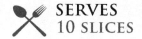 **SERVES** 10 SLICES

DIRECTIONS

1. Gather all the ingredients for the bread and plug in the bread machine having the capacity of 2 pounds of bread recipe.
2. Take a large bowl, crack eggs in it, beat in vinegar, oil, and water until blended and stir in walnuts until just mixed.
3. Take a separate large bowl, place flour in it, and then stir in baking powder, husk powder, and salt until mixed.
4. Add egg mixture into the bread bucket, top with flour mixture, shut the lid, select the "basic/white"

cycle setting and then press the up/down arrow button to adjust baking time according to your bread machine; it will take 3 to 4 hours.

5. Then press the crust button to select light crust if available, and press the "start/stop" button to switch on the bread machine.
6. When the bread machine beeps, open the lid, then take out the bread basket and lift out the bread.
7. Let bread cool on a wire rack for 1 hour, then cut it into ten slices and serve.

Nutrition: Cal 201, Fat 8.1 g, Protein 6 g, Carb 7.5 g, Fiber 4.7 g, Net Carb 2.8

64. ALMOND BUTTER BREAD

INGREDIENTS

- 3 eggs, pasteurized
- 1 cup / 225 grams almond butter
- 1 tablespoon apple cider vinegar
- ½ teaspoon baking soda

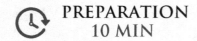 **PREPARATION**
10 MIN

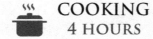 **COOKING**
4 HOURS

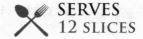 **SERVES**
12 SLICES

DIRECTIONS

1. Gather all the ingredients for the bread and plug in the bread machine having the capacity of 1 pound of bread recipe.
2. Crack eggs in a bowl and then beat in butter, vinegar, and baking soda until combined.
3. Add egg mixture into the bread bucket, shut the lid, select the "basic/white" cycle setting and then press the up/down arrow button to adjust baking time according to your bread machine; it will take 3 to 4 hours.
4. Then press the crust button to select light crust if available, and press the "start/stop" button to switch on the bread machine.
5. When the bread machine beeps, open the lid, then take out the bread basket and lift out the bread.
6. Let bread cool on a wire rack for 1 hour, then cut it into twelve slices and serve.

Nutrition: Cal 152, Fat 13 g, Protein 6.4 g, Carb 5.6 g, Fiber 3.1 g, Net Carb 2.1 g

65. CHOCOLATE ZUCCHINI BREAD

INGREDIENTS

- 1 cup / 200 grams grated zucchini, moisture squeezed thoroughly
- 1/3 cup / 60 grams ground flaxseed
- ½ cup / 100 grams almond flour
- ½ teaspoon salt
- 2 ½ teaspoons baking powder
- 1 ¼ tablespoon psyllium husk powder
- 1/3 cup / 60 grams of cocoa powder

- 4 eggs, pasteurized
- 1 tablespoon coconut cream
- 5 tablespoons coconut oil
- ¾ cup / 150 grams erythritol sweetener
- 1 teaspoon vanilla extract, unsweetened
- ½ cup / 115 grams sour cream
- ½ cup / 100 grams chocolate chips, unsweetened

 PREPARATION
10 MIN

 COOKING
4 HOURS

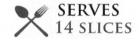 **SERVES**
14 SLICES

DIRECTIONS

1. Wrap zucchini in cheesecloth and twist well until all the moisture is released, set aside until required.

2. Gather all the ingredients for the bread and plug in the bread machine having the capacity of 2 pounds of bread recipe.

3. Take a large bowl, place flaxseed and flour in it, and then stir salt, baking powder, husk, and cocoa powder in it until mixed.

4. Take a separate large bowl, crack eggs in it and then beat in coconut cream, coconut oil, sweetener, and vanilla until combined.

5. Blend in half of the flour mixture, then sour cream and remaining half of flour mixture until incorporated and then fold in chocolate chips until mixed.

6. Add batter into the bread bucket, shut the lid, select the "basic/white" cycle setting and then press the up/down arrow button to adjust baking time according to your bread machine; it will take 3 to 4 hours.

7. Then press the crust button to select light crust if available, and press the "start/stop" button to switch on the bread machine.

8. When the bread machine beeps, open the lid, then take out the bread basket and lift out the bread.

9. Let bread cool on a wire rack for 1 hour, then cut it into fourteen slices and serve.

Nutrition: Cal 187, Fat 15.9 g, Protein 6.2 g, Carb 8.8 g, Fiber 5.2 g, Net Carb 3.6 g

66. PUMPKIN BREAD

INGREDIENTS

- 2 eggs, pasteurized
- 1 cup / 225 grams almond butter, unsweetened
- 2/3 cup / 130 grams erythritol sweetener
- 2/3 cup / 150 grams pumpkin puree
- 1/8 teaspoon ground cloves
- 1/2 teaspoon ground cinnamon
- 1/8 teaspoon ground ginger
- 1 teaspoon baking powder
- 1/2 teaspoon ground nutmeg

 PREPARATION 10 MIN

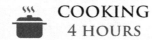 **COOKING** 4 HOURS

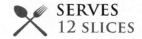 **SERVES** 12 SLICES

DIRECTIONS

1. Gather all the ingredients for the bread and plug in the bread machine having the capacity of 2 pounds of bread recipe.
2. Take a large bowl, crack eggs in it and then beat in remaining ingredients in it in the order described in the ingredients until incorporated.
3. Add batter into the bread bucket, shut the lid, select the "basic/white" cycle setting and then press the up/down arrow button to adjust baking time according to your bread machine; it will take 3 to 4 hours.
4. Then press the crust button to select light crust if available, and press the "start/stop" button to switch on the bread machine.
5. When the bread machine beeps, open the lid, then take out the bread basket and lift out the bread.
6. Let bread cool on a wire rack for 1 hour, then cut it into twelve slices and serve.

Nutrition: Cal 150, Fat 12.9 g, Protein 6.7 g, Carb 7 g, Fiber 2 g, Net Carb 5 g

67. STRAWBERRY BREAD

INGREDIENTS

- 5 eggs, pasteurized
- 1 egg white, pasteurized
- 1 ½ teaspoons vanilla extract, unsweetened
- 2 tablespoons heavy whipping cream
- 2 tablespoons sour cream
- 1 cup monk fruit powder
- 1 ½ teaspoons baking powder
- ½ teaspoon salt
- ½ teaspoon cinnamon
- 8 tablespoons butter, melted
- ¾ cup / 100 grams coconut flour
- ¾ cup / 150 grams chopped strawberries

 PREPARATION 10 MIN   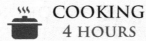 **COOKING** 4 HOURS   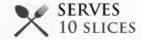 **SERVES** 10 SLICES

DIRECTIONS

1. Gather all the ingredients for the bread and plug in the bread machine having the capacity of 2 pounds of bread recipe.
2. Take a large bowl, crack eggs in it and then beat in egg white, vanilla, heavy cream, sour cream, baking powder, salt, and cinnamon until well combined.
3. Then stir in coconut flour and fold in strawberries until mixed.
4. Add batter into the bread bucket, shut the lid, select the "basic/white" cycle or "low-carb" setting and then press the up/down arrow button to adjust baking time according to your bread machine; it will take 3 to 4 hours.
5. Then press the crust button to select light crust if available, and press the "start/stop" button to switch on the bread machine.
6. When the bread machine beeps, open the lid, then take out the bread basket and lift out the bread.
7. Let bread cool on a wire rack for 1 hour, then cut it into ten slices and serve.

Nutrition: Cal 201, Fat 16.4 g, Protein 4.7 g, Carb 6.1 g, Fiber 3 g, Net Carb 3.1 g

68. BLUEBERRY BREAD LOAF

INGREDIENTS

For the bread dough:
- 10 tbsp. coconut flour
- 9 tbsp. melted butter
- 2/3 cup granulates swerve sweetener
- ½ tsp. baking powder
- 1 tbsp. heavy whipping cream
- 1 ½ tsp. vanilla extract
- ½ tsp. cinnamon
- 3 tbsp. sour cream
- 6 large eggs
- ½ tsp. salt
- ¾ cup blueberries

For the topping:
- 2 tbsp. heavy whipping cream
- 1 tbsp. swerve sweetener
- 1 tsp. melted butter
- 1/8 tsp. vanilla extract
- ¼ tsp. lemon zest

 PREPARATION 20 MIN

 COOKING 65 MIN

 SERVES 12

DIRECTIONS

1. Gather all the ingredients for the bread and plug in the bread machine having the capacity of 2 pounds of bread recipe.
2. Take a large bowl, crack eggs in it and then beat in cream, butter, and vanilla until combined.
3. Take a separate large bowl, place coconut flour in it, then stir in sweetener and baking powder until mixed and fold in blueberries.
4. Add egg mixture into the bread bucket, top with flour mixture, shut the lid, select the "basic/white" cycle or "low-carb" setting and then press the up/down arrow button to adjust baking time according to your bread machine; it will take 3 to 4 hours.
5. Then press the crust button to select light crust if available, and press the "start/stop" button to switch on the bread machine.
6. When the bread machine beeps, open the lid, then take out the bread basket and lift out the bread.
7. Meanwhile, in a bowl, beat the vanilla extract, butter, heavy whipping cream, lemon zest, and confectioner swerve. Mix until creamy.

8. Then drizzle the icing topping on the bread.

9. Enjoy.

Nutrition: Calories 155, Fat 13 g, Carb 4 g, Protein 3 g

69. CRANBERRY AND ORANGE BREAD

INGREDIENTS

- 1 cup / 200 grams chopped cranberries
- 2/3 cup and 3 tablespoons / 175 grams monk fruit powder, divided
- 5 eggs, pasteurized
- 1 egg white, pasteurized
- 2 tablespoons sour cream
- 1 ½ teaspoons orange extract, unsweetened
- 1 teaspoon vanilla extract, unsweetened
- 9 tablespoons butter, grass-fed, unsalted, melted
- 9 tablespoons coconut flour
- 1 ½ teaspoons baking powder
- ¼ teaspoon salt

 PREPARATION 10 MIN   **COOKING** 4 HOURS   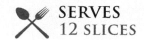 **SERVES** 12 SLICES

DIRECTIONS

1. Take a small bowl, place cranberries in it, and then stir in 4 tablespoons of monk fruit powder until combined, set aside until required.

2. Gather all the ingredients for the bread and plug in the bread machine having the capacity of 2 pounds of bread recipe.

3. Take a large bowl, crack eggs in it, beat in remaining ingredients in it in the order described in the ingredients until incorporated and then fold in cranberries until just mixed.

4. Add batter into the bread bucket, shut the lid, select the "basic/white" cycle or "low-carb" setting and then press the up/down arrow button to adjust baking time according to your bread machine; it will take 3 to 4 hours.

5. Then press the crust button to select light crust if available, and press the "start/stop" button to switch on the bread machine.

6. When the bread machine beeps, open the lid, then take out the bread basket and lift out the bread.

7. Let bread cool on a wire rack for 1 hour, then cut it into twelve slices and serve

Nutrition: Cal 149, Fat 13.1 g, Protein 3.9 g, Carb 4 g, Fiber 1.5 g, Net Carb 2.5 g

70. BLUEBERRY BREAD

INGREDIENTS

- 4 eggs, pasteurized
- 3 tablespoons heavy whipping cream
- 3 tablespoons butter, grass-fed, unsalted, melted
- 1 teaspoon vanilla extract, unsweetened
- 2 tablespoons coconut flour
- 2 cups / 200 grams almond flour
- ½ cup / 100 grams erythritol
- 1 ½ teaspoons baking powder
- 1 cup / 200 grams blueberries

 PREPARATION
10 MIN

 COOKING
4 HOURS

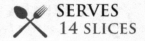 **SERVES**
14 SLICES

DIRECTIONS

1. Gather all the ingredients for the bread and plug in the bread machine having the capacity of 2 pounds of bread recipe.
2. Take a large bowl, crack eggs in it and then beat in cream, butter, and vanilla until combined.
3. Take a separate large bowl, place flours in it, then stir in sweetener and baking powder until mixed and fold in blueberries.
4. Add egg mixture into the bread bucket, top with flour mixture, shut the lid, select the "basic/white" cycle or "low-carb" setting and then press the up/down arrow button to adjust baking time according to your bread machine; it will take 3 to 4 hours.
5. Then press the crust button to select light crust if available, and press the "start/stop" button to switch on the bread machine.
6. When the bread machine beeps, open the lid, then take out the bread basket and lift out the bread.
7. Let bread cool on a wire rack for 1 hour, then cut it into eleven slices and serve.

Nutrition: Cal 211, Fat 18.2 g, Protein 7.7 g, Carb 8.9 g, Fiber 3.7 g, Net Carb 5.2 g

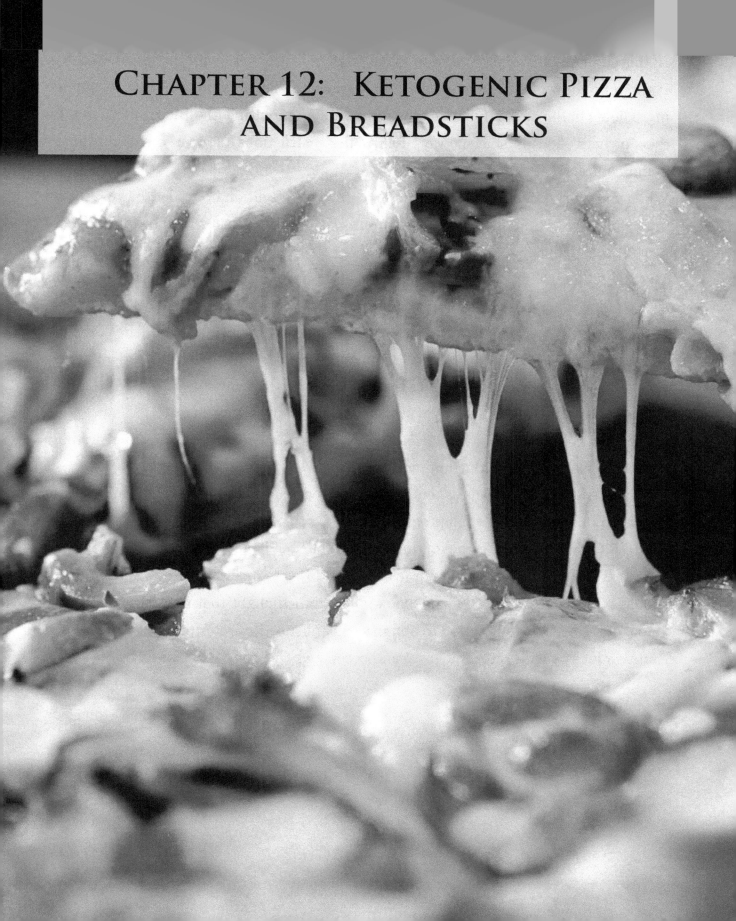

CHAPTER 12: KETOGENIC PIZZA AND BREADSTICKS

In this chapter I will explain how to make pizza or breadsticks with the bread machine. It's a very convenient and easy method, because as usual, you just need to put the ingredients in the basket following the right sequence, putting first the liquids and then the powders (at this stage always follow the instructions of your bread machine's manufacturer).

When you make pizza with your bread machine, pay attention not to let the yeast come into contact with the salt (it could compromise leavening), the rest will be taken care of by your bread maker.

The only difference is the cooking you have to do in your kitchen oven., because in this case you can't do it with the bread machine... unless you want to get a tasty loaf of bread.

Generally, every bread machine has a program for pizza dough, make your checks before you start baking. It's a very interesting function that lasts 45-60 minutes and alternates processing phases with pause phases to allow leavening. It's one of my favorite programs because it's really amazing to make pizza to bake then in your oven.

Using this program has a great advantage, it allows you to dough and leaven everything in a single place and at a constant temperature.

For breadsticks many bread makers have also a specific setting. If it is not available, you can use cookies or pasta dough program.

IMPORTANT: in some recipes of this chapter, the bread maker will not be used because there are no ingredients to knead or leaven. For this reason, at first, I was undecided if I should put this section in the cookbook, but then I thought that it is still about tasty ketogenic recipes that allow you to obtain excellent substitutes for pizza. Try them!

And now let's go with ketogenic pizza and breadstick recipes!

71. DOUGH FOR YEAST KETO PIZZA (WITH GLUTEN)

INGREDIENTS

- 1 ¼ cup super fine almond flour
- 1 cup plus 2 tablespoons warm (like bath water) water, divided
- 1 teaspoon sugar (needed to activate yeast)
- ½ teaspoon ground ginger
- ½ teaspoons active dry yeast
- 1 cup vital wheat gluten

- ½ teaspoon salt
- 1 ½ teaspoon baking powder
- 3 tablespoons extra virgin olive oil
- ½ tablespoon butter, melted

 PREPARATION 75 MIN

 COOKING 33 MIN

 SERVES 8

DIRECTIONS

1. Add all ingredients to bread machine pan following order in your bread machine's manual instructions, taking care on how to mix in the yeast.
2. Place the bread pan in the machine, and select the dough cycle setting, or specific pizza program, if available.
3. Then press start once you have closed the lid of the machine.
4. Remove dough from bread machine when cycle is complete.
5. Cover a large cookie sheet with parchment paper.
6. Form the dough into a ball and place it on the parchment covered cookie sheet. Press the dough and form it into a large circular crust (about 10 inches wide).
7. Pre-heat the oven for 2 minutes until the temperature reaches 100-110 degrees F.
8. Place the crust in the warm oven and allow to rise for 45 minutes.
9. Remove from the oven and pre-heat the oven to 375 degrees F.
10. Brush the crust with melted butter and bake for 12-15 minutes until crust is firm and just beginning to brown.

11. Remove the crust from the oven and turn the heat up to 450 degrees F.
12. Top your pizza with whatever you like and then pop it back into the 450 degree oven for another 6-8 minutes until the crust has browned and the cheese has melted.
13. Allow the pizza to cool on the pan for 10 minutes before cutting into 8 slices.

IMPORTANT: this recipe contains gluten, so be careful if you are intolerant or have celiac disease. Immediately after this, you will find the recipe for gluten-free version. However, if gluten doesn't bother you, the keto pizza you are going to obtain will be indistinguishable from the original version!

Nutrition: Calories 216, Fat 15 g, Carbohydrates 7 g, Fiber 3 g, Protein 16 g

72. GLUTEN-FREE KETO PIZZA YEAST DOUGH

INGREDIENTS

- 1 ½ cups Almond Flour
- 1 ¼ tsp Xanthan Gum
- ¼ tsp Baking Powder
- 1 tsp Salt
- ½ tbsp Apple Cider Vinegar
- 1 tbsp Active Yeast
- ¼ cup Warm Water *for yeast
- 2 Egg Whites, room temperature
- 1 whole Egg, room temperature

 PREPARATION 30 MIN   **COOKING** 10 MIN   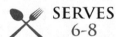 **SERVES** 6-8

DIRECTIONS

1. Add all ingredients to bread machine pan fruit following order in your bread machine's manual instructions, taking care on how to mix in the yeast.

2. Place the bread pan in the machine, and select the dough cycle setting, or specific pizza program, if available.

3. Then press start once you have closed the lid of the machine.

4. Remove dough from bread machine when cycle is complete.

5. Place the dough onto a pizza pan lined with parchment and cover it with cling wrap, gently pressing into a flat round. You can roll up the edges for a high crust if you'd like.

6. Tent the dough with a clean cloth towel and allow to rise in a warm spot for 10-15 minutes.

7. Bake at 375° for 10-15 minutes or until the crust is golden.

8. If the sides are browning before the center, cover the edges with a bit of foil to prevent burning OR reduce the temperature to 325°/350° and bake an extra 5 minutes.

9. Add pizza toppings and return to a HOT oven (375) for 10-15 minutes.

Nutrition: Calories 180, Total Fat 15 g, Carbohydrates 7 g, Net Carbohydrates 4 g, Fiber 3 g, Protein 8 g

73. KETO UNLEAVENED PIZZA

INGREDIENTS

- 2 eggs
- 2 tbsp. parmesan cheese
- 1 tbsp. psyllium husk powder
- ½ tsp. Italian seasoning
- salt
- 2 tsp. frying oil
- 1 ½ ounce mozzarella cheese
- 3 tbsp. tomato sauce
- 1 tbsp. chopped basil

 PREPARATION
10 MIN

 COOKING
20 MIN

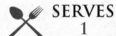 **SERVES**
1

DIRECTIONS

NOTE: bread machine not required

1. In a blender, place the parmesan, psyllium husk powder, Italian seasoning, salt, and two eggs and blend.
2. Heat a large frying pan and add the oil.
3. Add the mixture to the pan in a large circular shape.
4. Flip once the underside is browning and then remove from the pan.
5. Spoon the tomato sauce onto the pizza crust and spread.
6. Add the cheese and spread over the top of the pizza.
7. Place the pizza into the oven – it is done once the cheese is melted.
8. Top the pizza with basil.

Nutrition: Calories 459, Fat 35 g, Carb 3.5 g, Protein 27 g

74. EASY ALMOND FLOUR PIZZA CRUST

INGREDIENTS

- 2 cups almond flour
- 2 eggs
- 2 tbsp. coconut oil, melted
- ½ tsp. sea salt

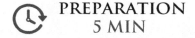 **PREPARATION**
5 MIN

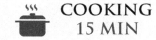 **COOKING**
15 MIN

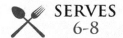 **SERVES**
6-8

DIRECTIONS

1. Preheat the oven to 350F. Line a baking sheet with parchment paper.
2. Add all ingredients to bread machine pan fruit following order in your bread machine's manual instructions.
3. Place the bread pan in the machine, and select the dough cycle setting, or specific pizza program, if available.
4. Then press start once you have closed the lid of the machine.
5. Remove dough from bread machine when cycle is complete.
6. Form the dough into a ball. Put in between two parchment paper sheets, and roll out the dough to ¼ inch thick.
7. Remove the parchment paper piece on top. Place the crust on a pizza pan. Poke the crust with a toothpick a few times to prevent bubbling.
8. Bake for 15 to 20 minutes or until golden.
9. Top with your preferred toppings.
10. Return to the oven and bake for 10 to 15 minutes.
11. Serve.

Nutrition: Calories 211, Fat 19 g, Carb 3 g, Protein 8 g

75. PIZZA WITH A CHICKEN CRUST

INGREDIENTS

- 7 ounces chicken breast meat, ground
- 7 ounces mozzarella cheese, grated
- 1 tsp. garlic salt
- 1 tsp. dried basil
- 4 tbsp. pizza topping sauce, no sugar added
- 4 ounces cheddar cheese, grated

- 12 slices pepperoni
- Fresh basil leaves

 PREPARATION 10 MIN

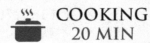 **COOKING** 20 MIN

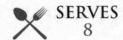 **SERVES** 8

DIRECTIONS

NOTE: bread machine not required

1. Pre-heat the oven to 450F.
2. Line a 12-inch pizza pan with parchment.
3. Mix the chicken, cheese, garlic salt, and dried basil together.
4. Spread into the pizza pan in an even layer and bake in the preheated oven for 10 to 12 minutes.
5. Remove from the oven and cool a little before adding the topping of sauce, cheddar cheese, and pepperoni.
6. Once the topping is on, replace it in the hot oven and cook for 5 to 7 minutes or until hot and bubbly.
7. Remove from the oven and top with torn basil leaves.
8. Cut and serve.

Nutrition: Calories 228, Fat 14.6 g, Carb 3 g, Protein 20.2 g

76. KETO BREAKFAST PIZZA

INGREDIENTS

- ½ tsp. salt
- 1 tbsp. psyllium husk powder
- 2 cups cauliflower florets, riced
- 2 tbsp. coconut flour
- 3 eggs

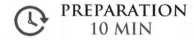
PREPARATION
10 MIN

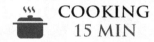
COOKING
15 MIN

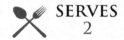
SERVES
2

DIRECTIONS

NOTE: bread machine not required

1. Preheat the oven to 350F and line a baking tray with parchment paper.
2. In a bowl, add everything and mix well. Set aside for 5 minutes.
3. Then transfer into the baking tray. Flatten to give pizza dough shape.
4. Bake until golden brown, about 15 minutes.
5. Remove and top with toppings of your choice.
6. Serve.

Nutrition: Calories 454, Fat 31 g, Carb 8 g, Protein 22 g

77. THE BEST KETO PULL APART PIZZA BREAD RECIPE

INGREDIENTS

- 2 ½ cups mozzarella cheese shredded
- 3 eggs beaten
- 1 ½ cup almond flour
- 1 tablespoon baking powder
- 2 oz. cream cheese
- ½ cup grated Parmesan cheese
- 1 teaspoon rosemary seasoning
- ½ cup shredded mild cheddar or a cheese or your choice
- ½ cup mini pepperoni slices
- 3-4 Sliced jalapeños
- Non-stick cooking spray

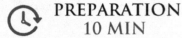 **PREPARATION** 10 MIN 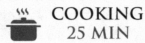 **COOKING** 25 MIN 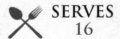 **SERVES** 16

DIRECTIONS

1. Melt the Mozzarella cheese and cream cheese. You can do this on the stove top or for 1 minute in the microwave.
2. Add all ingredients to bread machine pan following order in your bread machine's manual instructions.
3. Place the bread pan in the machine, and select the dough cycle setting, or specific pizza program, if available.
4. Then press start once you have closed the lid of the machine.
5. Remove dough from bread machine when cycle is complete.
6. knead it until it forms into a sticky ball. I always use a silicone mat on the countertop to do this step.
7. Sprinkle the top of the dough with a small amount of parmesan cheese. This will help the dough not be so sticky when you start to handle it. I flip the dough over and sprinkle a small amount on the back side of the dough too.
8. Form the dough into a ball and cut it in half. Continue cutting the dough until you get about 16 pieces from each side, a total of 32 pieces total (give or take).

9. Roll the pieces of dough into equal sized balls then roll them in a plate of parmesan cheese that has been topped with a teaspoon of Rosemary seasoning. (This is the secret to forming the pull apart bread because the parmesan cheese coats each dough ball allowing it not to fully combine while it's baking. Plus, it adds an amazing flavor also.)

10. Spray the bundt pan with non-stick cooking spray.

11. Place the first layer of 16 prepared dough balls into a non-stick bundt pan.

12. Then add a layer of your favorite shredded cheese, mini pepperoni slices, and jalapeño if desired.

13. Add the next layer of 16 prepared dough balls on top of the first layer.

14. Top the last layer with the rest of the shredded cheese, mini pepperoni slices, and jalapeños.

15. Bake at 350°F for 25 minutes or until golden brown. It may take a bit longer if your bundt pan is thicker than the one I used.

Nutrition: Calories 142, Total Fat 9.4 g, Protein 11.1 g, Carbohydrates 3.5 g, Dietary Fiber 1.5 g, Sugar 0.8 g

78. MICROWAVE PEPPERONI PIZZA BREAD

INGREDIENTS

- 1 tablespoon unsalted butter melted
- 1 large egg
- 1 tablespoon almond milk
- 1 tablespoon superfine almond flour
- 1 tablespoon coconut flour (not substitute with almond flour)
- 1/8 teaspoon baking powder
- 1/8 teaspoon Italian seasoning
- 1 tablespoon shredded parmesan cheese
- 1 tablespoon shredded mozzarella cheese
- 1 tablespoon low sugar tomato sauce optional
- 6-8 mini pepperoni

 PREPARATION 10 MIN

 COOKING 2 MIN

 SERVES 1

DIRECTIONS

NOTE: bread machine not required

1. In a large and wide (about 4 inches wide) microwave safe mug, add butter, egg, milk, almond flour, coconut flour, baking powder. Whisk until the batter is smooth.
2. Stir in Italian seasoning and Parmesan cheese.
3. Cook in the microwave at full power for about 90 seconds, or until the bread has cooked.
4. Spread tomato sauce (if using) over surface of bread.
5. Sprinkle mozzarella cheese over sauce.
6. Place mini pepperoni on top of the cheese.
7. Cook for an additional 30 seconds or until the cheese has melted.
8. Enjoy while still warm.

Nutrition: Nutrition: Calories 332, Total Fat 25.5 g, Saturated Fat 12.5 g, Protein 16.1 g, Carbohydrates 10.4 g, Dietary Fiber 4.3 g, Sugars 3.6 g

79. 5 MINUTES KETO PIZZA

INGREDIENTS

Pizza Crust:
- 2 large eggs
- 2 tablespoons parmesan cheese
- 1 tablespoon psyllium husk powder
- ½ teaspoon Italian seasoning
- Salt to taste
- 2 teaspoons frying oil (you can use bacon fat)

Topping:
- 1 ½ oz. Mozzarella Cheese
- 3 tablespoons Rao's Tomato Sauce
- 1 tablespoon Freshly Chopped Basil

 PREPARATION 5 MIN

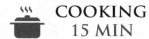 **COOKING** 15 MIN

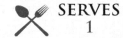 **SERVES** 1

DIRECTIONS

NOTE: bread machine not required

1. In a bowl or container, use an immersion blender to mix together all the pizza crust ingredients.
2. Heat frying oil in a pan until hot, then spoon the mixture into the pan.
3. Spread out into a cirlce.
4. Once the edges have browned, flip and cook for 30-60 seconds on the other side.
5. Turn the stove off, and turn the broiler on.
6. Add tomato sauce and cheese, then broil for 1-2 minutes or until cheese is bubbling.

Nutrition: Calories 459, Total Fat 35 g, Protein 27 g, Carbohydrates 3.5 g, Dietary Fiber 9 g

80. ITSY BITSY PIZZA CRUSTS

INGREDIENTS

For dough:
- 5 whole eggs and 3 egg whites
- ½ tsp. baking powder
- ¼ cup coconut flour sifted, with more for dusting
- Salt, pepper, Italian spices

For sauce:
- 2 garlic cloves, minced
- ½ cup organic tomato sauce
- 1 tsp. dried basil
- ¼ tsp. pink sea salt

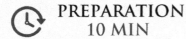 **PREPARATION**
10 MIN

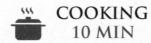 **COOKING**
10 MIN

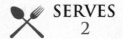 **SERVES**
2

DIRECTIONS

1. Preheat oven to 350°F.
2. Add all dough ingredients to bread machine pan fruit following order in your bread machine's manual instructions.
3. Place the bread pan in the machine, and select the dough cycle setting, or specific pizza program, if available.
4. Then press start once you have closed the lid of the machine.
5. Remove dough from bread machine when cycle is complete.
6. Lightly grease a small pan and place over medium-low heat. Pour some of the batter evenly once the pan is hot.
7.
8. Cover and let cook in oven for about 3-5minutes or until bubbles form on top. Flip the other side and cook for 2 minutes.
9. Transfer to a platter and repeat this for the remaining batter.
10. Once the crusts are cool, use a fork to roughly poke holes on the crusts. This will help them cook evenly.
11. Lightly dust with coconut flour and set aside.

12. For the sauce, whisk all the ingredients together then let stand for 30 minutes to allow thickening.

13. Spread the pizza bases with the sauce and top with your favorite toppings and bake for about 3-5 minutes or until done to desire.

Nutrition: Calories 125, Total Fat 1 g, Carb 6, Dietary Fiber 3 g, Protein 8 g, Cholesterol 34 mg, Sodium 89 mg

81. SIMPLE KETO PIZZA CRUST

INGREDIENTS

- 100 g blanched almond flour
- 3 tablespoons coconut flour
- 2 tapioca flour
- 2 teaspoons baking powder
- ¼ teaspoon pink sea salt
- 2 teaspoons apple cider vinegar
- ¼ cup water
- 1 egg

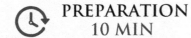 **PREPARATION**
10 MIN

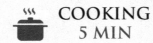 **COOKING**
5 MIN

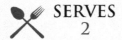 **SERVES**
2

DIRECTIONS

1. Add all ingredients to bread machine pan fruit following order in your bread machine's manual instructions.
2. Place the bread pan in the machine, and select the dough cycle setting, or specific pizza program, if available.
3. Then press start once you have closed the lid of the machine.
4. Remove dough from bread machine when cycle is complete.
5. Set your oven to 350 degrees F and line a baking tray with parchment paper.
6. Flatten the dough and spread it on the prepared tray and bake for 5-7 minutes on each side or until browned.
7. Top with your favorite topping and return to the oven for about 3-5 more minutes or store it in the freezer for later use.

Nutrition: Calories 118, Total Fat 9 g, Carb 6, Dietary Fiber 3 g, Protein 5 g, Cholesterol 27 mg, Sodium 116 mg

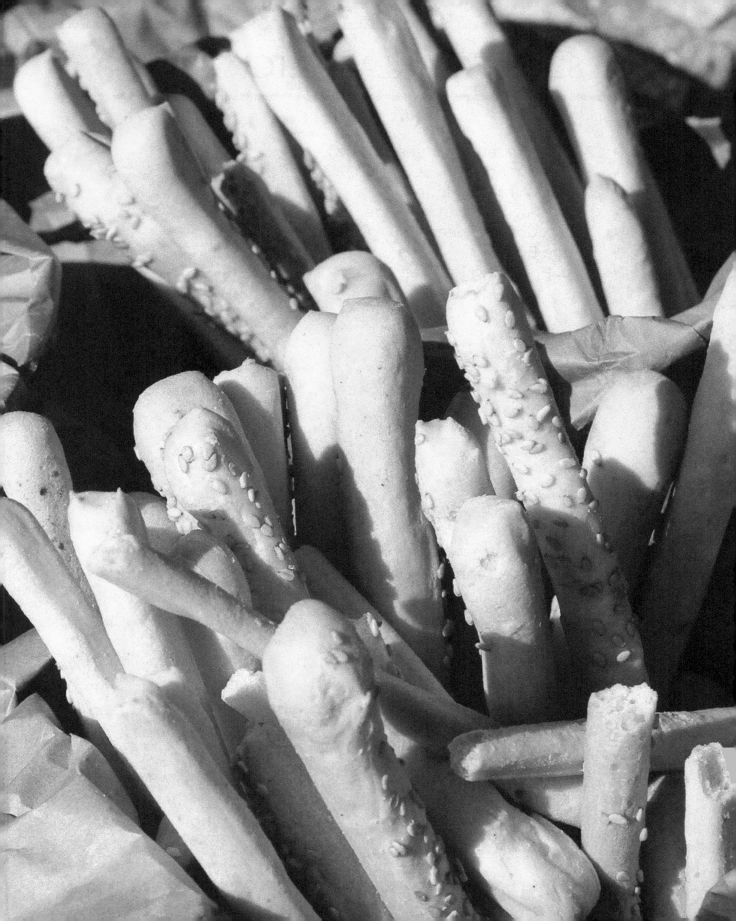

82. KETO BREADSTICKS BASE

INGREDIENTS

- 2 cups Mozzarella Cheese (~8 oz.)
- ¾ cup Cheddar Cheese (~3 oz.)
- 3/4 cup Almond Flour
- 1 tbsp. Psyllium Husk Powder
- 3 tbsp. Cream Cheese (~1.5 oz.)
- 1 huge Egg
- 1 tsp. Preparing Powder

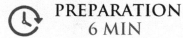 **PREPARATION**
6 MIN

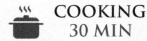 **COOKING**
30 MIN

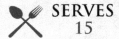 **SERVES**
15

DIRECTIONS

1. Pre-heat stove to 400F.
2. Combine egg and cream cheddar until somewhat joined. In another bowl, consolidate all the dry fixings following order in your bread machine's manual instructions.
3. Measure out the mozzarella cheddar and microwave in 20-second interims until sizzling.
4. Add the egg, cream cheddar, and dry fixings into the mozzarella cheddar and combine.
5. Pour mixture in the bread machine loaf pan.
6. Place the bread pan in the machine, and select the breadstick setting. If not available use cookies or pasta dough program.
7. Then press start once you have closed the lid of the machine.
8. Remove dough from bread machine when cycle is complete.
9. Divide the dough into 15 equal pieces and roll them with your hands forming breadsticks.

10. At that point season the mixture with the flavorings you like.
11. Arrange the breadsticks on the baking sheet and brush them with the egg yolks.
12. Bake 13-15 minutes on top rack until fresh.
13. Serve while warm!

Nutrition: Cal 60, Carb 4 g, Net Carb 2.5 g, Fiber 4.5 g, Fat 6 g, Protein 4 g, Sugars 3 g

83. ALMOND FLOUR BREADSTICKS

INGREDIENTS

For Breadstick:
- 2 eggs
- 1 ½ tbsp. Olive oil
- ½ tsp. Oregano
- ½ tsp. Parsley
- ½ tsp. Basil
- ½ tsp. Garlic powder
- ½ tsp. Onion powder
- 2 ½ tbsp. Coconut flour
- 2 cups almond flour

For Topping:
- ¼ tsp. Salt
- ½ tsp. Garlic powder
- 2 tsp. Parmesan grated
- 1 tbsp. Olive oil

 PREPARATION 5 MIN

 COOKING 15 MIN

 SERVES 10

DIRECTIONS

1. Preheat the oven to 350 F and line a baking pan with parchment paper.
2. In a bowl, whisk almond flour, olive oil, and seasoning.
3. Whisk the eggs in another bowl, mix into the almond flour.
4. Add 1 tbsp. Coconut flour to the mixture at a time, stirring to combine.
5. Allow dough to rest for 1 to 2 minutes after each tbsp. Once the mixture gets thick, add the remaining coconut flour.
6. Pour mixture in the bread machine loaf pan.
7. Place the bread pan in the machine, and select the breadstick setting. If not available use cookies or pasta dough program.
8. Then press start once you have closed the lid of the machine.
9. Remove dough from bread machine when cycle is complete.
10. Form dough into a ball. And roll out into 1.5-inch wide rope-like sticks.

11. Transfer to the prepared baking sheet, place in the oven, and bake for 10 minutes.
12. Meanwhile, mix together salt, parmesan, and garlic.
13. Once baked, carefully brush the tops of breadsticks with oil, then sprinkle with garlic parmesan mix.
14. Bake for 5 minutes more.

Nutrition: Calories 169, Fat 15 g, Carb 6.14 g, Protein 7 g

84. CHEESY BREADSTICKS

INGREDIENTS

For breadsticks:
- ½ cup of parmesan cheese, shredded
- 1 cups of mozzarella cheese, shredded
- ½ teaspoon of garlic powder
- 1 teaspoon of Italian seasoning
- ¼ teaspoon of baking powder
- ½ teaspoon of salt
- 4 eggs
- 1 oz of cream cheese, softened
- 1/3 cup of coconut flour
- 4 ½ tablespoons of butter (melted and cooled)

For topping:
- 12 teaspoons of Italian seasoning
- ¼ cup of parmesan cheese, shredded

 PREPARATION 10 MIN

 COOKING 15 MIN

 SERVES 8

DIRECTIONS

1. Preheat your oven to 400 degrees F.
2. Prepare a 7x11 baking pan by greasing it with cooking spray.
3. Combine the cream cheese, salt, eggs and melted butter then mix.
4. Add the spices, baking powder and coconut flour to the butter mixture and stir until combined then stir in the parmesan and mozzarella.
5. Pour mixture in the bread machine loaf pan.
6. Place the bread pan in the machine, and select the breadstick setting. If not available use cookies or pasta dough program.
7. Then press start once you have closed the lid of the machine.
8. Remove dough from bread machine when cycle is complete.
9. Transfer the batter to a casserole dish then top with the additional Italian spices, parmesan cheese and mozzarella.
10. Bake until the breadsticks are done for 15 minutes. Halfway through baking, use a pizza cutter to create individual breadsticks.
11. Transfer the pan to the top rack of your oven and broil until the cheese is bubbly and brown for around 1-2 minutes
12. Serve with keto friendly marinara sauce.

Nutrition: Calories 299, Protein 17 g, Carb 4 g, Fat 23 g

85. ITALIAN BREADSTICKS

INGREDIENTS

- 1 tbsp. of pulverized psyllium husk
- 3/4 cup of almond flour
- 1 tbsp. of flaxseed meal
- 3 tbsp. of cream cheese
- 1 tsp. baking powder—gluten-free
- 2 cups mozzarella cheese—shredded
- 2 medium eggs
- 1 tsp. of pepper
- 2 tsp. of Italian seasoning
- 1 tsp. of salt

 PREPARATION
10 MIN

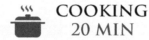 **COOKING**
20 MIN

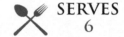 **SERVES**
6

DIRECTIONS

1. Make sure that the oven is set to heat at 400°F. Use a silicone baking mat or cover a standard sized baking sheet with baking paper.
2. Place 2 pieces of parchment paper to the side or you can use aluminum foil instead.
3. On medium heat, use a double boiler to melt the mozzarella cheese completely.
4. Meanwhile, in another bowl, combine the eggs and cream cheese until mixed thoroughly. Set to the side.
5. Whisk the psyllium husk & baking powders & almond flour into the large-sized bowl together, removing any lumps.
6. Add in the mixture of cheese to the bowl of dry ingredient and mix thoroughly. Next, add the melted mozzarella cheese to the batter.
7. Pour mixture in the bread machine loaf pan.
8. Place the bread pan in the machine, and select the breadstick setting. If not available use cookies or pasta dough program.
9. Then press start once you have closed the lid of the machine.

10. Remove dough from bread machine when cycle is complete.
11. Use a rolling pin to press the dough flat on parchment paper, keeping an even thickness throughout.
12. Transfer the flattened dough to a piece of aluminum foil or the additional piece of parchment paper to cut into strips with a pizza cutter.
13. Sprinkle the salt, Italian seasoning and pepper on each breadstick.
14. Put it on a piece of cookie sheet & then you need to bake it for 13-15 mins. and serve warm.

Nutrition: Calories 238, Net Carb 2.8 g, Fat 19 g, Protein 13 g

86. ULTIMATE KETO BREADSTICKS

INGREDIENTS

For breadsticks:
- ¼ cup coconut flour
- ¾ cup ground flax seeds
- 1 tbsp. psyllium husk powder
- 1 cup almond flour
- 2 tbsp. ground chia seeds
- 1 tsp. salt
- 1 cup lukewarm water, plus more if needed

For topping:
- 2 egg yolks, for brushing
- 4 tbsp. mixed seeds
- 1 tsp. coarse sea salt

 PREPARATION 10 MIN

 COOKING 40 MIN

 SERVES 20

DIRECTIONS

1. Preheat the oven to 350F.
2. Combine the almond flour, psyllium husks, flax seeds, and coconut flour to bread machine pan following order in your bread machine's manual instructions. Add the chia seeds, salt, and the water.
3. Place the bread pan in the machine, and select the breadstick setting. If not available use cookies or pasta dough program.
4. Then press start once you have closed the lid of the machine.
5. Remove dough from bread machine when cycle is complete.
6. Cover and place in the fridge for 20-30 minutes.
7. Line a baking sheet with parchment paper.
8. Divide the dough into 20 equal pieces and roll them with your hands forming breadsticks.
9. Arrange the breadsticks on the baking sheet and brush them with the egg yolks.
10. Sprinkle with seeds and salt and bake for 20 minutes.
11. Serve.

Nutrition: Calories 75, Fat 9.6 g, Carb 4.1 g, Protein 3.5 g

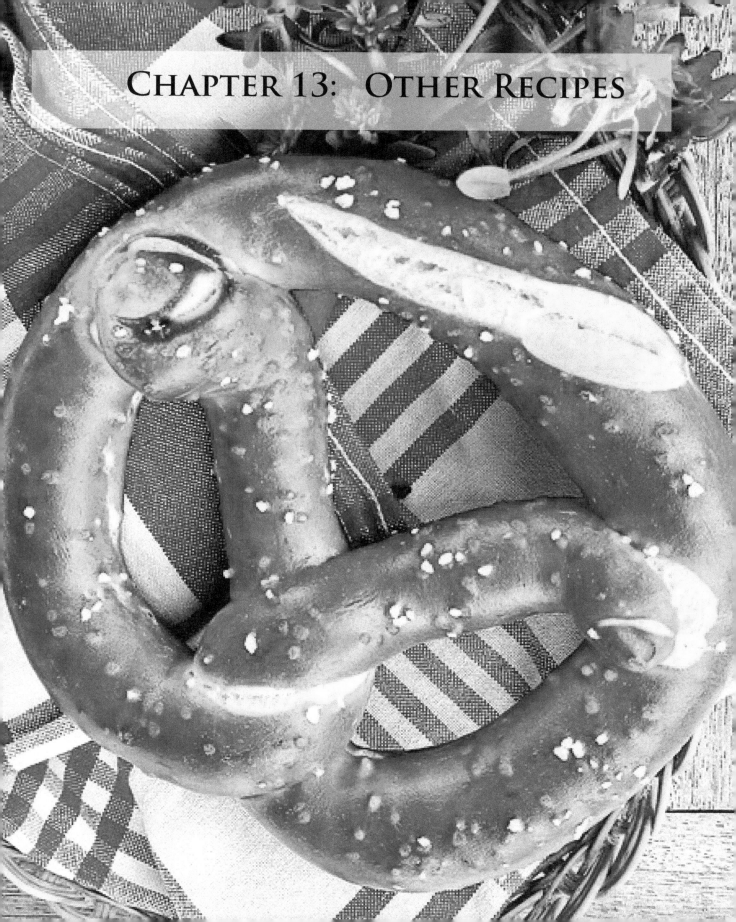

CHAPTER 13:   OTHER RECIPES

87. PUMPKIN PECAN BREAD

INGREDIENTS

- ½ cup almond milk
- ½ cup canned pumpkin
- 1 egg
- 2 tablespoons margarine or butter, cut up
- 3 cups almond flour
- 3 tablespoons erythritol
- 1 tablespoon inulin
- ¾ tsp salt
- ¼ tsp ground nutmeg
- ¼ tsp ground ginger
- 1/8 tsp ground cloves
- 1 tsp active dry yeast or bread machine yeast
- ¾ cup coarsely chopped pecans

 PREPARATION 10 MIN

 COOKING 3 HOURS

 SERVES 16

DIRECTIONS

1. Add ingredients to bread machine pan following bread machine's manual instructions, taking care on how to mix in the yeast.
2. Place the bread pan in the machine, and select the basic bread setting, together with the bread size and light/medium crust type, if available, then press start once you have closed the lid of the machine.
3. When the bread is ready, using oven mitts, remove the bread pan from the machine.
4. Use a stainless spatula to extract the bread from the pan and turn the pan upside down on a metallic rack where the bread will cool off before slicing it.

Nutrition: Calories 183, Fat 12 g sat. fat), Sodium 126 mg, Carb 7 g, Fiber 2 g, Protein 6.5 g

88. RED HOT CINNAMON BREAD

INGREDIENTS

- ¼ cup lukewarm water
- ½ cup lukewarm almond milk
- ¼ cup softened butter
- 2 ¼ tsp instant yeast
- 1 ¼ tsp salt
- ¼ cup Swerve
- 1 teaspoon honey or sugar (or Inulin)
- 1 tsp vanilla
- 1 large egg, lightly beaten
- 3 cups almond flour
- ½ cup Cinnamon Red Hot candies

 PREPARATION 5 MIN   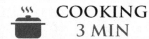 **COOKING** 3 MIN   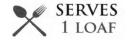 **SERVES** 1 LOAF

DIRECTIONS

1. Add ingredients to bread machine pan except candy.
2. Choose dough setting.
3. After cycle is over, turn dough out into bowl and cover, let rise for 45 minutes to one hour.
4. Gently punch down dough and shape into a rectangle.
5. Knead in the cinnamon candies in 1/3 at a t time.
6. Shape the dough into a loaf and place in a greased or parchment lined loaf pan.
7. Tent the pan loosely with lightly greased plastic wrap, and allow a second rise for 40-50 minutes.
8. Preheat oven 350 degrees.
9. Bake 30-40 minutes.
10. Remove and cool on wire rack before slicing.

Nutrition: Calories 207, Total fat 6.9 g (4.1 g sat. fat), Sodium 317 mg, Carb 4 g, Fiber 1 g, Protein 7.6 g

89. HEARTY SEEDED BREAD LOAF

INGREDIENTS

- ½ cups pumpkin seeds (1 cup finely chopped with a food processor)
- ½ cup whole psyllium husks
- ½ cup flax seeds
- ½ cup chia seeds
- ½ cups warm water
- 1 tsp. pink salt
- 1 cup raw sunflower seeds

- 1 tbsp. sugar-free maple syrup
- 1 tbsp. melted coconut oil

 PREPARATION 70 MIN

 COOKING 60 MIN

 SERVES 16

DIRECTIONS

1. Prepare bread machine loaf pan greasing it with cooking spray.
2. In a bowl, mix together dry Ingredients until well combined.
3. Pour the maple syrup, warm water, and melted coconut oil into another bowl and continue stirring until the batter becomes thick.
4. Following the instructions on your machine's manual, mix the dry ingredients into the wet ingredients and pour in the bread machine loaf pan, taking care to follow how to mix in the baking powder.
5. Place the bread pan in the machine, and select the basic bread setting, together with the bread size, if available, then press start once you have closed the lid of the machine.
6. When the bread is ready, using oven mitts, remove the bread pan from the machine.
7. Let it cool before slicing.
8. Cool, slice, and serve.

Nutrition: Calories 172, Fat 6 g, Carb 2 g, Protein 7 g

90. EGGY COCONUT BREAD

INGREDIENTS

- ½ cup coconut flour
- 4 eggs
- 1 cup water
- 1 tbsp. apple cider vinegar
- ¼ cup coconut oil, plus 1 tsp. melted
- ½ tsp. garlic powder
- ½ tsp. baking soda
- ¼ tsp. salt

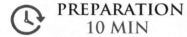 **PREPARATION** 10 MIN
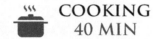 **COOKING** 40 MIN
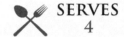 **SERVES** 4

DIRECTIONS

1. Prepare bread machine loaf pan greasing it with cooking spray.
2. In a bowl, mix together coconut flour, baking soda, garlic powder, and salt. Until well combined.
3. Into another bowl, add eggs to a blender along with vinegar, water, and ¼-cup coconut oil. Blend for 30 seconds.
4. Following the instructions on your machine's manual, mix the dry ingredients into the wet ingredients and pour in the bread machine loaf pan, taking care to follow how to mix in the baking powder.
5. Place the bread pan in the machine, and select the basic bread setting, together with the bread size and crust type, if available, then press start once you have closed the lid of the machine.
6. When the bread is ready, using oven mitts, remove the bread pan from the machine.
7. Let it cool before slicing.
8. Cool, slice, and enjoy.

Nutrition: Calories 297, Fat 14 g, Carb 9 g, Protein 15 g

91. SPICY BREAD

INGREDIENTS

- ½ cup coconut flour
- 6 eggs
- 3 large jalapenos, sliced
- 4 ounces turkey bacon, sliced
- ½ cup ghee
- ¼ tsp. baking soda
- ¼ tsp. salt
- ¼ cup water

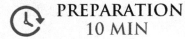 **PREPARATION** 10 MIN

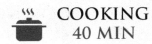 **COOKING** 40 MIN

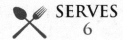 **SERVES** 6

DIRECTIONS

1. Cut bacon and jalapenos on a baking tray and roast for 10 minutes.
2. Flip and bake for 5 more minutes.
3. Remove seeds from the jalapenos.
4. Place jalapenos and bacon slices in a food processor and blend until smooth.
5. In a bowl, mix together add the coconut flour, baking soda, and salt. Stir until well combined.
6. Into another bowl, add ghee, eggs, and ¼-cup water. Mix well.
7. Add bacon and jalapeno mix.
8. Grease the machine loaf pan with ghee.
9. Following the instructions on your machine's manual, mix the dry ingredients into the wet ingredients and pour in the bread machine loaf pan, taking care to follow how to mix in the baking powder.
10. Place the bread pan in the machine, and select the basic bread setting, together with the bread size and crust type, if available, then press start once you have closed the lid of the machine.
11. When the bread is ready, using oven mitts, remove the bread pan from the machine.
12. Let it cool before slicing.

Nutrition: Calories 240, Fat 20 g, Carb 5 g, Protein 9 g

92. CHOCOLATE CHIP SCONES

INGREDIENTS

- 2 cups almond flour
- 1 tsp. baking soda
- ¼ tsp. sea salt
- 1 egg
- 2 tbsp. low-carb sweetener
- 2 tbsp. milk, cream or yogurt
- ½ cup sugar-free chocolate chips

 PREPARATION
10 MIN

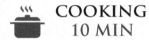 **COOKING**
10 MIN

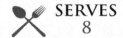 **SERVES**
8

DIRECTIONS

1. Preheat the oven to 350F.
2. In a bowl, add almond flour, baking soda, and salt and blend.
3. Then add the egg, sweetener, milk, and chocolate chips. Blend well.
4. Pour mixture in the bread machine loaf pan.
5. Place the bread pan in the machine, and select the cookies setting. If not available use pasta dough program.
6. Then press start once you have closed the lid of the machine.
7. Remove dough from bread machine when cycle is complete.
8. Pat the dough into a ball and place it on parchment paper.
9. Roll the dough with a rolling pin into a large circle. Slice it into 8 triangular pieces.
10. Place the scones and parchment paper on a baking sheet and separate the scones about 1 inch or so apart.
11. Bake for 7 to 10 minutes or until lightly browned.
12. Cool and serve.

Nutrition: Calories 213, Fat 18 g, Carb 10 g, Protein 8 g

93. FATHEAD ROLLS

INGREDIENTS

- ¾ cup shredded mozzarella cheese
- 3 oz. cream cheese
- ½ cup shredded cheddar cheese
- 2 beaten egg
- ¼ tsp. garlic powder
- 1/3 cup almond flour
- 2 tsp. baking powder

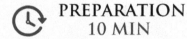 **PREPARATION** 10 MIN

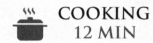 **COOKING** 12 MIN

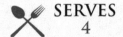 **SERVES** 4

DIRECTIONS

1. Preheat the oven to 425F.
2. Combine the cream cheese and mozzarella. Place in the microwave and cook for 20 seconds at a time until cheese melts.
3. Beat the eggs in another bowl, add all the dry ingredients (set aside 1.5 tablespoons of almond flour) and stir in cheddar cheese.
4. Pour the mixture into bread machine pan following order in your bread machine's manual instructions.
5. Place the bread pan in the machine, and select the dough program.
6. Then press start once you have closed the lid of the machine.
7. Remove dough from bread machine when cycle is complete.
8. Gently start working the dough into a ball. Cover and place in the fridge for ½ hour.
9. Sprinkle the top of the bread with remaining almond flour.

10. Slice the dough ball into four parts and roll each one into a ball. Cut the ball in half.

11. Place the cut side down onto a well-greased sheet pan.

12. Bake for 10 to 12 minutes.

Nutrition: Calories 160, Fat 13 g, Carb 2.5 g, Protein 7 g

94. LOW-CARB PRETZELS

INGREDIENTS

- 1 tbsp. pretzel salt
- 2 tbsp. butter, melted
- 2 tbsp. warm water
- 2 tsp. dried yeast
- 2 eggs
- 2 tsp. xanthan gum
- 1 ½ cups almond flour
- 4 tbsp. cream cheese
- 3 cups of shredded mozzarella cheese

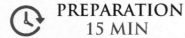 **PREPARATION**
15 MIN

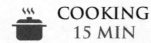 **COOKING**
15 MIN

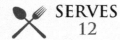 **SERVES**
12

DIRECTIONS

1. Preheat the oven to 390F.
2. Melt the mozzarella cheese and cream cheese in the microwave.
3. Mix the almond meal and xanthan gum with a hand mixer.
4. Add all ingredients to bread machine pan following order in your bread machine's manual instructions, taking care on how to mix in the yeast.
5. Place the bread pan in the machine, and select the dough cycle setting.
6. Then press start once you have closed the lid of the machine.
7. Remove dough from bread machine when cycle is complete.
8. Divide into 12 balls while the dough is still warm, then roll into a long, thin log and then twist to form a pretzel shape.
9. Cover a large cookie sheet with parchment paper.
10. Transfer onto a lined cookie sheet, leaving small space between them.
11. Brush the remaining butter on top the pretzels and sprinkle with the salt.
12. Bake for 12 to 15 minutes in the oven or until golden brown.

Nutrition: Calories 217, Fat 18 g, Carb: 3 g, Protein 11 g

95. IRANIAN FLAT BREAD (SANGAK)

INGREDIENTS

- 4 cups almond flour
- 2 ½ cups warm water
- 1 tbsp. instant yeast
- 12 tsp. sesame seeds
- Salt to taste

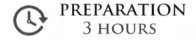 **PREPARATION**
3 HOURS

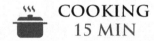 **COOKING**
15 MIN

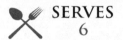 **SERVES**
6

DIRECTIONS

1. Add all ingredients to bread machine pan following order in your bread machine's manual instructions, taking care on how to mix in the yeast.
2. Place the bread pan in the machine, and select the dough cycle setting.
3. Then press start once you have closed the lid of the machine.
4. Remove dough from bread machine when cycle is complete.
5. Shape the dough into a ball and let stand for 3 hours covered.

6. Preheat the oven to 480F.
7. With a rolling pin, roll out the dough, and divide into 6 balls.
8. Roll each ball into ½ inch thick rounds.
9. Line a baking sheet with parchment paper and place the rolled rounds on it.
10. With a finger, make a small hole in the middle and add 2 tsp sesame seeds in each hole.
11. Bake for 3 to 4 minutes, then flip over and bake for 2 minutes more.
12. Serve.

Nutrition: Calories 26, Fat 1 g, Carb 3.5 g, Protein 0.7 g

96. SNICKERDOODLES

INGREDIENTS

- 2 cups almond flour
- 2 tbsp. coconut flour
- ¼ tsp. baking soda
- ¼ tsp. salt
- 3 tbsp. unsalted butter, melted
- 1/3 cup low-carb sweetener
- ¼ cup coconut milk
- 1 tbsp. vanilla extract
- 2 tbsp. ground cinnamon
- 2 tbsp. low-carb granulated sweetener

 PREPARATION
10 MIN

 COOKING
10 MIN

 SERVES
20

DIRECTIONS

1. Preheat the oven to 350F.
2. Whisk together the coconut flour, almond flour, baking soda, and salt in a bowl.
3. In another bowl, cream the butter, sweetener, milk and vanilla.
4. Add all ingredients to bread machine pan following order in your bread machine's manual instructions.
5. Place the bread pan in the machine, and select the cookies dough setting. If not available use pasta dough program.
6. Then press start once you have closed the lid of the machine.
7. Remove dough from bread machine when cycle is complete.
8. Line baking sheets with parchment paper.
9. Blend the ground cinnamon and low-carb granulated sweetener together in a bowl. With your hands, roll a tbsp. of dough into a ball.
10. Roll the dough ball in the cinnamon mixture to fully coat.

11. Place the dough balls on the cookie sheet, spread about an inch apart, and flatten with the underside of a jar.

12. Bake for 8 to 10 minutes.
13. Cool and serve.

Nutrition: Calories 86, Fat 7 g, Carb 3 g, Protein 3 g

97. PARMESAN-THYME POPOVERS

INGREDIENTS

- 4 eggs
- ½ cup coconut milk
- 2 tbsp. coconut flour
- Pinch salt
- 1 tbsp. parmesan cheese
- 1 tbsp. chopped fresh thyme

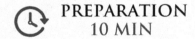 **PREPARATION** 10 MIN

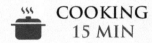 **COOKING** 15 MIN

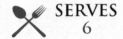 **SERVES** 6

DIRECTIONS

1. Preheat the oven to 425F.
2. Pre-grease a 12 cupcake pan with butter or oil
3. Add all ingredients to bread machine pan following order in your bread machine's manual instructions.
4. Place the bread pan in the machine, and select the cookies dough setting. If not available use pasta dough program.
5. Then press start once you have closed the lid of the machine.
6. Remove dough from bread machine when cycle is complete.
7. Fill greased nonstick cupcake pan at 2/3 level with dough.
8. Bake for 15 minutes, or until they begin to brown on top.
9. Cool and serve.

Nutrition: Calories 64, Fat 34 g, Carb 2 g, Protein 3 g

98. KETO-BREAD TWISTS

INGREDIENTS

- ¼ cup almond flour
- 2 tbsp. coconut flour
- ½ tsp. salt
- ½ tbsp. baking powder
- ½ cup cheese, shredded
- 2 tbsp. butter
- 2 eggs
- ¼ cup green pesto

 PREPARATION
20 MIN

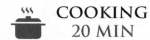 **COOKING**
20 MIN

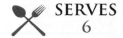 **SERVES**
6

DIRECTIONS

1. Preheat the oven to 350F and prepare a baking tray.
2. Combine coconut flour, almond flour, baking powder, and salt in a bowl.
3. Mix butter, cheese, and egg in another bowl.
4. Combine the flour mixture with the butter mixture pour it to bread machine pan following order in your bread machine's manual instructions.
5. Place the bread pan in the machine, and select the cookies dough setting. If not available use pasta dough program.
6. Then press start once you have closed the lid of the machine.
7. Remove dough from bread machine when cycle is complete.
8. Take 2 parchment sheets and place the dough in between them.
9. Form the dough into a rectangular shape with a rolling pin and remove the parchment paper from one side.
10. Drizzle the green pesto on the loaf and cut it into strips and twist them.
11. Put the baking tray in the oven and bake for 20 minutes.
12. Remove from oven and serve.

Nutrition: Calories 151, Fat 12.9 g, Carb 3.5 g, Protein 5.8 g

99. MUSTARD BEER BREAD

INGREDIENTS

- 1 ¼ cups dark beer
- 2 1/3 cups almond flour
- ¾ cup whole almond meal
- 1 tablespoon olive oil
- 3 teaspoons mustard seeds
- 1 ½ teaspoons dry yeast
- 1 teaspoon salt
- 2 teaspoons brown sugar

 PREPARATION
60 MIN

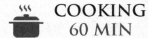 **COOKING**
60 MIN

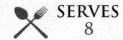 **SERVES**
8

DIRECTIONS

1. Open a bottle of beer and let it stand for 30 minutes to get out the gas.
2. In a bread maker's bucket, add the beer, mustard seeds, butter, amond flour, and almond meal.
3. From different angles in the bucket, put salt and sugar. In the center of the flour, make a groove and fill with the mustard seeds.
4. Start the baking program.
5. When cycle in finished and bread in ready, remove it from the pan and let cool in a banneton.
6. Enjoy!

Nutrition: Calories 148, Carbohydrates 4.2 g, Fats 21 g, Protein 4.1 g

100. LIKE-POTATO ROSEMARY KETO-BREAD

INGREDIENTS

- 3 jicama root (like potatoes replacement)
- 4 cups almond flour
- 1 tablespoon sugar (needed to activate yeast)
- 1 tablespoon oil
- 3 ½ teaspoons salt
- 1 ½ cups water
- 1 teaspoon dry yeast
- 1 cup mashed potatoes, ground through a sieve
- crushed rosemary

 PREPARATION 60 MIN   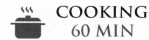 **COOKING** 60 MIN   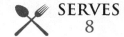 **SERVES** 8

DIRECTIONS

1. Peel the jicama root and shred it using a food processor.
2. Place the shredded jicama root in a colander to allow the water to drain. Mix in 2 tsp of salt as well.
3. Squeeze out the remaining liquid.
4. Microwave the shredded jicama for 5-8 minutes. This step pre-cooks it.
5. Measure the required amount of ingredients. Install the mixing paddle in the baking container.
6. Fill with flour, remaining salt, and sugar.
7. Add sunflower oil and water.
8. Close the lid, and put the yeast in the specially designated hole.
9. Set the mode of baking bread with a filling, according to the instructions of the bread maker.
10. When the dough knits and comes up the right number of times, a beep will sound, which means that you can add additional ingredients. Open the lid of the bread maker and pour in the jicama mixture and chopped rosemary. Close and press the "Start" button.
11. After the oven is finished, immediately remove the bread from the baking container.
12. Let cool down.
13. Serve and enjoy.

Nutrition: Calories 276, Carbohydrates 5 g, Fats 2.8 g, Protein 7.4 g

101. HOMEMADE OMEGA-3 BREAD

INGREDIENTS

- 3/5 cup almond milk
- ½ cup water
- 2 eggs
- 2 tablespoons rapeseed oil
- 3 cups almond flour
- 1 cup flax flour
- 2 teaspoons dry yeast
- 2 teaspoons salt
- 1 tablespoons cane sugar (needed for yeast activation)

- 3 tablespoons flaxseeds
- 1 tablespoon sesame seeds

PREPARATION 60 MIN

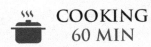 **COOKING** 60 MIN

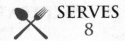 **SERVES** 8

DIRECTIONS

1. Soak the flaxseeds in cool water for 30 minutes.
2. Combine all the liquid ingredients in the bread pan
3. Add sifted almond flour, flaxseed flour, yeast, sugar, and salt.
4. Set it to the Basic program.
5. After the signal sounds, remove from pan
6. Add sesame seeds and strained flaxseeds.

Nutrition: Calories 289, Carbohydrates 4.5 g, Fats 9 g, Protein 11.1 g

CONCLUSION

Thank you for reaching the end of this book. A bread machine and this book is really a perfect couple in your kitchen. Finally, you can have lots of choices of keto bread you can make and serve for your beloved ones.

Bread is staple food that is consumed daily. Since health is the first number of investments in life, it is a good thing if you can prepare it from home. That means everything contained in the bread you and your beloved eat almost every day is under control.

Every recipe in this book is specially created for those who concern not only to health but also taste. However, consume the keto bread with several additional nourishing food, such as vegetables, meat, cheese, and many other healthy food options is totally great since it will enhance the nutritious content of the food.

For sure, every single recipe in this book has been tried in our kitchen and all of them are superb. However, as practice always makes perfect, it is suggested to you to make the bread as often as possible and to engage with your bread machine.

Cutting a lot of foods that are favorites is one of the main struggles that people go through when on keto diet.

Concentrate on the positives and you will succeed. Keto diet helps in prevention of some diseases such as respiratory problems, heart diseases and diabetes.

It does not matter if you want to start the keto lifestyle yourself or you are in search of traditional bread, there are suitable recipes for your every need. They range from sweet to savory and they are healthy and so satisfying. There is little effort needed to make these recipes using the bread machine.

Have wonderful and amazing experiences with your bread machine and enjoy baking, healthy people!

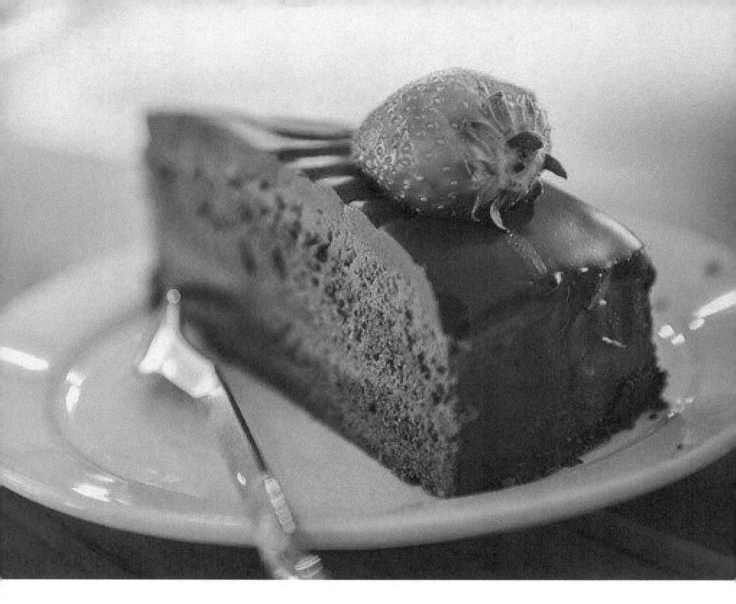

KETO SWEET SNACKS AND DESSERTS

THE ULTIMATE KETOGENIC COOKBOOK WITH 101 DELICIOUS RECIPES FOR YOUR LOW-CARB HIGH-FAT DIET THAT HELP YOU TO BOOST METABOLISM AND INCREASE WEIGHT LOSS

Amanda White

217

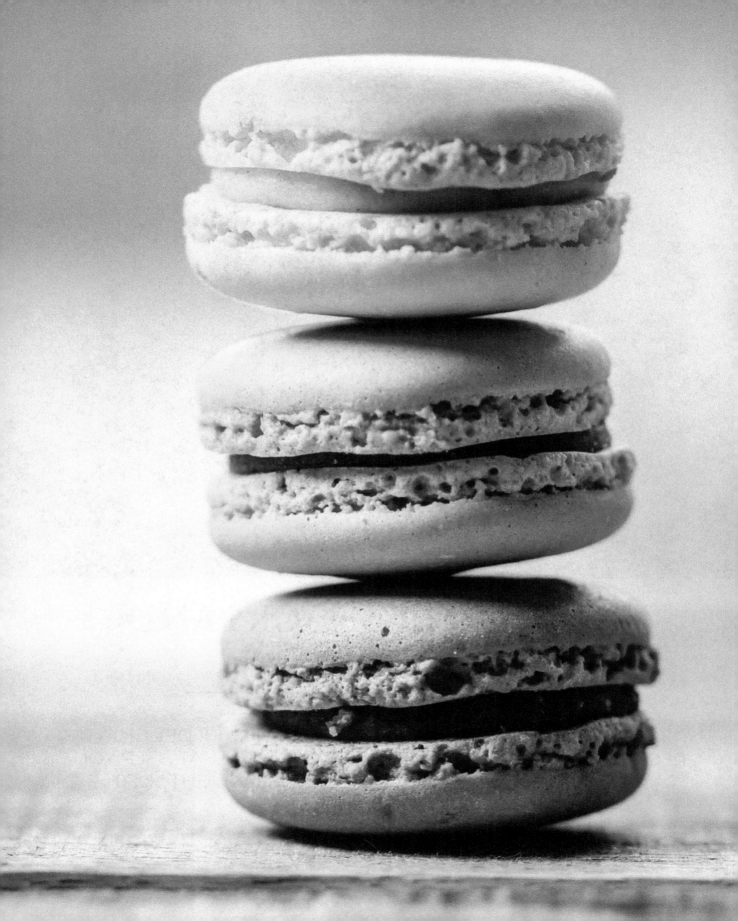

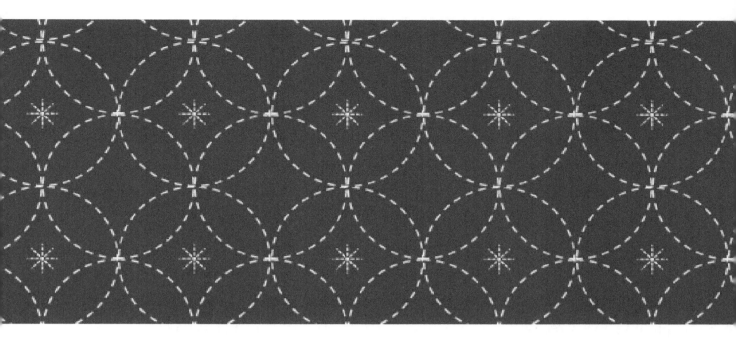

INTRODUCTION

It is absolutely true that there are several restrictions that one has to face while living a keto lifestyle, and one of them is avoiding food that contains sweetness obtained from sugar as it is very dangerous for ketosis.

Sugar is a key ingredient in any dessert, and in a normal eating lifestyle, one cannot imagine making any dessert without sugar. Still, in a keto lifestyle, this ingredient is strictly banned. This does not mean that one cannot enjoy the sweetness in desserts as there are substitutes available that can replace sugar while maintaining the same taste and texture that sugar creates in a recipe. Desserts made with such substitutes are called keto desserts.

Craving for eating sweet things is greatly suppressed when the body enters into ketosis. So people that are not much fond of eating desserts don't encounter any issue, but if you are one of those who are addicted to eating sweet things all the time, especially the desserts, then the knowledge about keto desserts is a must for you.

There are a lot of options in keto desserts you can go for when you want to satisfy your sweet tooth craving. Keto dieticians have come up with so many delicious and super healthy dessert recipes that you can easily make in your kitchen to enjoy the sweet taste while staying in ketosis.

There are dessert recipes that need some baking for their preparation, there are ones that do not require any baking but only blending of ingredients and chilling in freezer, and there are also some special desserts, making which demands both baking and chilling. Every recipe has its own taste and texture, so it depends on your mood that what you are feeling like to eat at a particular time.

The taste generated by the combination of chocolate and peanut butter is something you must try in your keto desserts, and once you do, you will realize that these two ingredients are meant to be together.

It has been proven through research that including desserts in your daily meals leaves several positive impacts on your health. Let's see how eating desserts can benefit us and help us improve our health.

Protection from stroke

Eating desserts that contain dark chocolate as an ingredient is greatly helpful in reducing the risk of strokes and keeping the blood vessels strong that carry the nutrients and oxygen to the brain.

A study was done on a group of people that were asked to eat desserts containing dark chocolate for a specific time period, and their comparison was made with another group, the members of which did not eat anything like that. The results showed that the dark chocolate dessert eating people were less likely to suffer from stroke.

Healthy breakfast

Including a dessert in your breakfast is a good step in moving towards a fitter and healthier lifestyle as eating cake, cookie, or a doughnut early in the morning helps in losing weight.

Another great benefit of having a desert in the breakfast is that it helps stay fuller for longer as compared to some high-calorie foods. It has been proven through research that taking a low-calorie diet in the form of cake and cookies in breakfast satisfies the appetite for a longer part of the day compared to a high-calorie diet containing cheese and milk.

Blood pressure control

High blood pressure is one of the major health issues all over the world, but you will be glad to know that keeping a desert in your daily diet plan helps you lower it.

Taking 100g of cocoa powder or dark chocolate on a daily basis brings a reduction of 2-3 mg Hg in your blood pressure.

So it will not be wrong to say that desserts can play their role in protecting you from a very dangerous brain disease "dementia" which is mostly caused by high blood pressure.

Enriched with nutrients

The nutrients like vitamins, antioxidants, and fiber are very essential for a healthy body, and they also play their role in preventing several diseases.

The desserts containing pumpkin as the main ingredient are really powerful in this regard as they are very enriched with all the healthy nutrients needed by the body, and they are also a great source of fuel for the brain.

Positive Emotions

People are mostly concerned about their physical and mental health, but emotional health is a crucial part of overall health that should never be ignored for happy living. It has been proven scientifically that taking your favorite dessert on a specific day positively impacts your body and mind creating the feelings of happiness, and that helps in inculcating positive emotions.

What happens is that certain types of chemicals are produced in our body and mind as a result of eating our favorite dessert, and this leads to improving emotional health.

Weight control

Many people think that eating desserts causes an increase in their body's weight, so the fear of being overweight makes them exclude desserts from their diet plan. Doing this might benefit them on a short term basis, but several health benefits can be achieved by adopting a different strategy in the long term.

Results gained through including desserts in a diet enriched with nutrients are much better than just excluding them, and weight loss happens quickly as, in keto diet, this strategy works the best.

So we come to the conclusion that avoiding desserts for the purpose of achieving short term weight loss goals leads to overconsumption and binge eating.

Fruits consumption

Eating desserts allows your body to consume fruits in a healthy way. Putting blueberries and raspberries in your dessert gives you a combination of healthy fats, vitamins, and many healthy nutrients that not only improve your immune system to fight against diseases but also keep your body strong and healthy.

The good thing is that there are countless options of ingredient combinations with keto fruits you can go for to make delicious and super healthy keto desserts.

So now, you know that there are several benefits we can get from desserts, and keto desserts are much more beneficial for health in keto diet that one should not forget while preparing the meal plan.

Choosing Keto Sweeteners

As you already know that you have to use sugar substitutes to make desserts when you are on keto diet, and these substitutes are different kinds of sweeteners. The low carb sweeteners used in keto recipes are actually called keto sweeteners.

There are different types of keto sweeteners that you can choose from depending on what dessert you are making.

Stevia

Stevia is a popular sweetener used as sugar substitute in keto recipes, and it is extracted from the leaves of stevia plant. It is available in three forms, granulated, powdered, and drops.

Stevia is a much powerful sweetener as compared to sugar, only few drops of it are enough to create sweetness in a keto recipe because it is 300 times more sweeter than sugar.

One thing that you have to be very careful about while using stevia is that you have to use it in the right proportion as using too much in your desert will create a bitter aftertaste, and this will ultimately destroy the taste and texture of your recipe.

If you are a beginner, then you must have complete knowledge of what quantity of it suits the best in a certain recipe. The best thing to do is that you go on, adding slowly and keep checking the taste to see if you need to add more. This way, you will easily get the taste you need without over adding and spoiling everything.

Erythritol

Erythritol is another very popular sweetener used by keto dieters, and it is extracted from glucose through the process of fermentation with the microorganism in a honeycomb.

One great benefit that all keto dieters get from this amazing sweetener that it does not create any problems in our digestive system like other sweeteners do in certain situations, but the condition is that it has to be consumed in balanced quality because it's overconsumption does create problems in the digestive system especially the side effects like bloating, cramps and diarrhea occur if its large quantities are consumed in a very short period of time.

The reason behind this is that erythritol takes some time to be broken down in the water, so our body is not able to digest a large quantity of erythritol quickly.

Erythritol is really helpful in creating resistance against bacteria in our mouth because it behaves differently from normal sugar as bacteria are mostly capable of breaking down sugar in our mouth. This helps them increase their population resulting in spreading more secretions and damaging our teeth, but in erythritol's case, this does not happen because bacteria are not able to break it down and no damages occur, so we can say that this sweetener is great for improving the health of our teeth.

It is very low in calories like in 1 gram of erythritol you get 0.21 calories. As far as sweetness is concerned, it is less sweet than sugar like its certain quantity is 70% sweet compared to the sugar with the same quantity, and this is the reason that it is not used mostly in its pure form. It is rather mixed with other sweeteners to generate the desired taste in keto desserts.

Some brands include artificial additives like aspartame to maintain the sweetness of erythritol, but this could be really dangerous for your mental health as well as your physical health. Such artificial additions cause short term memory loss and also depression and anxiety issues.

Regarding your physical health, you are likely to encounter fatigue, muscle weakness, and weight gain issues. So you have to be very careful while purchasing that if your brand is adding something artificial in your erythritol.

It does not have any effect on blood glucose levels in your body, so if you have diabetes, then this is a perfect choice for you.

On the other hand, erythritol is not a good option for you if you are facing irritable bowel syndrome because it has been proven medically that people using erythritol with this syndrome face further complicated issues.

So we reach to a conclusion that one has to make a decision depending on their body's need and compatibility, as everyone's body is different. If one thing is suiting to a certain person, that might not necessarily suit another person's health.

Swerve

Swerve is another natural sweetener that keto dieters love to use in their recipes. It not only contains zero net carbs and zero calories, but it is also non-glycemic, which shows that it has no impact on blood glucose levels in your body.

All the natural ingredients are involved in the preparation of swerve, and these are some natural flavors, oligosaccharides, and erythritol. Oligosaccharides found naturally in starchy vegetables and fruits are actually carbohydrates that are made up of sugar chains. Most enzymes are added to starchy root vegetables for their preparation. They fall into the category of prebiotic fibers that are not digestible by the human body.

All the natural flavors used in the formation of Swerve are manufactured in laboratories through natural methods.

Swerve is likely to cause digestive issues when fermented by bacteria in the colon as its both components oligosaccharides and erythritol are high in food maps, which are carbohydrates made up of short chains.

Monk Fruit

Monk fruit is extracted from dried small green melon fruit cultivated in southern China centuries ago by monks, and so it is named after them.

This keto sweetener is also calorie and carb-free, and it does not affect blood glucose levels in our body. Another good thing about this sweetener is that it does not create any issues like bloating and gas in the digestive system.

The sweetness in monk fruit is generated by mogrosides, which are natural compounds, and they are anti-inflammatory, play their role in keeping the blood sugar level in a stable position, and also prevent cancer in the body.

The process of cultivating, harvesting, and drawing the monk fruit is not easy, and there are several challenges in the way. It is also imported from the selected regions of the world where it is grown, so these factors make it an expensive ingredient as compared to other sweeteners available in the market.

Monk fruit is rarely observed as allergic, but there are still chances of it, and the possible allergic reactions from the monk fruit are dizziness, stomach pain, difficulty breathing, and swollen tongue. You should not ignore this if you are allergic to gourds as you might be at risk of getting an allergic reaction from this sweetener.

Chapter 1: Basic Of Ketogenic Diet And Benefits Of Keto Desserts

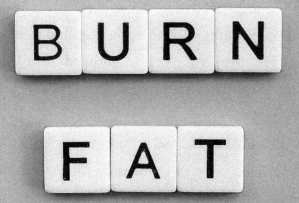

The ketogenic diet, or keto diet, is a high-fat diet that promotes a healthy lifestyle san any carbs and sugar. A food with super-low or no amount of carbs gets the body into ketosis, which is the primary goal of the ketogenic diet. Ketosis is a metabolic process in which the body switch to fats to get energy when carbs reserves are finished. The following are some proven benefits of the ketogenic diet:

- Weight loss
- Clear skin
- Reduced inflammation
- Mental clarity and focused
- More energy
- Reduced cravings
- Reduce the risk of chronic and metabolic diseases

Let's go into some more details of the ketogenic diet.

So, whatever you eat on a ketogenic diet, be it has carbs or sugar; just make sure that the body stays into ketosis process and doesn't spike its blood sugar level. Sugar is also a form of carbohydrate, and the amount of carbs allowed for a keto-er is about 50 grams or below this threshold per day. This amount includes refined sugar and all the sources of carbs.

So does this mean that you have to cut back on desserts? Absolutely not. Being on the Keto diet, you can still satisfy your sweet tooth and enjoy sweet treats. All you need to do is to prepare those desserts that don't bring your body out of ketosis. And there are two keys to doing this. Firstly, you need to choose keto-friendly ingredients that are high in fats to support ketone formation in the body. And secondly, use a sweetener that doesn't spike blood glucose level to a critical level. Luckily, as we have seen in the introduction, there are many sweeteners available in the market that add flavor to your desserts, without increasing carbs and sugar in it. Below we summarize them briefly:

- Stevia: This natural sweetener is nonnutritive, and this means it has no carbs or calories. Stevia is a great option to control and lower your blood sugar levels. It is available in both powdered and syrup form, but it is much sweeter than table sugar. Therefore use less stevia quantity to achieve the same sweetness – 1 teaspoon stevia for 1 cup sugar.

- Sucralose: This sucralose based artificial sweetener is indigestible and thus, provides no calories and carbs. Feel free to use this sweetener for any dessert except for those that require baking. Substitute it in the 1:1 ratio for most of the dessert recipes.

- Erythritol: It is a type of sugar alcohol that stimulates your taste buds, which gives you a taste of sugar. It can substitute sugar in a wide variety of dessert recipes, be it baking or cooking.

- Xylitol: This sugar alcohol is commonly found in gum and candies, and like other keto sweeteners, it has no carbs. Give a kick of flavor to your smoothies, shakes, tea, and coffee with this sweetener. Moreover, it also works well with baked desserts. However, do add a little bit of liquid when using xylitol as it absorbs moisture and increases dryness. Exchange xylitol in a 1:1 ratio with regular sugar.

- Monk Fruit Sweetener: As the name suggests, this sweetener is extracted from the monk fruit and, thus, contain natural sugar. And, since this extract contains no sugar and calorie, it is an excellent option for a ketogenic diet. Use it anywhere in place of regular sugar.

You can also use fruits to add sweetness to your desserts, such as:
- Strawberries
- Raspberries
- Blackberries
- Blueberries
- Lemon
- Lime
- Watermelon

- Cherries
- Peach
- Kiwi
- Cantaloupe
- Mandarin

Following are some sweeteners that are high in carbs, and you must avoid them.

- Honey
- Coconut sugar
- Maple syrup
- Agave nectar
- Dates

Here are some more tips that will help you satisfy your sweet tooth.

- It is normal to crave sugar in the initial days of Ketogenic dieting. You will have the temptation for sweet once in a while, and when this happens, Keto-friendly sweeteners can satisfy your sweet cravings without stalling your fat loss and maintaining the ketosis process in your body.

- Differentiate between the types of sweeteners that are available for the Ketogenic diet. There are three categories – natural sweeteners, sugar alcohols, and artificial sweeteners. Erythritol and stevia work just perfectly for any desserts without disturbing your insulin and blood sugar.

- Enhance your weight loss with Keto sweeteners. As mentioned before, sugar is also a form of carb, and therefore, using them in an appropriate amount not only led to shedding weight, it also optimizes your health.

Benefits of Keto Desserts

So, what's so great about low-carb desserts? Why should one have them?

Reason #1 – They contribute to weight loss. It turns out the limiting carbs in your desserts and emphasizing more on fats leads to more weight loss and improvement in overall health. The science behind this relates to the phenomenon of fuel for the body. For our body, carb is a go-to source for energy. And when it gets digested, it is converted into glucose and then burned for fuel. So, if you consume carb-filled food and no other nutrients like fat and protein, the fat in your body lingers and adds on if you fail, you burn all the carb reserve in your body.

Reason # 2 – When you restrict carb in your diet, the body switches to a fat-burning mood and creates ketones, which is another source of energy that the body can use. When this happens, the body enters into a metabolic state called ketosis, which will result in the burning and reduction of stored fat in the body. Moreover, this process will keep you energetic without spiking your blood sugar levels.

Reason # 3 – It improves your overall health. Beyond the significant benefit of keto desserts, which is weight loss, another advantage is substantial improvement in general health. It is proved scientifically that many ailments reduce significantly after eating low-carb consistently, like high blood pressure, coronary diseases, diabetes, epilepsy, dementia, and cancer.

With all these benefits, you might just forget about desserts, but the good news is that you don't have to.

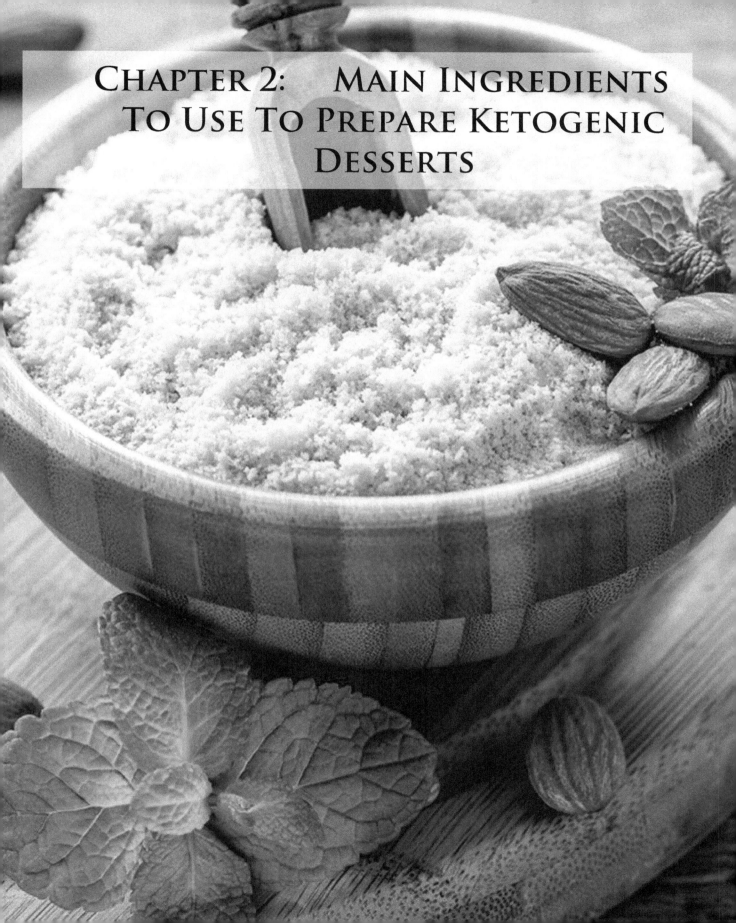

CHAPTER 2: MAIN INGREDIENTS TO USE TO PREPARE KETOGENIC DESSERTS

The keto-friendly "YES" foods

These are the low-carb foods that are permitted on the ketogenic diet. Some of them can be eaten liberally, such as leafy greens. Others can be eaten with a little more moderation, such as nuts and berries. Your calorie counter/macro calculator will let you know exactly how many net carbs are in each food, so you will soon learn the right quantities, and it will become second nature!

Nut and Seed Flour

- As grains are discouraged for the Keto Diet, you can make use of many different kinds of flour alternatives. Nut and seed flours can help you recreate your favorite dessert recipes. There are different types of seed flour that you can use, including the following:

- Almond flour: Almond flour is made from almonds that are ground into flour. Often, almond flour is made by removing the seed coat, which makes it better for baking. A quarter of a cup of almond flour contains 12 grams of fat, 5 grams of protein, and 2 grams of carbohydrates. It contains a lot of fat and does not contain any gluten at all, thus making it one of the best flour alternatives when making keto-friendly desserts. When using this flour, you may need to use additional eggs or baking powder in order to give it more volume and structure. Almond flour can be used to make cakes, pancakes, and bread, while almond meal can be used to make pie crusts and cookies.

- Almond meal: Almond meal should not be mistaken with almond flour that has a coarse texture and is often made together with the seed coat. It can also be used to thicken smoothies.

- Coconut flour: Coconut flour is rich in healthy fats, and it is made from dehydrated coconut meat. Unlike almond flour and other nut flours, it is denser, and it absorbs more liquid. When cooking with coconut flour, use more eggs and extra liquid than usual. In general, recipes that call for coconut flour use less of this ingredient. The correct substitution is to use ¼ or 1/3 cup of coconut flour for every cup of grain-based flour used.

- Seed flour: There is a variety of seed flour available in the market that can be used to make delicious keto-friendly desserts. These include those made from pumpkin seeds, sesame seeds, sunflower seeds, and others. Seed flour is perfect for making great keto-friendly pie crusts and bars.

- Chia and Flax seeds: Although not really used mainly as a keto-friendly flour substitute, both chia and flax seeds are used to bind ingredients together. It can be used as a substitute for eggs, especially for people who are following a Vegan Keto Diet. To use chia and flax as binders, use a ratio of 1:2 of chia or flax with water.

Oils and Fats

It is important to take note that oils and fats are not created equally. This means that some kinds of fats used in making desserts are not keto-friendly at all. This is especially true for butter made from grain-fed cattle. It is important to take note that a great keto-friendly dessert should contain healthy fat sources. Saturated fats or those that stay solid at room temperature are great fat sources. Another good fat to use is cold-pressed monosaturated fat. Thus, below are some of the best oils and fats that you can use when making keto-friendly desserts:

- Coconut oil: Cold-pressed, organic, and virgin coconut oil is a must-have in making keto-friendly meals, including desserts. It is a staple when making chocolate ganache as well as making rich and filling desserts.

- Butter: It is crucial to use butter sourced from grass-fed cows because its constitution does not contain too much lactose – a type of sugar or simple carbohydrate obtained from milk. Butter from grass-fed cows infuses a delicious and aromatic appeal to all kinds of food.

- Ghee: Ghee is clarified butter that is made by simmering butter in low heat to remove the milk solids and water. This is a preferred alternative to grass-fed butter, especially among people who suffer from dairy intolerance.
- Other types of oils: Aside from those mentioned above, other types of fats that can be used to make keto-friendly desserts include macadamia nut oil, hemp seed oil, and olive oil. However, they are ideal in garnishing meals than cooking.

Keto-Friendly Sweeteners

Perhaps one of the biggest hurdles when making keto-friendly desserts is how to make desserts sweet yet keto-friendly. Fortunately, there are many types of keto-friendly sweeteners that you can use to make your favorite desserts. It is important to take note that when it comes to using keto-friendly sweeteners, using artificial sweeteners should be avoided at all costs. Below are examples of guilt-free sweeteners that you can use. A table for the sweetener conversion is also listed thereafter.

- Lakanto: Lakanto is an all-natural sweetener made from the combination of erythritol and monk fruit extract. The sweet taste comes from the natural MoGro sides, thus making it low-carb and great for those following the Keto Diet. Aside from benefiting those following the Keto Diet, it can also benefit those who have diabetes. To use this sweetener, use in equal proportions as you would use white sugar.
- Stevia: Stevia is a marvelous leaf that is as sweet as sugar. You can grow the herb and use the leaves to make delicious desserts. You can also buy stevia sweeteners from your local health store.

Other Essential Ingredients

Aside from the basic ingredients already mentioned, it is also important to stock up on other keto-friendly items that will help you make great keto-friendly desserts. Below are other ingredients that you can use to make successful and delicious keto-friendly munchies.

- Psyllium husk powder: Aside from being used as a colon cleanser, psyllium husk powder can also give the finished product a crumb-like texture. It can be used to make pies and bread.
- Xanthan gum: Conventional thickeners are often starch-based. Instead of using cornstarch or cassava starch to thicken desserts, you can use xanthan gum as a carb-free substitute.

Oils:

- Olive oil
- Avocado oil
- Flaxseed oil
- MCT oil
- Coconut oil
- Walnut oil
- Nuts and seeds:
- Almonds
- Walnuts
- Pecans
- Brazil nuts
- Hazelnuts
- Macadamia nuts
- Cashews
- Pumpkin seeds
- Sunflower seeds
- Chia seeds
- Sesame seeds
- Nut and seed butters (plain, no flavors or sugars added)
- Low carb veggies such as: Lettuce, Spinach, Kale

- Avocado (technically a fruit...but it's an incredible keto food, full of healthy fats and fiber)
- Asparagus
- Artichokes
- Cabbage
- Broccoli
- Cauliflower
- Bok choy
- Chard
- Celery
- Green beans
- Mushrooms
- Mustard greens
- Tomatoes
- Zucchini
- Spaghetti squash
- Mung beans
- Cucumber

Alcohol

All spirits are okay on keto, in moderation. Note: this does not include liqueurs or sugary drinks such as Kahlua or Baileys Irish Cream. Plain, pure spirits such as vodka, gin, whiskey, rum, and tequila are all zero-carb as long as you mix them with water, plain soda or zero-carb soda. Champagne, dry white wine, and red wine are all fine in moderation.

For example, one glass of champagne (around 5 oz) has a maximum of 2 grams of net carbs.

Mixers: plain, unflavored soda with fresh citrus is best

Sauces and condiments

Full-fat mayonnaise and fresh guacamole are permitted the keto diet as long as they do not contain sugar. Salad dressing made from oil and vinegar is fine, but watch out for store-bought salad dressings which are often packed with sugar.

The keto-banned "NO WAY" foods

Pasta, noodles, bread and rice

All pasta, noodles, bread, and rice are off-limits. Basically, anything made from flour or grains is out of bounds.

Beans, lentils, chickpeas

Unfortunately, beans, lentils, and chickpeas are all prohibited on the keto diet because of their high carb content. These foods are in the legume food group and are all banned on keto. This also includes peas and peanuts.

Baked goods

Traditional baked goods such as cakes, cookies, bars, breads, scones, and cupcakes are all out of the question on keto. If they contain flour and sugar, get rid of them.

Sugary treats

Candy, chocolate (except 72% cocoa dark chocolate), ice cream, and all things in the candy aisle are not allowed on keto.

Juice, soda, premixed alcoholic drinks

Fruit juices, sodas, and premixed alcoholic drinks ("alcopops") are filled with sugar and are not ketogenic-approved. Stick to water, plain soda water, tea, and coffee.

Grains

Grains such as rice, quinoa, oats, and barley are all ruled out on keto because they are high-carb foods. You can use cauliflower and broccoli as rice substitutes.

Milk

Milk contains sugar and is therefore not permitted on keto. Stick to full-fat cream or unsweetened nut milk such as almond milk.

Most fruits

The only fruits you can eat on keto are avocados and berries (in moderation). Avoid all other fruits, especially bananas. Fruits are high-carb, high-sugar foods. While fruits are not unhealthy, they're simply too carb-rich and therefore negate the ketogenic process.

Starchy veggies

Starchy veggies such as potato, sweet potato, corn, yams, peas, carrots, and beets are not keto-friendly as they are high in carbs. Stick to leafy greens and low-carb veggies, as listed above.

Sauces and condiments

Stay away from store-bought sauces, condiments, and marinades as they are often packed with sugars. Make your own dressings, sauces, and marinades at home so you know exactly what's in them.

Can you really eat dessert on keto?

Uh, YES! Of course. Keto isn't about cutting out certain meals or recipes... it's about sticking to the correct macros. This means that as long as your dessert is within the parameters of your macros, it's completely permitted! Luckily for us, ingredients such as butter, cream, sour cream, mascarpone, cream cheese, and eggs are all wonderfully keto-friendly foods...and perfect dessert ingredients too. When it comes to sugar, there are many non-sugar sweeteners out there, which are 100% keto-approved.

Stevia, erythritol, and xylitol are the most popular sweeteners as they don't spike the blood sugar at all. I think that Stevia is the best sweetener as you only need a very small amount, and it contains barely any carbs or calories.

Note: these recipes were all formulated using STEVIA, which is extremely sweet and only requires 1 tsp per 1 cup of regular sugar. Other sweeteners are less sweet and require a far larger measure. My advice is to use Stevia for these recipes to get the best result.

Concerned about the issue of flour? No worries! We use ground almonds and sometimes ground hazelnuts. Ground almonds provide great fat and protein, with more fiber than regular flour. Ground almonds do give a denser result, but to me, that's a great thing! A dense, fudgy cake is nothing to be mad about.

Keto dessert ingredient staples (staples in these recipes, at least!)

- Heavy cream
- Real butter (grass-fed butter, no margarine or butter substitutes, please!)
- Coconut oil, canola oil, olive oil, flaxseed oil
- Cocoa powder (unsweetened, always)
- Pure vanilla extract (no essence or imitations)
- Fresh mint
- Flavor essences (such as almond or caramel)
- Cream cheese (plain, full fat)
- Espresso powder
- Mascarpone cheese (plain, full fat)
- Keto sweeteners such as Stevia
- Almonds, hazelnuts, and walnuts (ground and whole)
- Salt (for bringing out chocolate flavor)
- Eggs (always free-range)
- Berries (frozen, fresh and freeze-dried)
- Lemon zest and juice
- 72% cocoa dark chocolate (a small amount, and it must be at least 72% cocoa!)

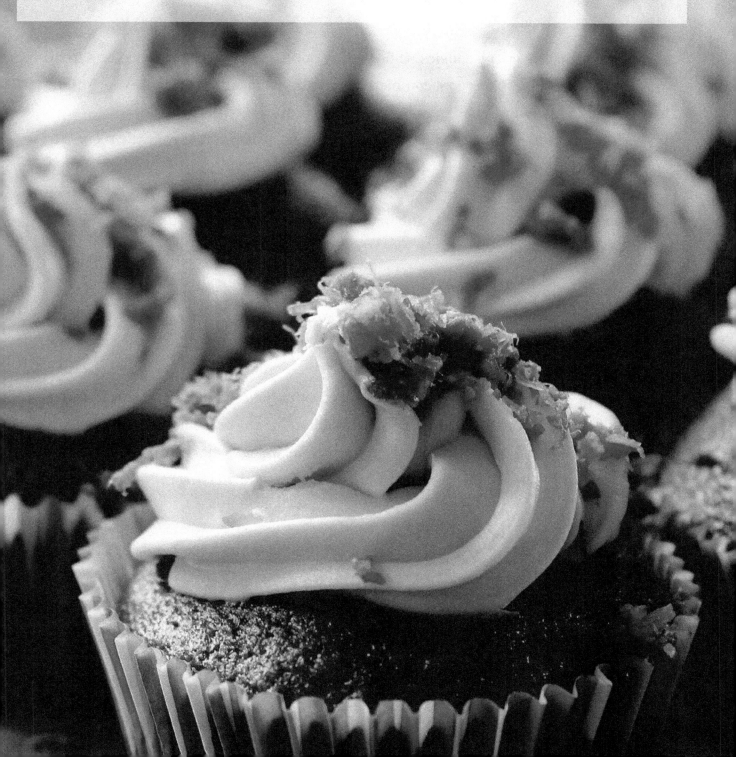

CHAPTER 3: MAIN TYPES OF KETO DESSERTS

Keto Dessert Essentials

There are many tips in helping you with these recipes and others that you find along your journey into the Keto diet. Here are some basic cooking tips for this cookbook that you will find helpful for the different types of recipes.

Cookies

If you prefer to have crispy cookies while you try out these Keto diet delights, be sure to make sure to let the cookies cool completely, even if this means overnight. They will be less crumbly, and you will not regret every crunch in your mouth.

If you prefer sweeter cookies, add 1/4 teaspoon stevia glycerite to any of the recipes to appease your sweet tooth.

If you find that you are not getting the fluffiness that you desire in your cookies, add 1/2 teaspoon of apple cider vinegar to the ingredients. It will alter the cookie texture, but it will give the cookies more rise.

Cakes

When you are frosting the cakes, be sure to make sure that the frosting is not applied to the cake while it is still warm. This will ensure that the frosting will not melt off as you are spreading it onto the cake.

You will find a sprinkle recipe that is based on coconut flakes. You can use this recipe to top any of your sweet treat desserts, and it is brilliant for any occasion.

If you dread cutting a cake into uniform pieces, there are cake markers and cutters that you can buy that will save you the hassle. Most come in 14 or 16 slices.

Mousses

Of the recipes that are served right away without the use of the freezer or fridge they are going to be more of the soft-serve consistency. If you prefer to have a more thick mousse, simply put it in the fridge or freezer to harden it up.

Frozen Desserts

You will find that many of the desserts can be transformed into other sweet frozen treats. Keep an eye out for Tricks and Tips at the end of recipes on how to add variety. You will find that you can get really creative with the recipes and still stay within the Keto diet guidelines.

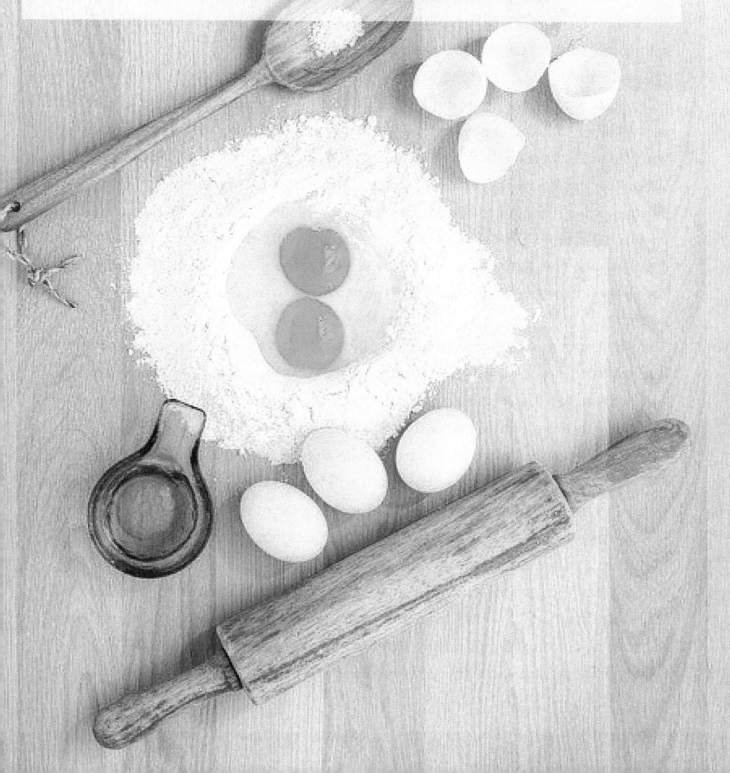

Chapter 4: What Kitchen Tools Do You Need?

You will have many of these cooking utensils in your kitchen already, but if you collect these tools ahead of time, it will save you time, and you will have what you need to make the Keto diet a lifestyle change for you.

The items that you will need that you probably already own are the absolute basics for cooking and baking. These include basic mixing dishes, electrical beater, stirring spoons, rolling pin, rubber scraper, fine mesh strainer, and a whisk.

If you already do not own a food processor or a high powered blender, you will find these will be fantastic additions to your kitchen, as these will help you to be able to bake these recipes much more quickly compared to mixing ingredients by hand. This will also leave you able to do other methods or tell the children to do their homework in the meantime. When you are baking sweet treats in the Keto diet, it is best to use baking paper or silicone-based pans and cooking trays because they tend to stick to the pan more so than traditional recipes. The silicone products are brilliant when it comes to baking and especially with the Keto diet, as nothing will stick to the silicone. If you choose to use the parchment paper liners, they also have the benefit of sweeties not getting too wet on the bottom.

The Silpat or non-stick mat will make your life so much grander when it comes to keeping it simple with cleanup for the sweeties. It is easy to wash, and nothing sticks to it. It is a good substitute for parchment paper, and it is reusable. The only downside is you cannot use sharp objects on the Silpat, as they will cause damage.

Cookie scoopers are a nice addition to the collection, as I can guarantee you will be using this tool a lot after tasting these recipes. It will help to keep your cookies in a uniform shape and makes baking much easier than scraping the dough off a spoon.

For the cakes, you can use a springform pan to release the baked loaf without a bunch of fuss. It is used specifically in the Birthday Cake Recipe, but you will find that you will need it when you gather even more recipes or convert your grandma's cheesecake recipe. If you are not familiar with springform pans, they come in two parts and are kept together by a spring lock mechanism. When you release the lock, the cake comes out rather easily, making these cake recipes a breeze.

You will find that many of these dishes you will want them to look like they came out of the bakery down the street. Many of the mousse and cake recipes call for having a pastry bag. You can find these in craft or baking good stores, or you can fashion one yourself rather quickly using a ziplock bag.

This will be a way to decorate and pipe the ingredients into serving dishes that is a lot more beautiful than just spooning the dishes in by hand. Although, these sweet dishes might not even make it out of the mixing bowl!

All ovens heat differently depending on if they are along an outside wall of your home. Keep this in mind, as you may need to raise or lower the oven temperature up or down by 25° Fahrenheit to get the desired time of baking.

Regular Electric Mixer

This is a basic tool that supplies you with a variety of speeds to be used as needed. Your mixes will be better blended, which will improve the quality of your baked goods. Forget the days of having to hand mix all of your raw baking items!

Regular or Mini-Food Processor

Prepare healthy options for nut butter using a processor. It is useful for many items, including preparing homemade hummus, delicious truffles, chopping nuts, and so much more.

Immersion or Stick Blender

You can prepare a high-quality latte at home using a stick blender and the microwave. Stick blenders are light, easy to handle, and are versatile. If it needs to be whipped, emulsified, beaten, or made into a smoothie or sauce, your stick blender can do the job. They're also easy to clean versus food processors and blenders.

Silicone Baking Mat

Make cleanup time simpler and keep your pans from slipping.

Colander

Use a metal or plastic colander rinsing fruits and other items prepared for your desserts. Mixing Bowls: Be sure to include a sturdy, four-quart capacity bowl, which is excellent for most baking needs. However, keep two or three others to prevent interruptions after you begin the dessert preparations.

Measuring Cups & Spoons

Purchase a measuring cup and spoon system that shows both the Metric and US standards of weight, so there is no confusion during prep. For dry ingredients, it's important to level off the product using a butter knife. When measuring liquids, be sure you have the measuring cup placed on a flat surface.

- Measuring Cups: You should purchase sturdy measuring cups for dry ingredients. The oval types are much easier to reach into boxes for measurement.
- Glass Measuring Cup: Two and four cup measurement cups can also be used for mixing the ingredients. It also provides you a clear image of the contents to ensure proper measurement; no more eyeballing for accuracy.
- Measuring Spoons: If possible, purchase spoons that have a magnet system, making storage much simpler. Never hunt for a spoon again!

Mini Whisk

You have three types you can use for baking; the mini, flat, and twirl whisk. Its balloon-type multi-purpose whisk that excels at aerating liquids and preparing the light thick whipped cream. You can also effectively blend dry fixings in your recipes. Save your cookware by using a flat silicone type on your more delicate nonstick surfaces.

Wire Cooling Rack

The rack helps bread cool down quickly. Eliminate the steam that will build up in the baking pan, which can make the bread loaves soggy on the bottom if cooled on a flat surface.

Baking Sheets

You will be using a baking sheet for many of your dessert items. Purchase a rimmed baking pan for any items that can easily slide off of the edges, such as cookies.

Square Baking Pans

You should check your recipes for specific sizes before baking. If you choose a smaller pan, it will take a bit longer to cook because it's deeper. The measurements should be a minimum of 2-inches deep. The sizes run from 8 to 9-inches and can be used for bar cakes and brownies

Muffin Pans

Muffin tins come in three popular sizes, including mini, standard, and jumbo. The standard-size offers a .5 cup capacity with either 6 or 12 count cups. Mini tins provide one- cup capacity in both the 12 or 24-count cups and jumbo ones also provide one-cup capacity with a 6-count tray. These are great for cupcakes and muffins. It's best to have a set of two, so you can make larger batches without wasted time and money.

Tart Pans

Prepare a delicious tart or quiche using a 9-inch round tart pan with a nonstick surface for quick clean up times.

Ramekins

Use ramekins for small portions such as the Chocolate Mini Cakes.

Cake Pans

Round cake pans work best and are at least 2-inches deep. Some recipes will suggest 6-inch pans, but the 8-inch and 9-inch versions are more popular. Layered cakes work best in the 8-inch pans, but always follow what is suggested in your recipe when possible for more accurate cooking times.

Bundt Cake Pans

You can prepare your favorite cake recipe in a beautifully shaped pan, making the Bundt pan an excellent to your kitchen supply.

Spring Form Pan

Some of your recipes will call for this leak-proof (10 cups) 9-inch pan for baking cakes. Its nonstick surface is excellent for preparing your favorite cheesecake.

TIPS & TRICKS

For the Best Results: Add MCT Oils to Your Keto Plan

Your ketogenic experience can improve with the use of medium-chain triglycerides (MCT oil). These exclusive fatty acids are found in their natural form in palm and coconut oil. You will notice some of the smoothies use this as a component. These are just a few of the examples:

- The oil helps lower your blood sugar.
- The use of MCTs makes it much easier to get into – and remain - in ketosis.
- It is a natural anti-convulsive.
- It is also excellent for appetite control and weight loss.

Important Note: Seek your doctor's advice before changing your eating patterns. In some cases, you could reduce the need for some medications.

Have these on hand:

- Plastic Wrap/Kitchen Towel: You should always have a clean kitchen towel handy for wiping your hands. You should have another towel set aside for covering your yeast bread products. If using plastic wrap, be sure to spray the side of the wrap facing the dough.

- Parchment Baking Paper & Aluminum Foil: You can save tons of time by covering your baking pans and other cooking pots.

CHAPTER 5:   KETO DESSERTS TIPS AND FAQS FOR BEGINNERS

In this day in age, we always lack time and money. Well, the good news is many of these recipes are quick and easy. You will not need to spend all day in the kitchen, struggling to make a healthy meal for yourself and your family. In fact, this is probably going to change the more you get involved in the Keto diet lifestyle as you start seeing how your body looks healthier, and you will feel it in your mind as well.

Time Saving Tips

The biggest time-saving tip is you can double or even triple these recipes as they all keep for many days either on the counter or an even longer time in your freezer or refrigerator. It can't get easier than that!

You will find that the unfrosted cakes can be kept in the freezer for up to 3 months. When you are ready to use them, simply move them from the freezer to the fridge the day before you want to serve the cake. This will give the cake time to thaw properly, and it will be a breeze to apply the frosting as well.

You can even keep the cakes in the refrigerator for up to a week before they will need to be eaten, although we would be surprised if they lasted that long!

If you are going to store your sweeties on the counter, keep them in an air-tight container as they will keep longer. As with the cookies, you can always keep them in the all familiar cookie jar as you know, this always brings back wonderful memories of childhood. This method will also keep your sweet treats even softer. Most cookies will need to be eaten within 5 days if stored on the counter.

Storing your Keto sweets in the freezer or the refrigerator is just as easy. Simply wrap each pastry securely in plastic wrap, put them in a sealed container (only if putting into the refrigerator), or throw them into a zip-lock plastic bag. If you are storing them in the freezer, be sure to put them in a freezer-safe container or zip lock bag.

Whenever you need to eat them, you can put them back into the oven to heat them up, throw them into the microwave, or even eat them straight out of the bag. This will make the cookies, in particular, crispier, as you have already learned.

If you keep your sweeties in the fridge, they will keep for a week, and in the freezer, they will keep up to one month's time.

The key before storing them away is to make sure that the sweets are completely cool beforehand. This will ensure that they will not end up crumbling to pieces, and the excess moisture from the heat will not cause condensation on the packaging.

One tip to use for any of the baked goods using a pan, melt 2 teaspoons of coconut oil and brush the inside of the pan. Freeze for at least 20 minutes for the coconut oil to harden, and this will ensure the baked goods do not stick. This will come in handy as many of the recipes in Keto stick to the pan due to the alternative ingredients used.

Money-Saving Tips

You will find that the ingredients that are called for in the Keto diet recipes are going to be more expensive. Mentally you will need to get past this fact because, again, you need to keep in mind why you have made the choice to begin this lifestyle change. Once you start seeing the benefits to your health, you will be hooked and try to find more ways to further your journey into this lifestyle change you have chosen.

Luckily, there are ways to ensure that you get the best bang for your buck when it comes to buying ingredients to stock your pantry. You will also find benefit in talking and researching on your own with what other people have found during their own personal journeys that it will help you on your own path. If this seems overwhelming at first, just take a deep breath. We have some good tips for you to follow, making this transition as easy as possible.

Be sure to shop around for the best prices and educate yourself on the prices of items, so you know you are getting the best deal, but know that the quality may vary. Read through the ingredients to make sure there are no other additives that are not specific to the Keto diet and do not ever lose hope.

To make sure that you are not wasting money, look through your kitchen and pantry, and see what you already have. Many times mason jars or cans get forgotten about or stuffed behind something that we rarely use. If you go through the pantry and get rid of all the sugary and processed foods, it will make this process easier. You can even donate the items that you are not going to be able to eat to the local food pantry, as this is another way to give back to the community.

Once you have an idea of what you already have, then just make sure that you try to use these items first and do not buy more unless it is an item that you will use regularly. When you throw food out, it is the same as throwing money out with it.

A good rule of thumb when you are shopping for Keto on a budget is to stray away from the prepackaged items that are labeled specifically Keto. You will find that if you look for these same products or ingredients that they will be cheaper. This is because with the Keto diet growing in popularity, the marketing corporations are trying to cash in. Do not be fooled!

Most times, these prepackaged and Keto labeled items can be made more cheaply in your kitchen and will not take that much time to make yourself. However, if you are able and you simply do not have the time, the pre-packed items are following the Keto diet. Just know that you will be spending more money on convenience.

One way to cut down costs is to make the almond and coconuts flour in your own kitchen. As stated before, the almond flour can be made at home using a high powered blender and buying raw almonds. This will also ensure the freshness of the final product, and you will feel even more empowered in your continued journey into the Keto diet.

Buying the ingredient components in bulk will also cut down on costs. For example, instead of buying the cheese already shredded, compare the prices to buying a block of the same cheese and grating it yourself. The time that it takes to accomplish this is minimal, and your pocket will feel the difference.

Another tip is to look for the sale prices and utilize weekly coupons in the Sunday paper or the deals offered by the grocery stores. Most items can be packed and stored in your freezer for later. This is especially true for fruits and vegetables as they are cheaper when they are in season. If you educate yourself on the options out there, you will find there are many shortcuts that will not hurt your waistline, and your wallet will be fatter.

Even looking for fruits, cheeses, milk, and eggs at the local farmers market is a great tip, as they are the mom and pop growers that rely on you to keep in business. They will even have organic and GMO-free options, most likely and might have some of the specialty items that you need. So shop locally whenever possible as you will feel better all-around inside and out for helping the local community to grow themselves.

For instance, when you purchase almond meal at the supermarket, it is going to be about 10 dollars for each pound. Do not fret! Many of these recipes call for smaller amounts compared to traditional recipes. Remember, a little bit goes a long way.

You can also look into other flour substitutes such as flax meal, which has better benefits compared to almond flour. First off is the cost, as it will usually run you about $4 a pound compared to $10 a pound for the almond flour.

Again, saving money on the Keto diet is all about education and knowing where to look. Be creative with the ingredients and find cheaper alternatives. Another suggestion is to buy almond meal rather than almond flour. This is an ingredient that is easily substituted for almond flour, and most recipes will have this ingredient.

Costs for the coconut flour are considerably cheaper than almond flour, and you end up using less in the recipes. You can find several brands of coconut flour that will average about $5 per pound. Again, if you take advantage of the online shopping networks, you will have them delivered straight to you without the hassle of driving to several supermarkets to find the best price for your budget.

If you do not have a nut allergy, these would also be a good addition to your pantry and would substitute for the almond or coconut flours in the recipes. You will find that these nut flours will cost about $4 a pound as well.

I know it may not seem like a money-saving tip at first glance, but if you plan your meals out ahead of time and make a shopping list, you are more likely to buy what you need. This cuts down on food waste and helps you to stay on track with your diet. When you shop, stay away from the isles that have been tempting in the past and certainly refrain from shopping while you are hungry. Although the more you get into the Keto diet, you will find that the hunger will not strike as much.

Even though we stress about the benefits of the specialty ingredients that are available on the Keto diet, do not feel pressured to buy specific items if they do not fit into your budget. Remember the end goal of you trying to better your health by making better food choices.

Ketogenic Diet FAQ

1. Will I Be Able to Eat Carbohydrates Again?

Yes, but it's important that you cut them out entirely when beginning this diet. A good time frame is about 2 to 3 months before you should have them again and then only on rare occasions. If you fall off the wagon, don't worry, just pick yourself up and continue onward.

2. How Much Protein Am I Allowed to Eat?

You should only eat protein in moderation. Having a higher intake of protein can lead to lower ketones and a spike in your insulin levels. About 35% of your total caloric intake is about the upper limit.

3. Do I need to Carb Load or Refeed On This Diet?

No. However, having a few days that are higher calorie can be beneficial to you every once in a while.

4. Will This Diet Cause Me to Lose Muscle?

Every diet comes with the risk of losing at least some of your muscles. Since this diet focuses on intaking high levels of protein, it may aid in minimizing your muscle loss. If you're that concerned, try lifting weights as one of your forms of exercise.

5. Am I Able to Build Muscle On A Keto Diet?

Yes, however, it can be harder to do than if you were on a diet with a moderate amount of carbs.

6. I Thought Ketosis Was Dangerous. Is That True?

Many people get ketosis confused with ketoacidosis. Ketosis is a natural and perfectly healthy when on this diet. The latter will only occur in people with a case of diabetes that has gone uncontrolled. Ketoacidosis can be very dangerous.

7. What If I Constantly Feel Weak, Fatigued, or Tired?

If you feel this way, your body may not be fully in ketosis and using your ketones and fats efficiently. To combat this, try lowering your intake of carbs. You may also want to try using an MCT oil supplement for additional help. Another good suggestion is to eat salty items and stay hydrated. This will help combat some of the side effects you're feeling.

8. My Breath Smells. Is There Anything I Can Do?

This reaction is a normal side effect. Chew sugar-free gum or drink water that is naturally flavored.

9. My Urine Has A Fruity Smell? Is This Normal?

Yes, this is normal. It is due to you excreting the byproducts that are created while in ketosis.

10. I Have Diarrhea and Digestion Problems. Can I Do Something?

This is a normal side effect. It will subside in 3 to 4 weeks. If it continues on past this, you should eat more vegetables high in fiber. You may also want to consider a magnesium supplement if you find yourself constipated.

11. How Long Does Ketosis Take to Occur?

A keto diet isn't something you can start and stop at a whim. Your body needs time to adjust if you want to reach the metabolic state of ketosis. This process may take between 2 and 7 days. It all depends on your activity level, body type, and foods you're eating. The quickest way into ketosis is by exercising while on an empty stomach. You'll also want to restrict your intake of carbs to less than 20g a day while drinking plenty of water.

12. How Do I Keep Track Of My Carbohydrates?

I use a free app called MyFitnessPal. It's both web-based and mobile, so I can track everything no matter what I'm doing. To track your net amount of carbs, subtract your total intake of fiber for the day from your total intake of carbs. I'm sure there's plenty of other apps and trackers you can use to do the same thing, but this is the one I have experience with. Look around and see if you find one more suited to you.

13. Will I Need Always to Count My Calories?

No matter what diet you're on, calories matter. That being said, with a keto diet, you rarely must worry about your calorie intake because the proteins and fats you consume will keep you feeling full for long periods of time. If you exercise frequently, remember that you're burning calories, so you must make sure you're eating enough to make up for this deficit.

14. How Much Weight Can I Expect to Lose?

The answer to this is dependent on you. Weight loss will fluctuate depending on your level of exercise and your specific metabolism. One tip to help you out is to try cutting out things that cause your weight loss to stall. These things are wheat products, dairy, and artificial sweeteners.

15. Is It Possible to Eat Too Much Fat?

Yes. When you eat too much fat, it will push you from being in a calorie deficit to a surplus. Most people find it's hard to overeat on a Keto diet, but it's possible. If you're worried about that, you can always use your keto calculator to figure out how many proteins, fats, and carbohydrates you need to eat each day.

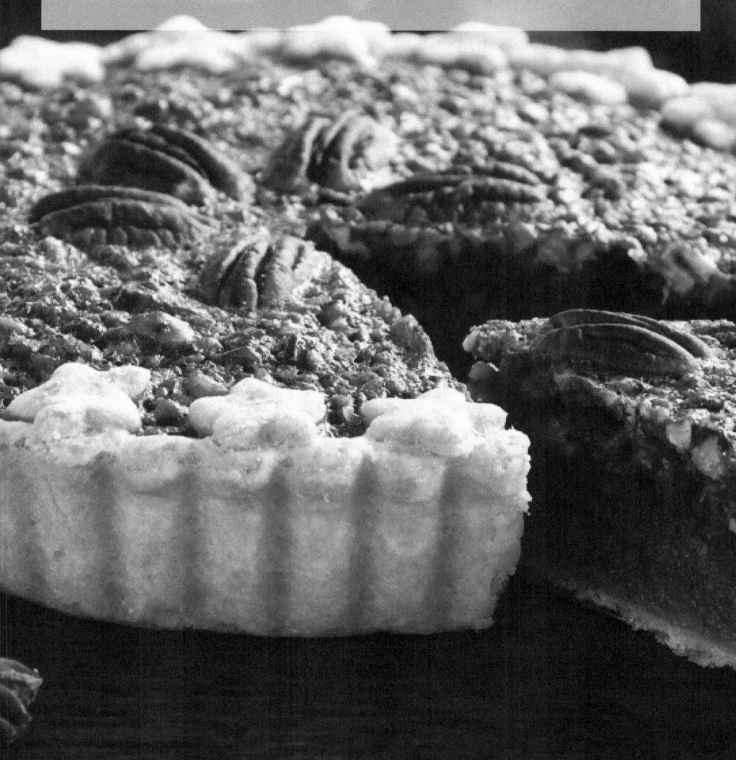

CHAPTER 6:   CAKE RECIPES

1. NO-BAKE BLUEBERRY CHEESECAKE BARS

INGREDIENTS

For Bar:
- 2 (8-oz.) softened packages of Cream Cheese
- 1 Easy Shortbread Crust
- ¼ cup heavy whipping cream kept at room temp
- ½ cup of powdered Erythritol-based Sweetener
- 1 tsp grated Lemon Zest

For Topping:
- ¼ cup of Water
- 1 cup of Blueberries
- 1 tbsp fresh Lemon juice
- ¼ cup of powdered Erythritol-based Sweetener
- ¼ tsp Xanthan gum for garnish (optional)

 PREPARATION 15

 COOKING 7 MIN

 SERVES 16

DIRECTIONS

Preparing the Bars:

9. Firmly press the crust mixture of the shortbread into the bottom of a baking pan.

10. Place the crust in the refrigerator.

11. Melt the chocolate in a bowl that you've set over a pan that is placed on a water that just began simmering.

12. Take the bowl out of the pan and allow it to cool for about 10 minutes.

13. With an electric mixer, beat the sweetener and the butter for 2 minutes until it is well incorporated and fluffy.

14. Carefully add the melted chocolate while the mixer is running and continue beating until smooth. Add the salt, espresso powder, and vanilla extract.

15. Add in the eggs one after the other and continue beating for 5 minutes.

16. Carefully pour the filling ingredients on the top of the chilled crust and make sure to smoothen the top.

17. Refrigerate for 2 hours.

Garnishing the Bars:

18. Carefully spread the whipped cream and chocolate on top.

Nutrition: Calories 255, Fat 23.7 g, Carbs 4.6 g, Protein 4.6 g, Erythritol 15 g, Fiber 2.2 g

2. CHOCOLATE-COVERED CHEESECAKE BITES

INGREDIENTS

- 1 (8 oz.) package of softened Cream Cheese
- ½ stick (¼ cup) unsalted softened Butter
- ½ cup of powdered Erythritol-based Sweetener
- ½ tsp. of vanilla extract
- 4 oz. of sugarless chopped dark Chocolate
- 1½ tbsp. of Coconut oil or ¾ oz. of Cacao Butter

 PREPARATION
20

 COOKING
5 MIN

 SERVES
2

DIRECTIONS

1. Line a baking sheet with parchment or wax paper.

2. Beat the butter and cream cheese with an electric mixer in a large bowl until it is thoroughly mixed. Beat in the vanilla extract and sweetener until smooth.

3. Form the mixture into 1-inch balls and position on the coated baking sheet. Place them in the fridge for 3-4 hours until it becomes firm.

4. Melt the cacao butter and chocolate together over water that just began simmering over a heatproof bowl. Stir until mixture becomes smooth. Remove from heat.

5. Dunk each ball into melted chocolate. Coat well and remove using a fork. Firmly tap the fork on the sides of the bowl to eliminate extra chocolate.

6. Position the ball on the baking sheet and let it set. Do the same for the rest of the cheesecake balls.

7. Decoratively sprinkle the rest of the chocolate over the lined balls.

Nutrition: Calories 148, Fat 13.5 g, Carb 5.2 g, Protein 1.7 g, Erythritol 12 g, Fiber 2.2 g

3. DELICIOUS ITALIAN CAKE

INGREDIENTS

For cake:
- 5 eggs
- 2½ cups almond flour
- 1 tsp baking powder
- 1 cup unsweetened coconut flakes
- 2 tsp vanilla extract
- 2 cups Swerve
- 1 cup butter
- 1 tsp baking soda
- 1 cup sour cream

For frosting:
- 1 cup unsweetened coconut flakes
- ½ cup walnuts, chopped
- 2 Tbsp unsweetened almond milk
- 2 cups Swerve confectioners sugar
- 1 tsp vanilla extract
- ½ cup butter
- 8 oz cream cheese

 PREPARATION
10

 COOKING
55 MIN

 SERVES
12

DIRECTIONS

1. Pour one cup of water into the Instant Pot and place a trivet in the pot.

2. Spray a 7-inch cake pan with cooking spray and set aside.

3. In a small bowl, mix together sour cream and baking soda and set aside.

4. In a large bowl, whisk together 1 cup butter and the sweetener until fluffy. Mix in the eggs, almond flour, baking powder, 1 cup coconut flakes, 2 tsp vanilla, and the sour cream mixture.

5. Pour batter in the prepared cake pan. Cover pan with aluminum foil.

6. Place cake pan on top of the trivet in the Instant Pot.

7. Seal pot with lid and cook on manual mode for 35 minutes.

8. When finished, allow pressure to release naturally for 20 minutes, and then release using the quick release method. Open the lid.

9. Remove cake from the pot and let it cool completely.

10. For frosting: In a mixing bowl, beat together ½ cup butter, Swerve, cream cheese, and vanilla until fluffy. Add almond milk, walnuts, and coconut flakes and stir well.

11. Spread frosting on top of the cake.

12. Slice and serve.

NOTE: This recipe calls for the use of an Instant Pot or Pressure Cooker.

Nutrition: Calories 591, Fat 57.6 g, Carb 11.3 g, Protein 11.9 g

4. TIRAMISU SHEET CAKE

INGREDIENTS

- ¾ cup granulated Erythritol
- 2 cups of blanched Almond flour
- ⅓ cup of unflavored Whey Protein powder
- 37g (⅓ cup) of Coconut flour
- 1 tbsp. of baking Powder
- ½ tsp. of salt
- 1 stick (½ cup) of unsalted and melted butter
- ¾ cup of unsweetened Almond Milk
- 1 tsp. of Vanilla extract
- 3 large eggs
- 1 tbs. of dark Rum (optional)

Mascarpone Frosting:
- 4 oz. (½ cup) of softened Cream Cheese
- 8 oz. of softened Mascarpone Cheese
- 1 tsp. of Vanilla extract
- ½-⅔ cup of heavy Whipping cream kept at room temp
- ½ cup of powdered Erythritol-based Sweetener

Garnishing:
- 1-oz. of sugarless dark Chocolate
- 1 tbsp. of Cocoa powder

 PREPARATION 25

 COOKING 22

 SERVES 20

DIRECTIONS

1. In a blender or food processor, grind the macadamia nuts to a fine texture.

2. Add all the cinnamon roll ingredients with the exception of for caramel sauce, and then put in the refrigerator to chill for an hour.

3. Heat the oven to 350° F. Line a baking tray with parchment paper.

4. Roll out the dough and make a large rectangle shape on a parchment-lined surface.

5. Spread Keto Caramel Sauce over the batter.

6. Carefully roll the dough into a log shape and seal the edge.

7. Place a sharp knife in a warm water and cut the log into about 10-12 rolls.

8. Position rolls on coated tray and place in the oven for 25 to 30 minutes, making sure that you check after 20 minutes to check if it is cooked through.

9. While the cinnamon rolls are baking in the oven, make the glaze. Combine all ingredients in a blender or mixing bowl.

10. Take keto cinnamon rolls out of the oven. Let it cool before you glaze. You can serve warm with glaze garnished on the top.

Nutrition: Calories 477, Fat 45.6 g, Carb 17.1 g, Fiber 7.1 g, Protein 5.6 g

5. CINNAMON CRUMB CAKE KETO DONUTS

INGREDIENTS

- ½ cup of Coconut flour
- ¼ cup of Almond flour
- 1 tbsp of Flaxseed meal
- 1 tsp of baking powder
- ¼ tsp salt
- 1 tsp of Cinnamon
- ¼ tsp of Nutmeg
- 2/3 cup of Erythritol Sweetener (e.g. Swerve)

- 6 large eggs
- ½ cup of Butter, melted
- 1 tsp of Vanilla
- ½ cup of Almond flour
- ¼ cup of diced pecans (optional)
- 1 pinch of salt
- 2 tbsp of softened Butter

 PREPARATION
10

 COOKING
15

 SERVES
1

DIRECTIONS

1. Heat the oven to 350° F.

2. Use a non-stick spray to spray a donut pan.

3. Whisk the coconut flour, almond flour, flax meal, sweetener, baking powder, salt, nutmeg, and cinnamon together inside a medium bowl. Set aside.

4. Whisk the eggs, vanilla, and melted butter until it appears. Add all the dry ingredients into wet ingredients and mix.

5. Spoon the batter into the donut space and fill it ¾ of the way full.

6. Preparing the crumb topping:

7. Stir together the sweetener, almond meal, and salt inside a small bowl. Add the butter and mix. Thoroughly mix until all of the flour is well combined and the mixture is moistened throughout.

8. Garnish the topping on the donuts, with fingers to break up the mixture until it is well mixed.

9. Place in the oven for 12-15 minutes or until the sides appear light brown.

Nutrition: Calories 138, Fat 12 g, Carb 3 g, Fiber 2 g, Protein 4 g

6. KETO ESPRESSO CHOCOLATE CHEESECAKE BARS

INGREDIENTS

Chocolate Crust:
- 7 tbsp. of melted Butter
- 2 cups of ultrafine, blanched Almond flour
- 3 tbsp. of Cocoa powder
- 1/3 cup granulated Erythritol sweetener

Cheesecake:
- 16 oz. of full fat Cream Cheese
- 2 large eggs
- ½ cup of granulated Erythritol sweetener
- 2 tbsp. of instant Espresso powder
- 1 tsp. of Vanilla extract
- Extra cocoa powder for dusting over the top.

 PREPARATION 10 MIN

 COOKING 35

 SERVES 16

DIRECTIONS

Preparation of the Chocolate Crust:

1. Heat the oven to 350° F.
2. Combine the almond flour, melted butter, cocoa powder and sweetener in a medium sized bowl.
3. Transfer the crust dough to a 9 x 9" pan coated with foil or parchment paper.
4. Firmly press the crust to the bottom of the pan.
5. Place the crust in the oven and bake for about 8 minutes.
6. Take out of the oven and set aside to cool.

Preparing the cheesecake filling:

7. Place the eggs, cream cheese, espresso powder, vanilla extract, and sweetener inside a blender and blend the mixture until smooth.
8. Pour over the crust and evenly spread out in the pan.

9. Bake for 25 minutes. Take out of the oven and allow it to cool. Dust it with the cocoa powder

10. Place in the refrigerator to chill. Afterwards, cut into four rows of squares to serve.

Nutrition: Calories 232, Fat 21 g, Carb 5 g, Fiber 1.5 g, Protein 6 g

7. MINI NO-BAKE LEMON CHEESECAKES

INGREDIENTS

Crust Ingredients:
- ½ cup of blanched Almond flour
- 2 tbsp. of powdered Erythritol
- ⅛ tsp. of salt
- 2 tbsp. unsalted and melted Butter

Filling:
- 1 tbs. plus ¼ cup powdered Erythritol-based Sweetener

- ¾ cup (6 oz.) of softened Cream Cheese
- ¼ cup of heavy whipping cream kept at room temp
- ½ tsp. of Lemon extract
- 2 tsp. of grated Lemon Zest
- 2 tbsp. of fresh Lemon juice

 PREPARATION 20 MIN   **COOKING** 0 MIN   **SERVES** 6

DIRECTIONS

Preparing the Crust:

1. Line muffin pan with parchment paper or silicone.
2. Whisk the sweetener, almond flour.
3. Add the melted butter and stir until mixture starts clumping together.
4. Place the crust in the muffin cups you've prepared and make sure to firmly press into the bottoms.

Preparing the Filling:

5. With an electric mixer, beat the cream cheese in a medium bowl.
6. Add the sweetener until it is well combined.
7. Beat in the lemon extract, lemon juice, lemon zest, and the cream until smooth.
8. Share the filling mixture into the muffin cups you prepared and fill all of the cups to almost the top. Also, smoothen the top. In order to

let go of air bubbles firmly tap the pan on a counter.

9. For 2 hours, place the pan in the fridge so that the filling becomes firm. Carefully remove the silicone layers or the parchment paper liners.

10. Serve when ready.

Nutrition: Calories 223, Fat 20.1 g, Carb 3.9 g, Protein 4 g, Erythritol 17.5 g, Fiber 1.1 g

8. ALMOND COCONUT CAKE

INGREDIENTS

- 2 eggs, lightly beaten
- ½ cup heavy cream
- ¼ cup coconut oil, melted
- 1 tsp cinnamon
- 1 tsp baking powder
- 1/3 cup Swerve
- ½ cup unsweetened shredded coconut
- 1 cup almond flour

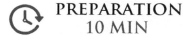 **PREPARATION**
10 MIN

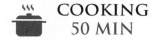 **COOKING**
50 MIN

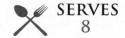 **SERVES**
8

DIRECTIONS

1. Spray a 6- inch cake pan with cooking spray and set aside.

2. In a large bowl, mix together the almond flour, cinnamon, baking powder, swerve, and shredded coconut.

3. Add eggs, heavy cream, and coconut oil into the almond flour mixture and mix until well combined.

4. Pour batter into the prepared cake pan and cover the pan with foil.

5. Add 2 cups of water into the instant pot then place a steamer rack in the pot.

6. Place cake pan on top of steamer rack.

7. Seal instant pot with lid and select manual high pressure and set the timer for 40 minutes.

8. Once the timer goes off then allow to release pressure naturally for 10 minutes then release using quick release method.

9. Open the lid carefully. Remove cake pan from the pot and let it cool for 20 minutes.

10. Cut cake into the slices and serve.

NOTE: This recipe calls for the use of an Instant Pot or Pressure Cooker.

Nutrition: Calories 228, Fat 21.7 g, Carb 5.2 g, Protein 5 g

9. TASTY CHOCOLATE CAKE

INGREDIENTS

- 3 large eggs
- ¼ cup butter, melted
- 1/3 cup heavy cream
- 1 tsp baking powder
- ¼ cup walnuts, chopped
- ¼ cup unsweetened cocoa powder
- 2/3 cup Swerve
- 1 cup almond flour

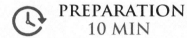 **PREPARATION**
10 MIN

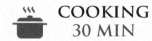 **COOKING**
30 MIN

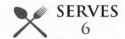 **SERVES**
6

DIRECTIONS

1. Spray cake pan with cooking spray and set aside.

2. Add all ingredients into a large mixing bowl and mix using a hand mixer until the mixture looks fluffy.

3. Pour batter into the prepared cake pan.

4. Pour 2 cups of water into the instant pot then place a steamer rack in the pot.

5. Place cake pan on top of steamer rack.

6. Seal instant pot with lid and cook on manual high pressure for 20 minutes.

7. Allow to release pressure naturally for 10 minutes then release using the quick release method.

8. Open the lid carefully. Remove cake pan from the pot and let it cool for 20 minutes.

9. Cut cake into the slices and serve.

Nutrition: Calories 275, Fat 25.5 g, Carb 7.5 g, Protein 9.3 g

10. WALNUT CARROT CAKE

INGREDIENTS

- 3 large eggs
- ½ cup walnuts, chopped
- 1 cup carrots, shredded
- ½ cup heavy cream
- ¼ cup butter, melted
- 1 ½ tsp apple pie spice
- 1 tsp baking powder
- 2/3 cup Swerve
- 1 cup almond flour

 PREPARATION 10 MIN

 COOKING 50 MIN

 SERVES 8

DIRECTIONS

1. Spray a 6-inch cake pan with cooking spray and set aside.

2. Add all ingredients into the large mixing bowl and mix using a hand mixer until mixture is well combined and looks fluffy.

3. Pour batter into the prepared cake pan and cover the pan with foil.

4. Pour 2 cups of water into the instant pot then place a trivet in the pot.

5. Place cake pan on top of the trivet.

6. Seal pot with lid and cook on manual high pressure for 40 minutes.

7. Allow to release pressure naturally for 10 minutes then release using the quick release method.

8. Open the lid carefully. Remove cake pan from the pot and let it cool for 20 minutes.

9. Slice and serve.

Nutrition: Calories 240, Fat 22 g, Carb 6.2 g, Protein 7.6 g

11. FUDGY CHOCOLATE CAKE

INGREDIENTS

- 2 eggs, lightly beaten
- 1 tsp vanilla extract
- 1 Tbsp coconut sugar
- ½ tsp baking soda
- 1 cup almond flour
- 2 Tbsp coconut oil, melted
- ¼ cup unsweetened almond milk
- 1 cup unsweetened chocolate chips
- Pinch of salt

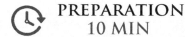 **PREPARATION**
10 MIN

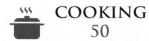 **COOKING**
50

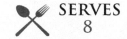 **SERVES**
8

DIRECTIONS

1. Spray a 6-inch cake pan with cooking spray and set aside.

2. Pour two cups of water into the Instant Pot and place a trivet in the pot.

3. Add chocolate chips and almond milk to a saucepan and heat over low heat until chocolate has melted. Stir frequently.

4. Once chocolate is melted, add coconut oil and stir to combine.

Remove saucepan from heat and let it cool completely.

5. In a large bowl, mix together all dry ingredients.

6. Add vanilla and eggs to the cool chocolate mixture and stir well.

7. Slowly add dry ingredients mixture and mix well.

8. Pour batter into the prepared cake pan and place cake pan on top of trivet in the pot.

9. Seal pot with lid and cook on manual mode for 40 minutes.

10. When finished, allow pressure to release naturally for 10 minutes, then release using the quick release method. Open the lid.

11. Remove cake from the pot and let it cool completely.

12. Slice and serve.

NOTE: This recipe calls for the use of an Instant Pot or Pressure Cooker.

Nutrition: Calories 344, Fat 29.2 g, Carb 11.6 g, Protein 8.6 g

12. MOIST AND DELICIOUS SPICE CAKE

INGREDIENTS

- 2 eggs
- 2 cups almond flour
- ½ tsp vanilla extract
- ⅓ cup water
- ⅓ cup coconut oil, melted
- ¼ tsp ground cloves
- 3 Tbsp walnuts, chopped
- ½ tsp ground ginger
- 1 tsp ground cinnamon
- 2 tsp baking powder
- ½ cup erythritol
- Pinch of salt

 PREPARATION
10 MIN

 COOKING
50 MIN

 SERVES
10

DIRECTIONS

1. Spray a 7-inch cake pan with cooking spray and set aside.

2. Pour one cup of water into the Instant Pot and place a trivet in the pot.

3. In a large bowl, mix together almond flour, cloves, ginger, cinnamon, baking powder, erythritol, and salt.

4. Stir in the eggs, vanilla, water, and coconut oil until well mix.

5. Pour batter into the prepared cake pan and sprinkle with chopped walnuts.

6. Cover cake pan with aluminum foil and place it on top of trivet in the Instant Pot.

7. Seal pot with lid and cook on manual mode for 40 minutes.

8. When finished, allow pressure to release naturally for 10 minutes, and then release using the quick release method. Open the lid.

9. Remove cake pan from pot carefully and let it cool completely.

10. Slice and serve.

Nutrition: Calories 220, Fat 20.8 g, Carb 5.9 g, Protein 6.5 g

13. CINNAMON ALMOND BUTTER CAKE

INGREDIENTS

- 2 large eggs
- ¼ tsp apple pie spice
- ¼ tsp cinnamon
- 1 tbsp unsweetened cocoa powder
- ½ cup cream cheese
- ¼ cup almond butter
- ½ cup Swerve
- ½ cup almond, minced
- 1 cup coconut flour
- Pinch of salt

 PREPARATION
10 MIN

 COOKING
35 MIN

 SERVES
8

DIRECTIONS

1. In a large bowl, mix together the coconut flour, apple pie spice, cinnamon, swerve, almonds, and salt until well combined.

2. Slowly, add the eggs, cream cheese, and almond butter and beat using a hand mixer until combined.

3. Pour 1 cup of water into the instant pot then place a trivet in the pot.

4. Line springform pan with parchment paper.

5. Pour the batter into the prepared pan and spread evenly. Cover the pan with foil and place on top of the trivet in the instant pot.

6. Seal pot with lid and cook on manual high pressure for 35 minutes.

7. Release pressure using the quick release method then open the lid.

8. Remove cake pan from the pot and let it cool for 30 minutes.

9. Sprinkle cocoa powder or chopped almonds on top of the cake.

10. Slice and serve.

Nutrition: Calories 116, Fat 9.9 g, Carb 3.4 g, Protein 4.4 g

14. CARROT CAKE

INGREDIENTS

- 4 eggs
- 1 cup pecans, chopped
- 2¼ cups carrots, grated
- ¼ tsp nutmeg
- 1 Tbsp cinnamon
- 1 Tbsp baking powder
- 1 cup almond flour
- 1½ cups coconut flour
- 1 tsp vanilla extract
- ¾ cup coconut oil, melted
- ½ cup stevia
- Pinch of salt

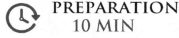 **PREPARATION** 10 MIN

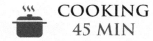 **COOKING** 45 MIN

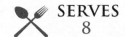 **SERVES** 8

DIRECTIONS

1. Spray a 7-inch cake pan with cooking spray and set aside.

2. Pour two cups of water into the Instant Pot and place a trivet in the pot.

3. In a mixing bowl, mix together sweetener, vanilla, and coconut oil.

4. Add eggs and stir well to combine.

5. Add coconut flour, nutmeg, cinnamon, baking powder, almond flour, and salt and stir to combine.

6. Add grated carrots and pecans and stir well.

7. Pour batter into the prepared cake pan. Cover cake pan with aluminum foil and place on top of the trivet.

8. Seal pot with lid and cook on steam mode for 45 minutes.

9. When finished, release pressure using the quick release method and then open the lid.

10. Remove cake from the pot and let it cool completely.

11. Slice and serve.

Nutrition: Calories 412, Fat 40.1 g, Carb 11.4 g, Sugar 3 g, Protein 7.9 g, Cholesterol 82 mg

15. CHOCOLATE CAKE

INGREDIENTS

- 3 eggs
- ¼ cup black coffee
- ½ stick (2 oz) butter
- 1 tsp baking powder
- ⅓ cup erythritol
- ⅓ cup cocoa powder
- ¼ cup coconut flour
- ¼ cup flaxseed meal
- ½ cup almond flour
- Pinch of salt

 PREPARATION
10 MIN

 COOKING
35 MIN

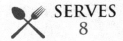 **SERVES**
8

DIRECTIONS

1. Spray a cake pan with cooking spray and set aside.

2. Pour one cup of water into the Instant Pot and place a trivet in the pot.

3. In a large bowl, mix together almond flour, sweetener, cocoa powder, flax seed meal, and coconut flour.

4. Add remaining ingredients and stir until well combined.

5. Pour batter into the prepared cake pan and cover the pan with aluminum foil.

6. Place the cake pan on top of the trivet.

7. Seal pot with lid and cook on manual mode for 35 minutes.

8. When finished, allow pressure to release naturally for 10 minutes, then release using the quick released method. Open the lid.

9. Remove cake from the pot and let it cool completely.

10. Serve and enjoy.

NOTE: This recipe calls for the use of an Instant Pot or Pressure Cooker.

Nutrition: Calories 143, Fat 12.5 g, Carb 5.1 g, Sugar 0.5 g, Protein 5 g, Cholesterol 77 mg

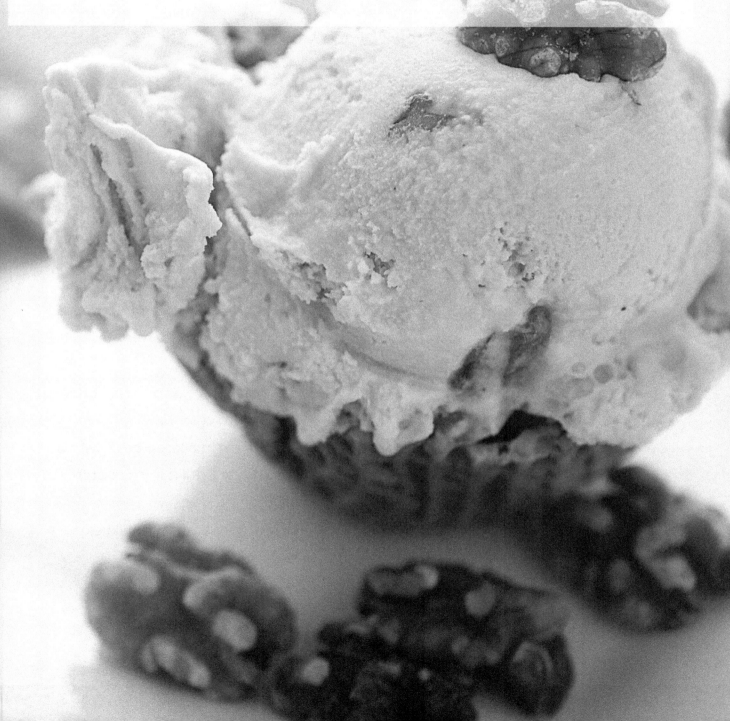

CHAPTER 7:   FROZEN DESSERTS RECIPES

16. COOKIE ICE CREAM

INGREDIENTS

- ¾ cup almond flour
- ¼ cup cocoa powder
- ¼ tsp baking soda
- ¼ cup erythritol
- ½ tsp vanilla extract
- 1 ½ tbsp coconut oil, softened
- 1 large egg, room temperature
- Pinch of salt
- 2 ½ cups whipping cream
- 1 tbsp vanilla extract
- ½ cup erythritol
- ½ cup almond milk, unsweetened

 PREPARATION 5 MIN

 FREEZING 120 MIN

 SERVES 2

DIRECTIONS

1. Preheat your oven at 300 °F and layer a 9-inch baking pan with wax paper.

2. Whisk almond flour with baking soda, cocoa powder, salt, and erythritol in a medium bowl.

3. Stir in coconut oil and vanilla extract then mix well until crumbly.

4. Whisk in egg and mix well to form the dough.

5. Spread this dough in the prepared pan and bake for 20 minutes in the preheated oven.

6. Allow the crust to cool then crush it finely into crumbles.

7. Beat cream in a large bowl with a hand mixer until it forms a stiff peak.

8. Stir in erythritol and vanilla extract then mix well until fully incorporated.

9. Pour in milk and blend well until smooth.

10. Add this mixture to an ice cream machine and churn as per the machine's instructions.

11. Add cookie crumbles to the ice cream in the machine and churn again.

12. Place the ice cream in a sealable container and freeze for 2 hours.

13. Scoop out the ice cream and serve.

Nutrition: Calories 214, Total Fat 19 g, Saturated Fat 5.8 g, Cholesterol 15 mg, Sodium 123 mg, Total Carbs 6.5 g, Sugar 1.9 g, Fiber 2.1 g, Protein 6.5 g

17. CHOCOLATE AVOCADO ICE CREAM

INGREDIENTS

- 2 large Hass avocados, flesh only
- 1 cup coconut milk
- ½ cup heavy whipping cream
- ½ cup unsweetened cocoa powder
- 2 tsp vanilla extract
- ½ cup erythritol, powdered
- 25 drops liquid stevia
- 6 squares unsweetened Baker's chocolate, chopped

 PREPARATION 5 MIN

 FREEZING 16 HOURS

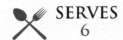 **SERVES** 6

DIRECTIONS

1. Mash avocado flesh in a bowl then add coconut milk, vanilla extract, and heavy cream.

2. Beat this mixture with an immersion blender (or another hand mixer) until smooth and creamy.

3. Stir in erythritol, cocoa powder, and stevia and mix well until fully incorporated.

4. Fold in chopped chocolate and mix well gently.

5. Refrigerate the avocado mixture for 12 hours.

6. Churn the ice cream mixture in an ice cream machine as per the machine's instructions.

7. Freeze it for 2 to 4 hours until it hardens.

8. Serve.

Nutrition: Calories 282, Total Fat 25.1 g, Saturated Fat 8.8 g, Cholesterol 100 mg, Sodium 117 mg, Total Carbs 6.4 g, Sugar 0.7 g, Fiber 3.2 g, Protein 8 g

18. PUMPKIN PECAN ICE CREAM

INGREDIENTS

- ½ cup cottage cheese
- ½ cup pumpkin puree
- 1 tsp pumpkin spice
- 2 cups unsweetened coconut milk
- ½ tsp xanthan gum
- 3 large egg yolks
- 1/3 cup erythritol
- 20 drops liquid stevia
- 1 tsp maple extract
- ½ cup chopped pecans, toasted
- 2 tbsp salted butter

 PREPARATION
5 MIN

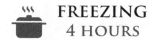 **FREEZING**
4 HOURS

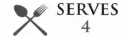 **SERVES**
4

DIRECTIONS

1. Add butter to a saucepan and place it over low heat until butter turns brown.

2. Whisk the remaining ingredients in a separate bowl using a hand mixer.

3. Churn this mixture in the ice cream mixture as per the machine's instructions.

4. Toss pecans with butter then add them to the ice cream.

5. Churn again then freeze for 4 hours.

6. Enjoy.

Nutrition: Calories 331, Total Fat 38.5 g, Saturated Fat 19.2 g, Cholesterol 141 mg, Sodium 283 mg, Total Carbs 6.2 g, Sugar 3 g, Fiber 1 g, Protein 2.1 g

19. MOCHA ICE CREAM (A)

INGREDIENTS

- 1 cup coconut milk
- ¼ cup heavy whipping cream
- 2 tbsp erythritol
- 15 drops liquid stevia
- 2 tbsp unsweetened cocoa powder
- 1 tbsp instant coffee
- ¼ tsp xanthan gum

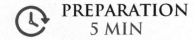 **PREPARATION**
5 MIN

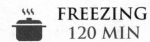 **FREEZING**
120 MIN

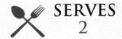 **SERVES**
2

DIRECTIONS

1. Whisk everything except xanthan gum in a bowl using a hand mixer.
2. Slowly add xanthan gum and stir well to make a thick mixture.
3. Churn the mixture in an ice cream machine as per the machine's instructions.
4. Freeze it for 2 hours then garnish with mint and instant coffee.
5. Serve.

Nutrition: Calories 267, Total Fat 44.5 g, Saturated Fat 17.4 g, Cholesterol 153 mg, Sodium 217 mg, Total Carbs 8.4 g, Sugar 2.3 g, Fiber 1.3 g, Protein 3.1 g

20. STRAWBERRY ICE CREAM

INGREDIENTS

- 1 cup heavy whipping cream
- 1/3 cup erythritol
- 3 large egg yolks
- ½ tsp vanilla extract
- 1/8 tsp xanthan gum
- 1 tbsp vodka
- 1 cup strawberries, pureed

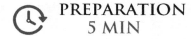 **PREPARATION 5 MIN**   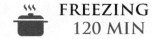 **FREEZING 120 MIN**   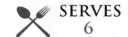 **SERVES 6**

DIRECTIONS

1. Add cream to a pot and place it over low heat and warm it up.
2. Stir in 1/3 cup erythritol and mix well to dissolve.
3. Beat in egg yolks and continue whisking until fluffy.
4. Stir in vanilla extract and mix well until smooth.
5. Lastly, add 1/8 tsp xanthan gum and the vodka.
6. Mix well then transfer the mixture to an ice cream machine and churn as per the machine's instructions.
7. Freeze it for 1 hour then add pureed strawberries.
8. Churn again and freeze for another 1 hour.
9. Serve.

Nutrition: Calories 259, Total Fat 34 g, Saturated Fat 10.3 g, Cholesterol 112 mg, Sodium 92 mg, Total Carbs 8.5 g, Sugar 2 g, Fiber 1.3 g, Protein 7.5 g

21. KETO VANILLA ICE CREAM

INGREDIENTS

- 2 (15-oz) cans coconut milk
- 2 cup heavy cream
- ¼ cup Swerve confectioner's sweetener
- 1 tsp pure vanilla extract
- Pinch kosher salt

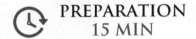 **PREPARATION** 15 MIN   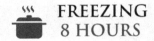 **FREEZING** 8 HOURS   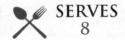 **SERVES** 8

DIRECTIONS

1. Refrigerate coconut milk for 3 hours or overnight and remove the cream from the top while leaving the liquid in the can. Place the cream in a bowl.

2. Beat the coconut cream using a hand mixer until it forms peaks.

3. Stir in vanilla, sweeteners, and whipped cream then beat well until fluffy.

4. Freeze this mixture for 5 hours.

5. Enjoy.

Nutrition: Calories 255, Total Fat 23.4 g, Saturated Fat 11.7 g, Cholesterol 135 mg, Sodium 112 mg, Carbs 6.5 g, Fiber 1 g, Protein 7.9 g

22. BUTTER PECAN ICE CREAM

INGREDIENTS

- 1 ½ cups unsweetened coconut milk
- ¼ cup heavy whipping cream
- 5 tbsp butter
- ¼ cup crushed pecans
- 25 drops liquid stevia
- ¼ tsp xanthan gum

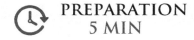 **PREPARATION**
5 MIN

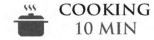 **COOKING**
10 MIN

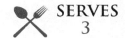 **SERVES**
3

DIRECTIONS

1. Place a pan over medium-low heat and melt butter in it until it turns brown.
2. Mix this butter with chopped pecans, heavy cream, and stevia in a bowl.
3. Stir in coconut milk then xanthan gum and mix well until fluffy.
4. Add this mixture to an ice cream machine and churn as per the machine's instructions.
5. Once done, serve.

Nutrition: Calories 251, Total Fat 24.5 g Saturated Fat 14.7 g, Cholesterol 165 mg, Sodium 142 mg, Total Carbs 4.3 g, Fiber 1 g, Protein 5.9 g

23. ANISE ICE CREAM

INGREDIENTS

- 3 ½ cups heavy whipping cream
- ¼ cup confectioners erythritol
- 1 ½ tsp vanilla
- 1 cup unsweetened flax milk
- 5 egg yolks
- 2 tbsp activated charcoal
- 1 ½ tsp anise oil

 PREPARATION 10

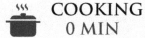 **COOKING** 0 MIN

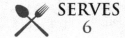 **SERVES** 6

DIRECTIONS

1. Take 2 cups of cream and erythritol in a saucepan and heat over low heat.

2. Mix well until sweetener is dissolved then set this mixture aside in a large bowl.

3. Stir cook 1.5 cups of cream with egg yolks and flax milk in the same saucepan.

4. Continue cooking until it's thick enough to coat the back of a spoon.

5. Pour this mixture into a bowl then stir in activated charcoal, anise oil, vanilla, and sweetener.

6. Mix well then transfer the mixture to an ice cream machine.

7. Churn as per the machine's instructions.

8. Freeze the ice cream until it's firm.

9. Serve.

Nutrition: Calories 153, Total Fat 13 g, Saturated Fat 9.2 g, Cholesterol 6.5 mg, Sodium 81 mg, Total Carbs 4.5 g, Fiber 0.4 g, Protein 5.8 g

24. KETO COOKIE AND CRÈME ICE CREAM

INGREDIENTS

For cookie crumbs:
- 1 ½ cups almond flour
- ½ teaspoon baking soda
- 1 teaspoon vanilla extract
- 2 eggs, at room temperature
- ½ cup cocoa powder
- ½ cup erythritol
- 3 tablespoons coconut oil, softened

- 1/8 teaspoon salt

For ice cream:
- 5 cups whipping cream
- 1 cup erythritol
- 2 tablespoons vanilla extract
- 1 cup almond milk, unsweetened

 PREPARATION
20 MIN

 COOKING
30 MIN

 SERVES
20

DIRECTIONS

1. Place a sheet of parchment paper in a large, round baking dish (10-12 inches). Spray some cooking spray in the pan.

2. Add almond flour, baking soda, salt, cocoa and erythritol into a mixing bowl and stir until well combined.

3. Stir in the oil and vanilla and mix with your hands until crumbly.

4. Mix in the eggs. Mix well into the dough.

5. Place the dough in the pan and press well into the bottom of the pan.

6. Bake in a preheated oven 350° F for about 25-30 minutes or until firm on top.

7. Remove the baking dish from the oven and cool completely.

8. Break the cookies into smaller pieces.

9. To make ice cream: Add whipping cream into a mixing bowl. Beat

with an electric hand mixer until stiff peaks are formed. Be careful as the cream can separate into small particles if you over beat.

10. Beat in the vanilla and erythritol until well combined.

11. Add almond milk and beat again until thick.

12. Pour into an ice cream maker and churn according to the manufacturer's instructions. Add cookie crumbs during the last 5 minutes of churning. Transfer into a freezer safe container. Freeze until set.

13. Alternately, pour the mixture into a freezer safe container after step 11 and freeze. After about an hour of freezing, remove the ice cream from the freezer and whisk well. Refreeze and beat again after 30-40 minutes.

14. Repeat the above steps a couple of times more until well frozen and without ice crystals.

Nutrition: Calories 285, Fat 30 g, Carb 5.3 g, Protein 3.7 g

25. MATCHA ICE CREAM

INGREDIENTS

- 1 cup heavy cream
- 1 tsp matcha powder
- 2 tbsp monk fruit, Swerve
- ½ tsp vanilla extract

 PREPARATION
10

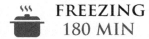 **FREEZING**
180 MIN

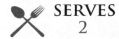 **SERVES**
2

DIRECTIONS

1. Start by throwing all the ingredients into a mason jar.

2. Shake it all well for 5 minutes then freeze for 3 hours.

3. Serve.

Nutrition: Calories 290, Total Fat 21.5 g, Saturated Fat 15.2 g, Cholesterol 12.1 mg, Sodium 9 mg, Total Carbs 6.5 g, Fiber 0.4 g, Protein 6.2 g

26. CHOCOLATE CHUNK AVOCADO ICE CREAM

INGREDIENTS

- 4 ripe Hass avocados, peeled, pitted, chopped
- 1 cup heavy cream
- 4 teaspoons vanilla extract
- 50 drops liquid stevia
- 2 cups coconut milk from carton
- 1 cup cocoa powder
- 1 cup powdered erythritol
- 12 squares unsweetened Baker's chocolate, chopped into chunks

 PREPARATION 10 MIN

 COOKING 0 MIN

 SERVES 12

DIRECTIONS

1. Add avocado, coconut milk, vanilla and heavy cream into a bowl.
2. Blend with an immersion blender until creamy.
3. Add erythritol, cocoa and stevia and blend until well incorporated.
4. Add chocolate and stir with a spoon.
5. Cover the bowl with cling wrap. Place in the refrigerator until very chilled.
6. Remove from the refrigerator 20 minutes before serving. Pour into an ice cream maker and churn according to the manufacturer's instructions.
7. Alternately, pour the mixture into a freezer safe container and freeze until firm. Stir a couple of times while freezing.

Nutrition: Calories 313, Fat 32 g, Carb 6.3 g, Protein 3.9 g

27. MOCHA ICE CREAM (B)

INGREDIENTS

- 2 cups coconut milk
- ¼ cup Erythritol
- ¼ cup cocoa powder
- ½ teaspoon xanthan gum
- ½ cup heavy cream
- 30 drops liquid stevia
- 2 tablespoons instant coffee

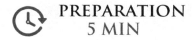 **PREPARATION** 5 MIN   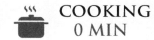 **COOKING** 0 MIN   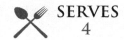 **SERVES** 4

DIRECTIONS

1. Mix together all the ingredients except xanthan gum in a mixing bowl. Using an immersion blender, blend until smooth.

2. Add the xanthan gum little by little, blending continuously.

3. Cover the bowl with cling wrap. Place in the refrigerator until very chilled.

4. Remove from the refrigerator 20 minutes before serving. Pour into an ice cream maker and churn the ice cream according to the manufacturer's instructions.

5. Alternately, pour into a freezer safe container and freeze until firm. Stir in between a couple of times while it is being frozen.

Nutrition: Calories 175, Fat 15 g, Carb 6.6 g, Protein 2.6 g

28. STRAWBERRY SWIRL ICE CREAM

INGREDIENTS

For vanilla ice cream:
- 2 cups heavy cream
- 2 tablespoons vodka (optional)
- 6 large egg yolks
- 2/3 cup erythritol
- ¼ teaspoon xanthan gum (optional)
- 1 teaspoon vanilla extract

For strawberry swirl ice cream:
- 2 cups strawberries, pureed

 PREPARATION 15 MIN

 COOKING 10 MIN

 SERVES 12

DIRECTIONS

1. Place a heavy bottomed pan over low heat. Add cream and erythritol. Stir frequently until erythritol dissolves completely. Remove from heat.

2. Add yolks into a mixing bowl and beat with an electric mixer until they double in volume.

3. Add about 2 tablespoons of the warm cream to the egg and beat constantly. Repeat this procedure until all the cream is added. Add vanilla and beat again.

4. Add vodka and xanthan gum if using and beat again. Cool completely. Transfer into a freezer safe bowl. Cover with cling wrap. Freeze for 30 minutes.

5. Pour into an ice cream maker and churn according to the manufacturer's instructions. Transfer into a freezer safe container. Follow step 8 onwards.

6. Alternately, pour into a freezer safe container and freeze until firm. Stir in between a couple of times while it is being frozen.

7. Remove ice cream from the freezer.

8. Swirl the strawberry puree all around on the top. With a knife, lightly mix to get a ripple effect. For making vanilla ice cream, do not add the strawberries. Freeze.

Nutrition: Calories 176, Fat 16.6 g, Carb 3 g, Protein 2.5 g

29. BROWN BUTTER PECAN KETO ICE CREAM

INGREDIENTS

- 3 cups coconut milk, unsweetened, from carton
- 10 tablespoons butter
- 50 drops liquid stevia
- ½ cup heavy cream
- ½ cup crushed pecans
- ½ teaspoon xanthan gum

 PREPARATION
10 MIN

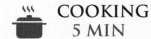 **COOKING**
5 MIN

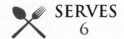 **SERVES**
6

DIRECTIONS

1. Place butter in a pan and cook until brown in color.
2. Stir in cream, pecans and stevia. Remove from heat.
3. Add coconut milk and xanthan gum and whisk well.
4. Cover the bowl with cling wrap. Place in the refrigerator until very chilled.
5. Remove from the refrigerator 20 minutes before serving. Pour into an ice cream maker and churn the ice cream according to the manufacturer's instructions.
6. Serve immediately for soft serve or if you like a more firm ice cream, freeze for 3-4 hours and serve.
7. Alternately, pour into a freezer safe container and freeze until firm. Stir in between a couple of times while it is being frozen.

Nutrition: Calories 355, Fat 36.4 g, Carb 4.5 g, Protein 2.1 g

30. PUMPKIN PECAN PIE ICE CREAM

INGREDIENTS

- 1 cup cottage cheese
- 2 teaspoons pumpkin pie spice
- 4 cups coconut milk, from carton
- ¼ cup Erythritol
- 1 cup pumpkin puree
- 1 teaspoon xanthan gum
- 4 tablespoons salted butter
- 6 large egg yolks
- 40 drops liquid stevia
- 1 cup chopped pecans
- 2 teaspoons maple extract

 PREPARATION
10 MIN

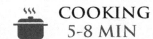 **COOKING**
5-8 MIN

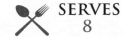 **SERVES**
8

DIRECTIONS

1. Place a pan over medium-low heat. Add butter and pecans and stir frequently until the pecans are toasted to desired doneness. Turn off the heat.

2. Add the rest of the ingredients into a bowl and blend with an immersion blender until well incorporated.

3. Add pecans along with butter and stir.

4. Pour into an ice cream maker and churn the ice cream according to the manufacturer's instructions.

5. Serve immediately for soft serve or if you like a more firm ice cream, freeze for 3-4 hours and serve.

6. Alternately, pour into a freezer safe container and freeze until firm. Stir in between a couple of times while it is being frozen.

Nutrition: Calories 287, Fat 23.7 g, Carb 6.9 g, Protein 7.5 g

31. BLUEBERRY ICE CREAM

INGREDIENTS

For Blueberry Puree:
- 2 cups blueberries, fresh or frozen
- 2 tbsp lemon juice
- 1 tbsp water
- 1/3 cup granulated erythritol or erythritol blend
- 1/8 tsp ground cinnamon
- 1/8 tsp almond extract
- ½ tsp vanilla extract

For Ice Cream Base:
- 1 cup almond milk, unsweetened
- 2 cups heavy cream
- ½ cup granulated erythritol
- 2 tbsp vodka
- ¼ tsp table salt

 PREPARATION 10 MIN

 COOKING 30 MIN

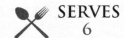 **SERVES** 6

DIRECTIONS

To Make the Blueberry Puree:

1. Add blueberries, water, lemon juice, cinnamon, and sweetener to a saucepan.
2. Cover the berries and cook on low heat for 10 minutes.
3. Mix well then puree the berries until smooth.
4. Return the mixture to the saucepan and cook for another 20 minutes until it thickens.

To Make the Ice Cream Base:

5. Add vodka, salt, sweetener, cream, and almond milk to a blender.
6. Pulse and blend well until combined.
7. Stir in the blueberry puree and blend well.
8. Transfer the blueberry mixture to an ice cream maker and churn as per the machine's instructions.
9. Freeze until it's firm then serve.

Nutrition: Calories 254, Total Fat 9 g, Saturated Fat 10.1 g, Cholesterol 13 mg, Sodium 179 mg, Total Carbs 7.5 g, Fiber 0.8 g, Protein 7.5 g

32. PEANUT BUTTER AND JELLY ICE CREAM SANDWICH

INGREDIENTS

- 4 bars Keto Watt peanut butter bars, halved (or use Perfect keto bars or Good Dee's peanut butter cookie mix)

For mixed berry jam:
- 1 cup mixed berries, thaw if frozen
- 2 tablespoons lemon juice
- 2 tablespoons sugar-free caramel syrup

For ice cream:
- 2 cups heavy cream
- 2 tablespoons sugar-free caramel syrup or 2 teaspoons vanilla extract
- ½ cup powdered monk fruit – erythritol blend
- 4 tablespoons salted peanut butter

 PREPARATION
10 MIN

 COOKING
10 MIN

 SERVES
8

DIRECTIONS

1. Reshape the Watt bar halves into balls.

2. Place the balls on a lined baking sheet. Press the balls with the back of a glass.

3. Bake in a preheated oven 350° F for about 8 – 10 minutes. Cool completely.

4. To make berry jam: Blend together all the ingredients in a blender until smooth.

5. To make ice cream: Place all the ingredients for ice cream into a blender and blend until smooth.

6. Pour into an ice cream maker and churn the ice cream according to the manufacturer's instructions.

7. Transfer into a freezer safe container and freeze until firm.

8. Alternately, pour into a freezer safe container and freeze until firm. Stir in between a couple of times while it is being frozen.

9. To assemble: Scoop ice cream and place on a cookie. Drizzle berry jam over it. Cover with another cookie and serve.

Nutrition: Calories 412, Fat 38.1 g, Carb 5.3 g, Protein 6 g

33. KETO NEAPOLITAN ICE CAKE

INGREDIENTS

For cake:
- ½ cup almond flour
- 2 tablespoons cocoa powder
- 1/8 teaspoon salt
- 2 tbsp Swerve sweetener
- ¾ teaspoon baking powder
- ¼ cup butter, melted
- 1-2 tbsp cold brewed coffee or water
- 1 large egg, at room temperature
- ¼ teaspoon vanilla extract

For ice cream:
- 1 cup heavy whipping cream
- 4 tablespoons powdered Swerve

- ½ teaspoon vanilla extract
- ½ cup chopped, fresh strawberries
- ¼ cup xylitol
- 1 ½ tablespoons butter
- ¼ teaspoon xanthan gum
- 6 ounces cream cheese, softened

For chocolate glaze:
- ¼ cup heavy whipping cream
- 2 tablespoons powdered Swerve
- 1 ounce unsweetened chocolate, cut into pieces
- ¼ teaspoon vanilla extract

 PREPARATION 30 MIN

 COOKING 45 MIN

 SERVES 8

DIRECTIONS

For cake:

1. Add all the dry ingredients into a mixing bowl and stir.

2. Add wet ingredients except coffee and mix well.

3. Stir in the coffee or water, about 2 teaspoons at a time and stir well each time. The batter should be thick and non-drippy -. e.g. you should be able to spread it.

4. Spoon the batter into a greased and lined springform pan (6 in).

5. Bake in a preheated oven at 325° F for about 20-25 minutes or until a toothpick when inserted in the center comes out clean. Cool completely.

6. Loosen the cake from the edges by passing a knife around the edges of the cake.

For ice cream:

7. Add cream and 3 tablespoons sweetener into a pan and place the pan over medium heat. When it

begins to boil, lower the heat and simmer for a couple of minutes. Turn off the heat.

8. Add xanthan gum and whisk constantly. Pour into a food processor bowl.

9. Add cream cheese and blend until smooth. Take out 1/3 of this mixture and place in a bowl. Spread the remaining mixture over the cake.

10. Add strawberries and 1-tablespoon sweetener into a blender and blend until smooth. Pour into the bowl of retained cream cheese mixture.

11. Mix well and spread over the cream cheese layer.

12. Place in the freezer until it sets.

For chocolate glaze:

13. Add cream into a saucepan and place over medium heat. When it begins to simmer, turn off the heat. Add chocolate and stir until it melts.

14. Add vanilla and sweetener after 10 minutes and stir. Let it rest for 5 minutes.

15. Pour over the frozen cake on top as well as a little on the sides.

16. Cut into slices and serve.

Nutrition: Calories 354, Fat 32.7 g, Carb 6.2 g, Protein 5.2 g

CHAPTER 8:   COOKIES RECIPES

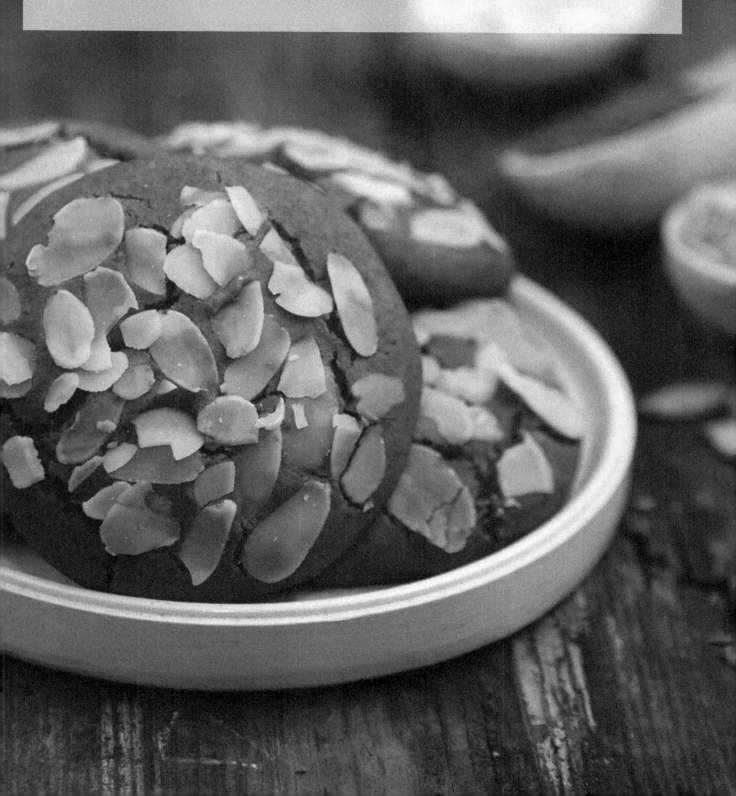

34. CHOCOLATE ALMOND COOKIES

INGREDIENTS

- ¼ cup unsweetened chocolate
- 2 tbsp heavy cream
- 2 tsp vanilla extract
- 2 egg yolks
- 1 egg (whole)
- 5 tbsp Splenda
- 3 tbsp xylitol
- ½ cup almond meal, blanched
- 1½ cups almond meal, whole
- ½ tbsp ground nutmeg
- ½ tbsp ground cloves
- 1 tbsp baking powder
- 2 tbsp ground cinnamon
- ½ cup soy protein powder
- 1 pinch of salt

 PREPARATION 30 MIN

 COOKING 14 MIN

 SERVES 18

DIRECTIONS

1. Preheat the oven to 350 °F and place a cookie sheet on top of a baking tray.

2. Put the chocolate and cream in a double boiler and simmer to melt the chocolate.

3. In a bowl, whisk together egg yolks, the egg, vanilla extract, melted chocolate, Splenda and xylitol in a bowl.

4. Combine and mix the remaining dry ingredients in another bowl.

5. Stir the dry mixture into the egg mixture gradually by dividing it into two equal parts.

6. Refrigerate the dough for about 15 minutes then form cookies with dough and place them onto the cookie sheet.

7. Transfer tray into the oven and bake for about 14 minutes.

8. Remove from the oven and serve and enjoy. You can add crushed almonds to the top if desired.

Nutrition: Calories 125 kcal, Total Fat 7.6 g, Saturated Fat 1.6 g, Cholesterol 35 mg, Sodium 16 mg, Carb 5.8 g, Fiber 1.9 g, Protein 5.8 g

35. CHOCOLATE CHIP COOKIES

INGREDIENTS

- 1/8 cup coconut flour
- 1/6 cup unsalted butter, melted
- 1 tbsp Swerve sweetener
- 1 egg, large
- 2 tbsp sugar-free chocolate chips
- 1/8 tsp vanilla extract
- 1 pinch salt

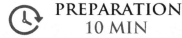 **PREPARATION**
10 MIN

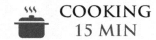 **COOKING**
15 MIN

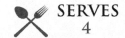 **SERVES**
4

DIRECTIONS

1. Preheat the oven to 350 °F and grease a cookie sheet.

2. Mix coconut flour, Swerve, and salt in a bowl.

3. Whisk egg with butter and vanilla extract in another bowl.

4. Combine the egg mixture with the flour mixture and fold in the chocolate chips.

5. Mix thoroughly and spoon the batter onto the cookie sheet to make individual cookies.

6. Transfer sheet into the oven and bake for about 15 minutes until golden brown.

7. Remove from the oven and serve.

Nutrition: Calories 106, Total Fat 9.5 g, Saturated Fat 5.6 g, Cholesterol 61 mg, Sodium 113 mg, Total Carbs 7.5 g, Fiber 1.5 g, Protein 2 g

36. SHORTBREAD COOKIES

INGREDIENTS

- 1 ¼ cups almond flour
- 3 tbsp butter
- 4 scoops stevia
- ½ tsp vanilla extract

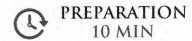 **PREPARATION** 10 MIN   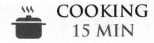 **COOKING** 15 MIN   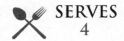 **SERVES** 4

DIRECTIONS

1. Preheat the oven to 350 °F and grease a cookie sheet lightly.
2. Whisk butter and stevia together in a bowl.
3. Combine almond flour and vanilla extract in another bowl to make a crumbly mixture. Then combine this with the butter mixture to form a dough.
4. Spoon out the batter onto the cookie sheet as individual cookies.
5. Transfer the sheet into the oven and bake for about 15 minutes.
6. Remove when done and serve.

Nutrition: Calories 288, Total Fat 25.3 g, Saturated Fat 6.7 g, Cholesterol 23 mg, Sodium 74 mg, Carb 7.6 g, Fiber 3.8 g, Protein 7.6 g

37. VANILLA COOKIES

INGREDIENTS

- 3 tbsp butter, unsalted
- 1 egg
- 2 ½ tbsp Splenda
- 1 ½ tbsp xylitol
- ½ tsp stevia
- 1 tsp vanilla
- ¾ cup almond meal
- ¼ cup oat flour
- ¼ cup soy protein powder
- ½ tsp baking powder
- 1 tsp lemon peel
- 1 pinch salt

 PREPARATION 20 MIN **COOKING** 20 MIN 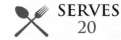 **SERVES** 20

DIRECTIONS

1. Preheat the oven to 350 °F and layer a cookie sheet on top of a baking tray.
2. Whisk together eggs, butter, sweeteners, and vanilla extract with a mixer in a bowl.
3. Blend all the dry ingredients in another bowl.
4. Stir the dry mixture into the egg mixture by dividing it into two halves.
5. Spoon out cookies onto the cookie sheet and transfer the tray into the oven.
6. Bake for about 20 minutes and remove from the oven.
7. Serve them to your guests.

Nutrition: Calories 58, Total Fat 3.9 g, Saturated Fat 1.3 g, Cholesterol 13 mg, Sodium 23 mg, Carb 3.4 g, Fiber 0.6 g, Protein 2.4 g

38. COCONUT CHIP COOKIES

INGREDIENTS

- ½ cup almond flour
- ¼ cup cacao nibs
- ¼ cup coconut flakes, unsweetened
- ¼ cup almond butter
- 1/8 cup butter, melted
- 1 large egg
- 4 scoops stevia
- 1/8 tsp salt

Glaze:
- 1/8 cup heavy whipping cream
- 1/8 tsp xanthan gum
- 2 scoops stevia
- ¼ tsp vanilla extract

 PREPARATION 15

 COOKING 25

 SERVES 4

DIRECTIONS

1. Preheat the oven to 350 °F and layer the baking tray with a cookie sheet.
2. Mix all the dry ingredients in a bowl.
3. Whisk together eggs with melted butter, stevia and almond butter in another bowl.
4. Combine the egg mixture with the dry mixture thoroughly.
5. Spoon out the batter onto a cookie sheet and press each cookie down slightly.
6. Place tray in the oven and bake for about 25 minutes.
7. Remove from the oven and let them cool for about 10 minutes.
8. Put a saucepan on the stove and add whipping cream, stevia, xanthan gum, and vanilla extract to it.
9. Cook until the mixture thickens then let it cool.
10. Pour glaze over the cookies and let them sit for about 15 minutes.
11. Serve them to your guests.

Nutrition: Calories 223, Fat 18.8 g, Sodium 142 mg, Carb 8.5 g, Fiber 4.9 g, Protein 6.1 g

39. GINGERSNAP COOKIES

INGREDIENTS

- 1 cup almond flour
- 1/8 cup butter, unsalted
- 4 scoops stevia
- 1 small egg
- ½ tsp vanilla extract
- 1/8 tsp salt
- 1 tsp ground ginger
- 1/8 tsp ground nutmeg
- 1/8 tsp ground cloves
- ¼ tsp ground cinnamon

 PREPARATION
10 MIN

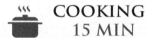 **COOKING**
15 MIN

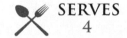 **SERVES**
4

DIRECTIONS

1. Preheat the oven to 350 °F and layer a cookie sheet on top of a baking tray.

2. Put all the dry ingredients in a blender and blend until smooth.

3. Mix rest of the ingredients in a bowl and combine with the dry mixture.

4. Spoon out the batter onto the cookie sheet to form individual cookies.

5. Bake for about 15 minutes then serve.

Nutrition: Calories 236, Total Fat 20 g, Cholesterol 50 mg, Sodium 138 mg, Carb 6.6 g, Fiber 3.2 g, Protein 7.3 g

40. NO-BAKE BUTTER COOKIES

INGREDIENTS

- ½ cup almond flour
- 1 ½ tbsp butter
- 1 tbsp Swerve
- ½ tsp vanilla extract
- 1 pinch salt

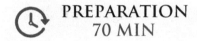 **PREPARATION**
70 MIN

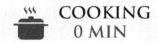 **COOKING**
0 MIN

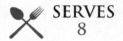 **SERVES**
8

DIRECTIONS

1. Mix all the ingredients in a bowl to prepare the cookie batter.

2. Spoon out the batter onto a cookie sheet positioned on a baking tray.

3. Put the tray in the refrigerator and refrigerate for about 1 hour 10 minutes.

4. Serve the cookies.

Nutrition: Calories 125, Total Fat 11 g, Cholesterol 11 mg, Sodium 75 mg, Carb 3.6 g, Fiber 1.5 g, Protein 3.1 g

41. CHOCOLATE COOKIES

INGREDIENTS

- 1/8 cup baking chocolate
- ¼ cup semi-sweet chocolate
- 2 tbsp butter, melted
- 2 tbsp heavy cream
- 1 egg
- 2 ½ tbsp Splenda
- 1 tsp vanilla extract
- ¾ cup almond meal
- ¼ cup soy protein powder
- ½ tsp baking powder
- 1 pinch of salt

 PREPARATION
30 MIN

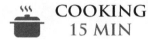 **COOKING**
15 MIN

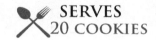 **SERVES**
20 COOKIES

DIRECTIONS

1. Preheat the oven to 350 °F and layer a cookie sheet on top of a baking tray.

2. Put the chocolate and cream in a double boiler and simmer until chocolate melts.

3. Whisk together eggs, butter, sweeteners, vanilla extract, and melted chocolate in a bowl.

4. Mix all the dry ingredients in another bowl.

5. Combine both mixtures and refrigerate for about 30 minutes.

6. Spoon out the batter onto the cookie sheet to form cookies and transfer into the oven.

7. Bake for about 15 minutes and place on a cooling rack to cool.

8. Serve or freeze the cookies to enjoy later.

Nutrition: Calories 75, Fat 4.9 g, Cholesterol 14 mg, Sodium 21 mg, Carb 5.3 g, Fiber 0.5 g, Protein 2.6 g

42. HAZELNUT COOKIES

INGREDIENTS

- 5 egg yolks
- 3 tbsp xylitol
- 1 tsp vanilla extract
- 2 cups hazelnut meal
- 2 tbsp protein powder
- 2 tbsp wheat protein powder
- 1 tbsp lemon peel
- 1 tsp baking powder
- 30 hazelnuts

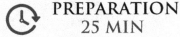 **PREPARATION** 25 MIN

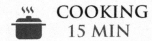 **COOKING** 15 MIN

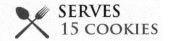 **SERVES** 15 COOKIES

DIRECTIONS

1. Preheat the oven to 350 °F and layer a cookie sheet on top of a baking tray.

2. Mix the egg yolks, xylitol, and vanilla extract in a bowl.

3. Mix rest of the ingredients together in another bowl.

4. Fold this mixture into the egg yolk mixture and refrigerate for about 30 minutes.

5. Spoon out the cookies onto the cookie sheet to form individual cookies and flatten each with your hand.

6. Top each with hazelnuts and place in the oven.

7. Bake for about 15 minutes and remove from the oven.

8. Let them cool on a cooling rack and serve.

Nutrition: Calories 134, Fat 10.9 g, Cholesterol 79 mg, Sodium 16 mg, Carb 3.9 g, Fiber 1.5 g, Protein 6.8 g

43. SNICKERDOODLE COOKIES

INGREDIENTS

For the cookies:
- 1 egg
- 1 tsp vanilla extract
- ½ cup almond butter
- ¼ cup almond milk
- 1/8 cup coconut oil, solid (at room temperature)
- 3 packets Monk fruit sweetener
- ¾ cup almond flour
- ½ cup coconut flour

- ½ tsp baking soda
- 1 tsp cream of tartar
- 1 pinch pink Himalayan salt
- ½ tsp cinnamon

For the coating:
- 2 packets Monk fruit sweetener
- ½ tbsp cinnamon

 PREPARATION 10 MIN   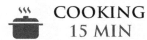 **COOKING** 15 MIN   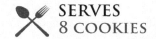 **SERVES** 8 COOKIES

DIRECTIONS

1. Preheat the oven to 350 °F and layer a cookie sheet on top of a baking tray.

2. Whisk together eggs, vanilla extract, almond butter, almond milk, coconut oil, sweetener, and cream of tartar in a bowl.

3. Mix almond flour, coconut flour, baking soda, salt, and cinnamon in another bowl.

4. Combine the two mixtures and transfer to the refrigerator for about 10 minutes.

5. Prepare small balls from the batter and coat the balls with monk fruit sweetener and cinnamon before arranging them on the prepared baking tray.

6. Bake for about 15 minutes.

7. Remove from the oven and serve.

Nutrition: Calories 157, Fat 12.1 g, Cholesterol 20 mg, Sodium 126 mg, Carb 8.6 g, Fiber 4.6 g, Protein 4.3 g

44. CREAM CHEESE COOKIES

INGREDIENTS

- 1/8 cup butter
- ¼ cup plain cream cheese + extra for topping
- ¼ cup xylitol
- 1 egg white
- 1 tsp vanilla extract
- 1 ½ cups almond flour
- 1/8 tsp sea salt

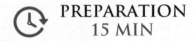 **PREPARATION** 15 MIN

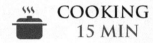 **COOKING** 15 MIN

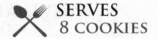 **SERVES** 8 COOKIES

DIRECTIONS

1. Preheat the oven to 350 °F and layer a cookie sheet on top of a baking tray.

2. Whisk together the egg white with butter, xylitol, and vanilla extract in a bowl.

3. Mix almond flour and sea salt in another bowl.

4. Combine the egg white mixture with the flour mixture.

5. Spoon out the mixture onto the cooking sheet forming the individual cookies.

6. Transfer tray into the oven and bake for about 15 minutes.

7. Remove from the oven and top each cookie with cream cheese to serve.

Nutrition: Calories 185, Fat 15.4 g, Cholesterol 16 mg, Sodium 85 mg, Carb 6 g, Fiber 2.3 g, Protein 5.5 g

45. COCONUT FLOUR COOKIES

INGREDIENTS

- ½ cup coconut flour, sifted
- ½ tsp baking powder
- ¼ tsp salt
- 3 tbsp butter
- 4 tbsp coconut oil
- 3 scoops stevia
- 2 large eggs
- ½ tbsp almond milk
- ½ tsp vanilla extract

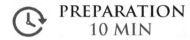 **PREPARATION** 10 MIN   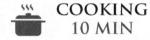 **COOKING** 10 MIN   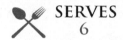 **SERVES** 6

DIRECTIONS

1. Preheat the oven to 375 °F and layer a cookie sheet on top of a baking tray.

2. Whisk together eggs, butter, coconut oil, stevia, almond milk, and vanilla extract in a bowl.

3. Mix coconut flour, baking powder, and salt in another bowl.

4. Stir the flour mixture into the egg mixture and spoon out the mixture onto the cookie sheet forming individual cookies.

5. Transfer tray into the oven and bake for about 15 minutes.

6. Remove from the oven and serve warm.

Nutrition: Calories 197, Fat 17.8 g, Cholesterol 77 mg, Sodium 162 mg, Carb 7.1 g, Fiber 4 g, Protein 3.5 g

46. KETO PEANUT BUTTER COOKIES

INGREDIENTS

- ½ cup peanut butter
- 1/3 cup powdered erythritol
- 1 egg

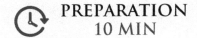 **PREPARATION**
10 MIN

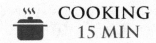 **COOKING**
15 MIN

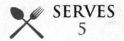 **SERVES**
5

DIRECTIONS

1. Preheat the oven to 350 °F and line a baking sheet with parchment paper.

2. Whisk together the egg, peanut butter, and erythritol in a bowl.

3. Spoon the batter forming individual cookies and arrange them on the prepared tray then press the cookie balls down with a fork.

4. Transfer tray into the oven.

5. Bake for about 15 minutes and remove from the oven.

6. Let the cookies cool for 10 minutes and serve.

Nutrition: Calories 175, Fat 13.9 g, Cholesterol 33 mg, Sodium 131 mg, Carb 7.8 g, Fiber 1.5 g, Protein 7.6 g

47. MACADAMIA NUT COOKIES

INGREDIENTS

- 3 tbsp butter
- 1 egg
- ½ tsp stevia
- 1 tsp vanilla extract
- ¾ cup macadamia nuts, roasted and chopped
- ¼ cup macadamia nut meal
- ¼ cup almond meal
- ¼ cup soy protein powder
- ½ tsp baking powder
- ¼ tsp nutmeg, ground

 PREPARATION 25 MIN

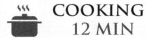 **COOKING** 12 MIN

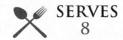 **SERVES** 8

DIRECTIONS

1. Preheat the oven to 350 °F and layer a cookie sheet on top of a baking tray.
2. Whisk together butter, egg, stevia, and vanilla extract in a bowl using a hand mixer.
3. Combine macadamia nuts, macadamia nut meal, almond meal, soy protein powder, baking powder, and nutmeg in another bowl.
4. Stir the dry mixture into the butter mixture and refrigerate the dough for about 15 minutes.
5. Scoop the batter to form individual cookies and place them on the cookie sheet and bake for about 12 minutes.
6. Remove from the oven and serve.

Nutrition: Calories, Fat 16.4 g, Cholesterol 32 mg, Sodium 39 mg, Carb 2.9 g, Fiber 1.5 g, Protein 5.6 g

48. PUMPKIN SEED COOKIES

INGREDIENTS

- 2 ½ tbsp butter, unsalted
- 1 egg
- 2 ½ tbsp Splenda
- ½ tsp stevia
- 1 tsp vanilla extract
- ¼ cup almond meal, blanched
- ¼ cup almond meal, whole
- ¼ cup soy protein powder
- 1/8 cup flaxseed meal
- ¼ cup pumpkin seeds, ground and roasted
- ½ tsp baking powder
- 1 pinch of salt

 PREPARATION
20 MIN

 COOKING
13 MIN

 SERVES
8

DIRECTIONS

1. Preheat the oven to 360 °F and layer a cookie sheet on top of a baking tray.

2. Mix the butter, egg, Splenda, stevia, and vanilla extract in a bowl using a mixer.

3. Combine almond meal, protein powder, flaxseed meal, pumpkin seeds, baking powder, and salt in another bowl.

4. Stir the almond meal mixture into the butter mixture and roll to form a dough.

5. Refrigerate the dough for about 30 minutes.

6. Scoop the batter out to form individual cookies and arrange them on the cookie sheet and place the tray in the oven.

7. Bake for about 13 minutes and remove from the oven to serve.

Nutrition: Calories 141, Fat 9.8 g, Cholesterol 30 mg, Sodium 54 mg, Carb 6.6 g, Fiber 1.4 g, Protein 6.5 g

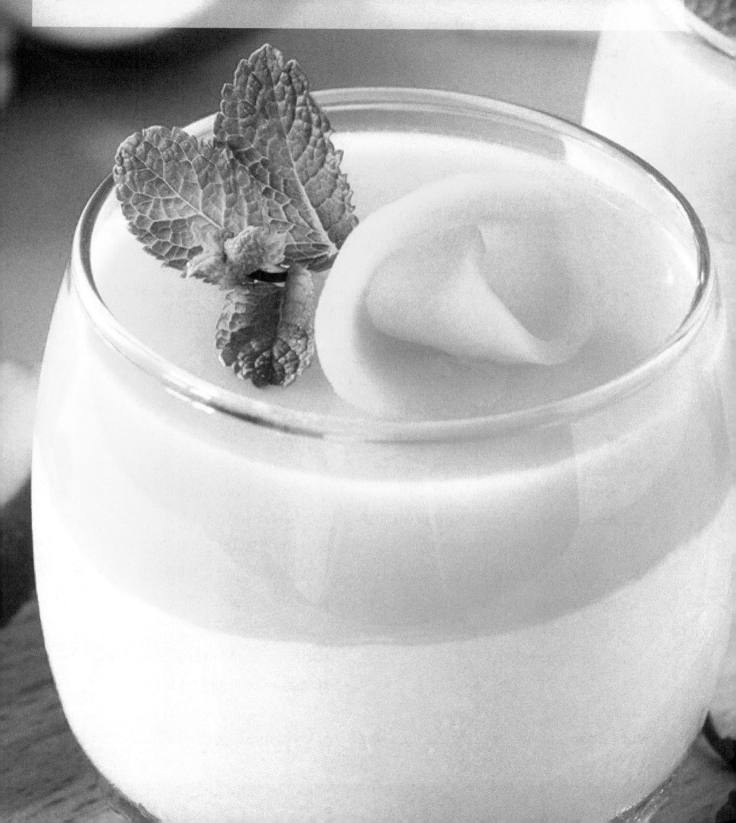

49. MOUSSES RECIPES

INGREDIENTS

For mousse:
- ¼ cup yogurt
- 1 cup whipping cream
- 2 cups mascarpone cheese
- ¼ tsp agar powder
- 1 tsp vanilla extract
- 3 Tbsp Swerve
- 1 Tbsp coconut oil, melted
- ½ cup coconut cream

For sauce:
- 2 Tbsp unsweetened cocoa powder
- 2 tsp Swerve
- ½ tsp vanilla extract
- ¼ cup coconut cream

 PREPARATION 10 MIN

 COOKING 5 MIN

 SERVES 8

DIRECTIONS

1. Add coconut oil to the Instant Pot and set the pot on sauté mode.
2. Add mascarpone, yogurt, Swerve, and vanilla. Stir well until warm.
3. Add agar powder and cook for 2–3 minutes. Stir continuously.
4. Transfer pot mixture to a bowl.
5. Add coconut cream and whipping cream to the bowl and beat using a hand mixer.
6. Divide mixture among serving bowls and set aside.
7. Again, set the instant pot on sauté mode. Start the sauce by adding the coconut cream to the pot.
8. Stir in Swerve, vanilla, and cocoa powder and cook for 1–2 minutes.
9. Remove sauce from pot and drizzle over mousse.
10. Place in refrigerator for 1 hour.
11. Serve chilled and enjoy.

Nutrition: Calories 266, Fat 23.3 g, Carb 6.9 g, Protein 8.9 g, Cholesterol 49 mg

50. ALMOND BERRY MOUSSE

INGREDIENTS

- 4 blueberries
- 4 strawberries, sliced
- ½ cup heavy cream
- 2 egg yolks
- ½ tsp vanilla extract
- ¼ cup almond milk
- ¼ cup Swerve
- 2 Tbsp water

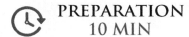 **PREPARATION** 10 MIN

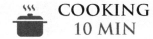 **COOKING** 10 MIN

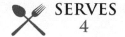 **SERVES** 4

DIRECTIONS

1. Pour 1 ½ cups of water into the Instant Pot and place a trivet in the pot.

2. In a small saucepan, add sweetener and 2 tablespoons water and heat over medium heat until sweetener is dissolved.

3. Remove pan from heat and whisk in vanilla, milk, and cream.

4. In a bowl, whisk egg yolks.

5. Slowly add cream mixture and stir into the eggs.

6. Pour mixture into 4 ramekins and place on top of the trivet.

7. Seal pot with lid and cook on high pressure for 6 minutes.

8. When finished, release pressure using quick release method and open the lid.

9. Remove ramekins from the pot and set aside to cool completely.

10. Place in refrigerator for 1–2 hours.

11. Top with blueberries and sliced strawberries and serve.

Nutrition: Calories 125, Fat 7.8 g, Carb 13 g, Protein 2.5 g, Cholesterol 111 mg

51. LEMON-YOGURT MOUSSE

INGREDIENTS

- 24 oz plain yogurt, strained overnight in a cheesecloth
- 2 cups swerve confectioner's sugar
- 2 lemons, juiced and zested
- Pink salt to taste
- 1 cup whipped cream + extra for garnish

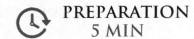 **PREPARATION** 5 MIN   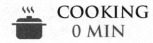 **COOKING** 0 MIN   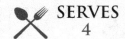 **SERVES** 4

DIRECTIONS

1. Whip the plain yogurt in a bowl with a hand mixer until light and fluffy.

2. Mix in the sugar, lemon juice, and salt.

3. Fold in the whipped cream to evenly combine.

4. Spoon the mousse into serving cups and refrigerate to thicken for 1 hour.

5. Swirl with extra whipped cream and garnish lightly with lemon zest.

6. Serve immediately.

Nutrition: Calories 223, Fat 18 g, Carb 3 g, Protein 12 g

52. BLUEBERRIES MOUSSE

INGREDIENTS

- 8 ounces heavy cream
- 1 teaspoon vanilla extract
- 1 tablespoon stevia
- 1 cup blueberries

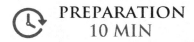 **PREPARATION**
10 MIN

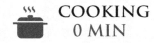 **COOKING**
0 MIN

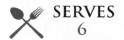 **SERVES**
6

DIRECTIONS

1. In a blender, combine the cream with the other ingredients, pulse well, divide into bowls and serve cold.

Nutrition: Calories 219, Fat 21.1 g, Fiber 0.9 g, Carb 7 g, Protein 1.4 g

53. EASY CITRUS MOUSSE WITH ALMONDS

INGREDIENTS

- ¾ lb cream cheese, softened
- 2 cups swerve confectioner's sugar
- 1 lemon, juiced and zested
- 1 lime, juice and zested
- Salt to taste
- 1 cup whipped cream + extra for garnish
- ¼ cup toasted almonds, chopped

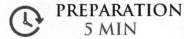 **PREPARATION** 5 MIN

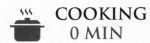 **COOKING** 0 MIN

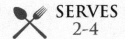 **SERVES** 2-4

DIRECTIONS

1. In a bowl and with a hand mixer, whip the cream cheese until light and fluffy.

2. Add in the sugar, lemon and lime juices and salt, and mix well.

3. Fold in the whipped cream to evenly combine.

4. Spoon the mousse into serving cups and refrigerate to thicken for 1 hour.

5. Swirl with extra whipped cream and garnish with lemon and lime zest.

6. Serve immediately topped with almonds.

Nutrition: Calories 242, Fat 18 g, Carb 3.3 g, Protein 6.5 g

54. CHOCOLATE MOUSSE WITH CHERRIES

INGREDIENTS

- 12 oz unsweetened dark chocolate
- 8 eggs, separated into yolks and whites
- 2 tbsp salt
- ¾ cup swerve sugar
- ½ cup olive oil
- 3 tbsp brewed coffee
- 1 cup cherries, pitted and halved
- ½ stick cinnamon
- ½ cup swerve sugar
- ½ cup water
- ½ lime, juiced

 PREPARATION 25 MIN   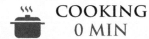 **COOKING** 0 MIN   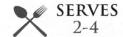 **SERVES** 2-4

DIRECTIONS

1. In a bowl, add the chocolate and melt in the microwave for 95 seconds.
2. In a separate bowl, whisk the yolks with half of the swerve sugar until a pale yellow has formed, then, beat in the salt, olive oil, and coffee.
3. Mix in the melted chocolate until smooth.
4. In a third bowl, whisk the whites with the hand mixer until a soft peak has formed.
5. Sprinkle the remaining swerve sugar over and gently fold in with a spatula.
6. Fetch a tablespoon of the chocolate mixture and fold in to combine.
7. Pour in the remaining chocolate mixture and whisk to mix.
8. Ladle the mousse into ramekins, cover with plastic wrap, and refrigerate overnight.

9. The next morning, pour ½ cup of water, ½ cup of swerve, ½ stick cinnamon, and the lime juice in a saucepan and bring to a simmer for 4 minutes, occasionally stirring to ensure the swerve has dissolved and a syrup has formed.

10. Add the cherries and poach in the sweetened water for 20 minutes until soft.

11. Turn the heat off and discard the cinnamon stick.

12. Spoon a plum each with syrup on the chocolate mousse and serve.

Nutrition: Calories 288, Fat 23.4 g, Carb 8.1 g, Protein 10 g

55. NO BAKE MOUSSE WITH STRAWBERRIES

INGREDIENTS

- 2 cups chilled heavy cream
- 2 cups fresh strawberries, hulled
- 4 tbsp xylitol
- 2 tbsp lime juice
- ¼ tsp strawberry extract
- 2 tbsp sugar-free strawberry preserves

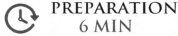 **PREPARATION**
6 MIN

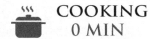 **COOKING**
0 MIN

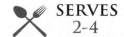 **SERVES**
2-4

DIRECTIONS

1. In a bowl, beat the heavy cream with a hand mixer at high speed until a stiff peak forms, for about 1 minute; refrigerate immediately.

2. Puree the strawberries in a blender and pour into a saucepan.

3. Stir in xylitol and lime juice, and cook on low heat for 3 minutes while stirring continuously.

4. Stir in the strawberry extract evenly, and turn off the heat to cool.

5. Fold in the cream until evenly incorporated, and spoon into ramekins.

6. Refrigerate for 3 hours, garnish with strawberry preserves and serve.

Nutrition: Calories 353, Fat 32.4 g, Carb 4.8 g, Protein 5.3 g

56. CHOCOLATE AND ORANGE MOUSSE

INGREDIENTS

- 2 egg yolks
- ¾ cup heavy cream
- 3 ounces Ricotta cheese, at room temperature
- 1 tablespoon freshly squeezed orange juice
- 1 ½ teaspoons orange zest
- ½ teaspoon ground cinnamon
- ¼ cup granulated stevia erythritol blend
- ¼ cup unsweetened cocoa powder

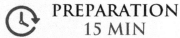 **PREPARATION**
15 MIN

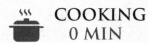 **COOKING**
0 MIN

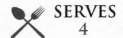 **SERVES**
4

DIRECTIONS

1. Beat egg yolks with your electric mixer until thick and pale.

2. Heat the cream in a pan over medium heat. Gradually stir hot cream into egg yolk mixture.

3. Turn the heat to low and cook for about 5 minutes, stirring constantly, until your mixture is thickened.

4. Now, beat the remaining ingredients with your electric mixer until everything is creamy.

5. Fold this mixture into cream mixture and serve well chilled.

Nutrition: Calories 154, Fat 13 g, Carb 7.1 g, Protein 5.3 g

57. DELICIOUS MOUSSE

INGREDIENTS

- 8 ounces mascarpone cheese
- ½ pint blueberries
- ½ pint strawberries
- 1 cup whipping cream
- ¾ teaspoon vanilla stevia

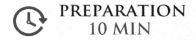 **PREPARATION**
10 MIN

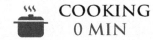 **COOKING**
0 MIN

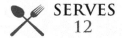 **SERVES**
12

DIRECTIONS

1. In a bowl, mix whipping cream with stevia and mascarpone and blend well using your mixer.

2. Arrange a layer of blueberries and strawberries in 12 glasses, then a layer of cream and so on.

3. Serve this mousse cold!

Nutrition: Calories 143, Fat 12 g, Fiber 1 g, Carb 3 g, Protein 2 g

58. SUGAR-FREE LOW CARB COFFEE RICOTTA MOUSSE

INGREDIENTS

- 1 ½ tsps. dry gelatin
- 1 tsp. vanilla liquid stevia
- ½ cup of hot brewed coffee
- pinch of salt
- 2 cups of Ricotta cheese
- 1 tsp. vanilla extract
- 1 tsp. instant espresso
- shaved sugar free chocolate to garnish (optional)
- 1 cup of heavy whipping cream

 PREPARATION
15 MIN

 COOKING
0 MIN

 SERVES
10

DIRECTIONS

1. Pour the gelatin into the hot coffee and stir properly until it dissolves. Set it aside and allow it to cool.

2. Add the ricotta, vanilla extract, salt, stevia, and espresso and blend the ingredients until combined.

3. Pour the cooled coffee-gelatin mixture and blend until smooth.

4. Pour in the whipping cream and blend on high until it's thickened and whipped.

5. Spoon into serving dishes then garnish with shaved chocolate if you wish.

6. Keep in the refrigerator for 2 hours and enjoy.

Nutrition: Calories 170, Fat 15.2 g, Carb 2.5 g, Protein 6.9 g

59. LEMON CHEESECAKE MOUSSE

INGREDIENTS

- 8 oz cream cheese, room temperature
- 1 cup heavy cream, cold
- 2/3 cup lemon curd
- 1/3 cup Swerve confectioners

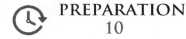 **PREPARATION** 10

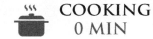 **COOKING** 0 MIN

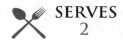 **SERVES** 2

DIRECTIONS

1. Beat cream in a bowl until it forms peaks.

2. Separately, beat cream cheese using a hand mixer then add the lemon curd and Swerve in a mixer.

3. Stir in the whipped cream then refrigerate for 10 minutes.

4. Garnish as desired.

5. Serve.

Nutrition: Calories 267, Fat 44.5 g, Cholesterol 153 mg, Sodium 217 mg, Carb 8.4 g, Fiber 1.3 g, Protein 3.1 g

60. CREAMY RICOTTA COFFEE MOUSSE

INGREDIENTS

- 2 cups ricotta cheese
- 1 cup heavy cream, chilled
- 1/3 cup monk fruit sweetener
- 1 ½ tbsp instant espresso powder
- 1 tbsp powdered gelatin
- tsp gelatin
- 1 tbsp orange zest, finely grated
- Shaved chocolate, for garnish

For Whipped Cream Topping:
- 1 cup heavy cream, chilled
- 1/3 cup monk fruit sweetener

 PREPARATION 10 MIN   **COOKING** 3 MIN 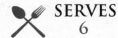 **SERVES** 6

DIRECTIONS

1. Add ricotta to a blender and blend until smooth.

2. Beat 1 cup heavy cream with 1/3 cup sweetener in a mixer until it forms peaks.

3. Heat ¼ cup water in a saucepan to boil then mix 2 tablespoons of this water with gelatin.

4. Mix well then set this mixture aside.

5. Mix ricotta with espresso, gelatin mixture, and whipped cream.

6. Divide this dessert into 6 serving glasses then refrigerate for 1 hour.

7. Beat a cup of cream with 1/3 cup sweetener, 2 tablespoons water, and 1 teaspoon gelatin in a bowl.

8. Place this bowl in the microwave and heat the cream mixture for 1 minute.

9. Beat well then fold in orange zest then transfer the mixture to a piping bag.

10. Pipe this mixture over the coffee mouse.

11. Refrigerate for 2 hours then garnish with chocolate shavings.

12. Serve.

Nutrition: Calories 259, Fat 34 g, Cholesterol 112 mg, Sodium 92 mg, Carb 8.5 g, Fiber 1.3 g, Protein 7.5 g

61. FROZEN RASPBERRY MOUSSE

INGREDIENTS

- 3 egg whites
- 2 cups raspberries, fresh
- 1 tbsp vodka or rum
- ½ cup Swerve

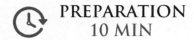 **PREPARATION**
10 MIN

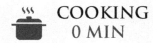 **COOKING**
0 MIN

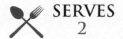 **SERVES**
2

DIRECTIONS

1. Start by blending the 3 egg whites in a blender until foamy and set aside.

2. Separately, blend the raspberries in a blender then add ½ cup sweetener and vodka/rum.

3. Mix well then fold in egg whites.

4. Divide this batter into the serving bowls.

5. Serve.

Nutrition: Calories 255, Fat 23.4 g, Cholesterol 135 mg, Sodium 112 mg, Carb 2.5 g, Fiber 1 g, Protein 7.9 g

62. PUMPKIN CHEESECAKE MOUSSE

INGREDIENTS

- 8 oz cream cheese, softened
- 1 cup canned pumpkin puree
- ½ cup Swerve sweetener
- 1 tsp pumpkin pie spice
- 1 tsp vanilla extract
- ¾ cup heavy whipping cream

 PREPARATION
10 MIN

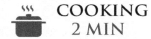 **COOKING**
2 MIN

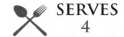 **SERVES**
4

DIRECTIONS

1. Start by adding cream cheese and pumpkin puree to a mixing bowl.
2. Mix until smooth then stir in remaining ingredients.
3. Transfer the mixture to a piping bag.
4. Pipe this mixture into small cups.
5. Refrigerate for 2 hours.
6. Serve.

Nutrition: Calories 251, Fat 24.5 g, Cholesterol 165 mg, Sodium 142 mg, Carb 4.3 g, Fiber 1 g, Protein 5.9 g

63. COCONUT CHOCOLATE MOUSSE

INGREDIENTS

- 1 cup heavy whipping cream
- 3 tablespoons raw cacao powder
- ½ teaspoon cinnamon
- Stevia extract, to taste
- Toasted flaked coconut or almonds for garnish

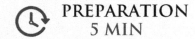 **PREPARATION**
5 MIN

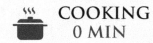 **COOKING**
0 MIN

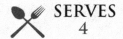 **SERVES**
4

DIRECTIONS

1. Beat cream with cacao powder in a suitable bowl until fluffy.

2. Stir in cinnamon and stevia.

3. Combine well then garnish with coconut.

4. Enjoy.

Nutrition: Calories 254, Fat 9 g, Cholesterol 13 mg, Sodium 179 mg, Carb 7.5 g, Fiber 0.8 g, Protein 7.5 g

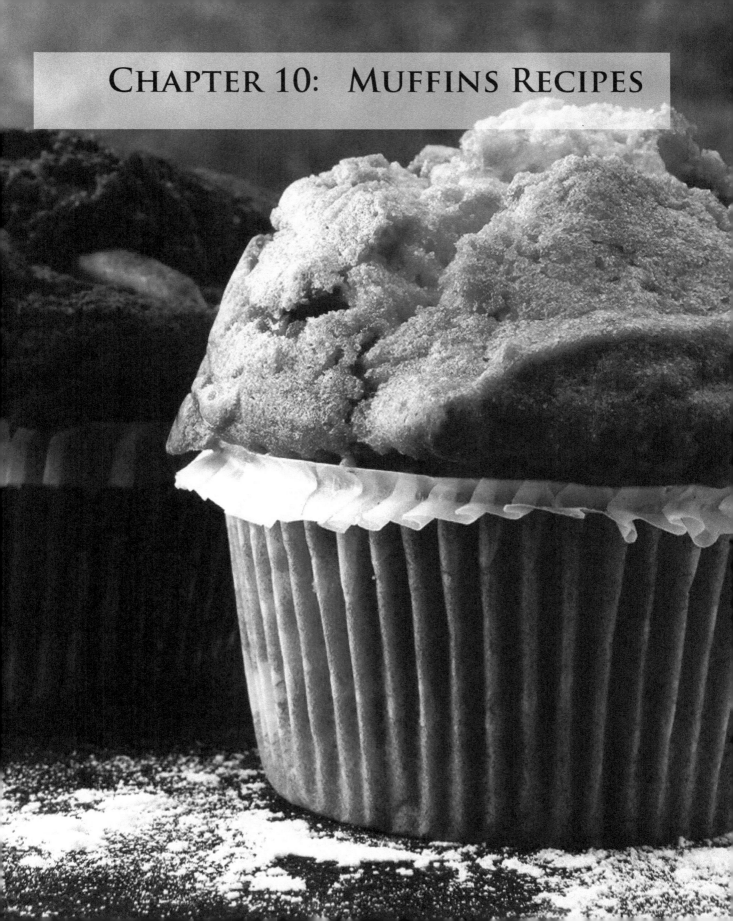

CHAPTER 10:   MUFFINS RECIPES

64. CINNAMON CHOCO ALMOND MUFFINS

INGREDIENTS

- 5 eggs
- 1 Tbsp dark chocolate chips
- 1 Tbsp butter
- ½ cup almond milk
- 1 Tbsp flax seed meal
- 1 Tbsp chia seeds
- ¼ cup almonds, chopped
- ½ cup almond flour

- ¼ tsp cinnamon
- 2 tsp Swerve
- 1 tsp orange extract
- ¼ tsp baking soda
- ½ tsp baking powder

 PREPARATION
10 MIN

 COOKING
30 MIN

 SERVES
5

DIRECTIONS

1. In a large bowl, mix together almond flour, baking soda, baking powder, flax seed meal, chia seeds, and almonds.

2. Add eggs, cinnamon, Swerve, orange extract, butter, and almond milk and beat using a hand mixer until well combined.

3. Pour batter evenly among silicone muffin molds. Top with chocolate chips.

4. Pour 1 cup of water into the Instant Pot and place a trivet in the pot.

5. Place muffin molds on top of the trivet.

6. Seal pot with lid and cook on high pressure for 30 minutes.

7. When finished, release pressure using quick release method and then open the lid.

8. Serve and enjoy.

Nutrition: Calories 208, Fat 17.5 g, Carb 6.2 g, Protein 8.4 g, Cholesterol 170 mg

65. CHOCO CHIP MUFFINS

INGREDIENTS

- 2 eggs
- ½ tsp baking soda
- 2 Tbsp butter, softened
- ½ cup Swerve
- 1 Tbsp vanilla extract
- ¾ cup unsweetened chocolate chips
- 1 cup almond flour
- Pinch of salt

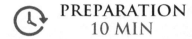 **PREPARATION** 10 MIN

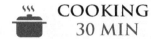 **COOKING** 30 MIN

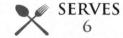 **SERVES** 6

DIRECTIONS

1. Pour 1 cup of water into the Instant Pot and place a trivet in the pot.
2. Add all ingredients to a bowl and mix until well combined.
3. Pour batter into greased muffin molds.
4. Place muffin molds in a pan and cover pan with foil.
5. Place pan on top of trivet in the pot.
6. Seal pot with lid and cook on manual at high pressure for 20 minutes.
7. When finished, allow pressure to release naturally for 10 minutes, and then release using the quick release method. Open the lid.
8. Remove pan from the pot and let it cool completely.
9. Serve and enjoy.

Nutrition: Calories 368, Fat 30.6 g, Carb 8.6 g, Protein 9.9 g, Cholesterol 65 mg

66. CINNAMON ROLL MUFFINS

INGREDIENTS

- ½ cup almond flour
- 2 scoops vanilla protein powder
- 1 tsp baking powder
- 1 tbsp cinnamon
- ½ cup almond butter
- ½ cup pumpkin puree
- ½ cup coconut oil
- ¼ cup coconut butter
- ¼ cup milk of choice
- 1 tbsp granulated sweetener
- 2 tsp lemon juice

 PREPARATION 5 MIN   **COOKING** 15 MIN   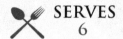 **SERVES** 6

DIRECTIONS

1. Let your oven preheat at 350 °F. Layer a 12-cup muffin tray with muffin liners.

2. Add all the dry ingredients to a suitable mixing bowl then whisk in all the wet ingredients.

3. Mix until well combined then divide the batter into the muffin cups.

4. Bake them for 15 minutes then allow the muffins to cool on a wire rack.

5. Prepare the cinnamon glaze in a small bowl then drizzle this glaze over the muffins.

6. Enjoy.

Nutrition: Calories 252, Fat 17.3 g, Cholesterol 141 mg, Sodium 153 mg, Carb 7.2 g, Fiber 1.4 g, Protein 5.2 g

67. CREAMY CHOCOLATE MUFFINS

INGREDIENTS

- 1 cup creamy almond butter
- 2/3 cup erythritol
- 2 tbsp unsweetened cocoa powder
- 2 tbsp peanut butter powder
- 2 large eggs
- 1 tbsp salted butter, melted
- 2 tbsp water
- 1 ½ tsp pure vanilla extract
- 1 tsp baking soda
- ¼ cup sugar-free dark chocolate baking chips

 PREPARATION 10 MIN

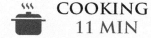 **COOKING** 11 MIN

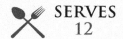 **SERVES** 12

DIRECTIONS

1. Start by preheating the oven to 350 °F.

2. Place a silicone muffin tray on a baking sheet.

3. Place almond butter in a mixing bowl and whisk in all other ingredients except chocolate chips.

4. Mix well until combined then fold in chocolate chips.

5. Divide the dough into 12 muffin cups.

6. Bake the muffins for 11 minutes, approximately.

7. Serve.

Nutrition: Calories 139, Total Fat 9.6 g, Carb 4.5 g, Protein 3.8 g

68. PUMPKIN SPICE MUFFINS

INGREDIENTS

- 2/3 cup almond flour
- 3 tbsp coconut flour
- 1 tbsp psyllium husk
- 1 tsp pumpkin pie spice
- ½ tsp xanthan gum
- ¼ tsp kosher salt
- ½ tsp baking powder
- ½ tsp baking soda
- 2 eggs, separated
- 1/3 cup golden erythritol

- 1 tsp vanilla extract
- 1 tsp apple cider vinegar
- ¼ cup unsalted butter, melted
- ¼ cup espresso, cooled

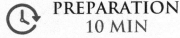 **PREPARATION** 10 MIN

 COOKING 20 MIN

 SERVES 6

DIRECTIONS

1. Start by preheating the oven to 350 °F.
2. Whisk all the dry ingredients in a bowl and beat the wet ingredients separately until fluffy.
3. Mix the two mixtures together then divide the batter into the muffin cups.
4. Bake them for 20 minutes or until golden brown.
5. Allow them to cool then serve.

Nutrition: Calories 261, Fat 13.4 g, Cholesterol 0.3 mg, Sodium 10 mg, Carb 4.1 g, Fiber 3.9 g, Protein 3.8 g

69. CHEESY HERB MUFFINS

INGREDIENTS

- 6 tbsp butter
- 1 tsp granulated erythritol sweetener
- 1 cup superfine blanched almond flour
- 3 tbsp coconut flour
- ¾ tsp kosher salt
- ¼ tsp garlic powder
- 2 tsp baking powder
- ¼ tsp xanthan gum
- 2 eggs
- ½ tsp fresh thyme leaves
- 1/3 cup unsweetened almond milk
- ½ cup cheddar cheese, shredded

 PREPARATION
10 MIN

 COOKING
22 MIN

 SERVES
12

DIRECTIONS

1. Start by preheating the oven to 375 °F. Grease a muffin tray with cooking spray.

2. Melt butter in a bowl by heating in a microwave for 30 seconds.

3. Stir in almond flour, sweetener, garlic powder, eggs, and all other remaining ingredients.

4. Divide the prepared batter into the muffin cups and bake for 22 minutes, approximately.

5. Serve.

Nutrition: Calories 195, Fat 14.3 g, Carb 4.5 g, Fiber 0.3 g, Protein 3.2 g

70. LEMON POPPY SEED MUFFINS

INGREDIENTS

- ¾ cup almond flour
- ¼ cup golden flaxseed meal
- 1/3 cup erythritol
- 1 tsp baking powder
- 2 tbsp poppy seeds
- ¼ cup salted butter, melted
- ¼ cup heavy cream
- 3 large eggs
- 2 lemons, zested
- 3 tbsp lemon juice
- 1 tsp vanilla extract
- 25 drops liquid Stevia

 PREPARATION
10 MIN

 COOKING
20 MIN

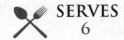 **SERVES**
6

DIRECTIONS

1. Start by preheating the oven to 350 °F.
2. Add poppy seeds, erythritol, flaxseed meal, and almond flour in a bowl.
3. Stir in eggs, cream, and melted butter then beat the mixture together.
4. Add Stevia, baking powder, lemon zest, lemon juice, and vanilla extract.
5. Divide the batter evenly into a muffin tray.
6. Bake them for 20 minutes or until golden brown on the top.
7. Serve.

Nutrition: Calories 252, Fat 17.3 g, Carbs 5.2 g, Fiber 1.4 g, Protein 5.2 g

71. MUFFINS WITH BLUEBERRIES

INGREDIENTS

- ¾ cup coconut flour
- 6 eggs
- ½ cup coconut oil, melted
- 1/3 cup unsweetened coconut milk
- ½ cup fresh blueberries
- 1/3 cup granulated sweetener
- 1 tsp vanilla extract
- 1 tsp baking powder

 PREPARATION
10 MIN

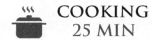 **COOKING**
25 MIN

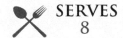 **SERVES**
8

DIRECTIONS

1. Preheat your oven at 350 °F.

2. Mix coconut flour with all the other ingredients except blueberries in a mixing bowl until smooth.

3. Stir in blueberries and mix gently.

4. Divide this batter in a greased muffin tray evenly.

5. Bake the muffins for 25 minutes until golden brown.

6. Enjoy.

Nutrition: Calories 195, Fat 14.3 g, Carbs 4.5 g, Fiber 0.3 g, Protein 3.2 g

72. CHOCOLATE ZUCCHINI MUFFINS

INGREDIENTS

- ½ cup coconut flour
- ¾ tsp baking soda
- 2 tbsp cocoa powder
- ½ tsp salt
- 1 tsp cinnamon
- ½ tsp nutmeg
- 3 large eggs
- 2/3 cup Swerve sweetener
- 2 tsp vanilla extract

- 1 tbsp oil
- 1 medium zucchini, grated
- ¼ cup heavy cream
- 1/3 cup Lily's chocolate baking chips

 PREPARATION 10 MIN

 COOKING 30 MIN

 SERVES 9

DIRECTIONS

1. Preheat your oven at 350 °F.
2. Layer a 9-cup o muffin tray with muffin liners then spray them with cooking oil.
3. Whisk coconut flour with salt, cinnamon, nutmeg, sweetener, baking soda, and cocoa powder in a bowl.
4. Beat eggs in a separate bowl then add oil, cream, vanilla, and zucchini.
5. Stir in the coconut flour mixture and mix well until fully incorporated.
6. Fold in chocolate chips then divide the batter into the lined muffin cups.
7. Bake these muffins for 30 minutes then allow them to cool on a wire rack.
8. Enjoy.

Nutrition: Calories 151, Fat 14.7 g, Carb 1.5 g, Fiber 0.1 g, Protein 0.8 g

73. BLACKBERRY-FILLED LEMON MUFFINS

INGREDIENTS

- 3 tbsp granulated stevia
- 1 tsp lemon juice
- ¼ tsp xanthan gum
- 2 tbsp water
- 1 cup fresh blackberries
- 2 ½ cups super fine almond flour
- ¾ cup granulated stevia
- 1 tsp fresh lemon zest

- ½ tsp sea salt
- 1 tsp grain-free baking powder
- 4 large eggs
- ¼ cup unsweetened almond milk
- ¼ cup butter
- 1 tsp vanilla extract
- ½ tsp lemon extract

 PREPARATION
5 MIN

 COOKING
30 MIN

 SERVES
12

DIRECTIONS

For the Blackberry Filling:

1. Add granulated sweetener and xanthan gum in a saucepan.

2. Stir in lemon juice and water then place it over the medium heat.

3. Add blackberries and stir cook on low heat for 10 minutes.

4. Remove the saucepan from the heat and allow the mixture to cool.

For the Muffin Batter:

5. Preheat your oven at 350 °F and layer a muffin tray with paper cups.

6. Mix almond flour with salt, baking powder, lemon zest, baking powder, and sweetener in a mixing bowl.

7. Whisk in eggs, vanilla extract, lemon extract, butter, and almond milk.

8. Beat well until smooth. Divide half of this batter into the muffin tray.

9. Make a depression at the center of each muffin.

10. Add a spoonful of blackberry jam mixture to each depression.

11. Cover the filling with remaining batter on top.

12. Bake the muffins for 30 minutes then allow them to cool.

13. Refrigerate for a few hours before serving.

14. Enjoy.

Nutrition: Calories 261, Fat 7.1 g, Carb 6.1 g, Fiber 3.9 g, Protein 1.8 g

74. BANANA MUFFINS

INGREDIENTS

- 3 large eggs
- 2 cups bananas, mashed (3-4 medium bananas)
- ½ cup almond butter (peanut butter can also be used)
- ¼ cup butter (olive oil can also be used)
- 1 tsp vanilla
- ½ cup coconut flour (almond flour can also be used)
- 1 tbsp cinnamon
- 1 tsp baking powder
- 1 tsp baking soda
- Pinch sea salt
- ½ cup chocolate chips

 PREPARATION 10 MIN

 COOKING 18 MIN

 SERVES 12

DIRECTIONS

1. Preheat your oven at 350 °F.
2. Line a 12-cup muffin tray with paper liners.
3. Whisk eggs with almond butter, vanilla, butter, and mashed bananas in a large bowl.
4. Stir in coconut flour, baking soda, cinnamon, baking powder, and salt. Mix well with a wooden spoon.
5. Divide this batter into the muffin cups then bake them for 18 minutes.
6. Allow them to cool then refrigerate for 30 minutes.
7. Enjoy.

Nutrition: Calories 139, Fat 8.6 g, Carb 5.5 g, Fiber 0.6 g, Protein 3.8 g

75. PLUM MUFFINS

INGREDIENTS

- 3 tablespoons coconut oil, melted
- ½ cup almond milk
- 4 eggs, whisked
- 1 teaspoon vanilla extract
- 1 cup almond flour
- 2 teaspoons cinnamon powder
- ½ teaspoon baking powder
- 1 cup plums, pitted and chopped

 PREPARATION 10 MIN

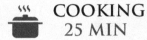 **COOKING** 25 MIN

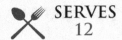 **SERVES** 12

DIRECTIONS

1. In a bowl, combine the coconut oil with the almond milk and the other ingredients and whisk well.

2. Divide into a muffin pan, introduce in the oven at 350 °F and bake for 25 minutes.

3. Serve the muffins cold.

Nutrition: Calories 270, Fat 6.4 g, Fiber 4.4 g, Carb 7 g, Protein 5 g

76. COCONUT MUFFINS

INGREDIENTS

- ½ cup ghee, melted
- 3 tablespoons swerve
- 1 cup coconut, unsweetened and shredded
- ¼ cup cocoa powder
- 2 eggs, whisked
- ¼ teaspoon vanilla extract
- 1 teaspoon baking powder

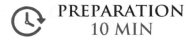 **PREPARATION** 10 MIN

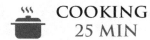 **COOKING** 25 MIN

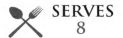 **SERVES** 8

DIRECTIONS

1. In bowl, combine the ghee with the swerve, coconut and the other ingredients.

2. Stir well and divide into a lined muffin pan.

3. Bake at 370 °F for 25 minutes.

4. Cool down and serve.

Nutrition: Calories 344, Fat 35.1 g, Fiber 3.4, Carb 8.3 g, Protein 4.5 g

77. CARROT FLOWERS MUFFINS

INGREDIENTS

- 2 eggs
- 2 cups shredded carrots
- ¼ cup coconut flour
- ½ cup coconut oil
- 1 tsp vanilla extract
- ¼ cup Erythritol
- 2 tsp ground cinnamon
- 1 tsp baking powder

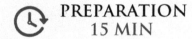 **PREPARATION** 15 MIN

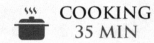 **COOKING** 35 MIN

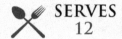 **SERVES** 12

DIRECTIONS

1. Preheat oven to 350 °F.

2. Prepare 12 muffin tins.

3. In your food processor, add in carrots, eggs, coconut oil, Erythritol, and vanilla. Blend together until combined.

4. In a separate bowl, mix together coconut flour, cinnamon, and baking powder.

5. Pour the carrot mixture into the dry ingredients and mix until completely combined.

6. Pour carrot mixture into the muffin tin and bake for about 30-35 minutes.

7. Remove from the oven, and let cool for at least 30 minutes. Serve.

Nutrition: Calories 127, Fat 10.4 g, Carb 3.8 g, Protein 6.5 g, Fiber 0.9 g

78. BLUEBERRY CHEESE MUFFINS

INGREDIENTS

- 16 oz. softened cream cheese
- ½ cup low-carb sweetener
- 2 eggs
- ¼ tsp. xanthan gum
- ½ tsp. vanilla extract
- ¼ cup blueberries
- ¼ cup sliced almonds
- 12-count muffin molds with paper liners

 PREPARATION 10 MIN   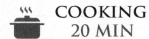 **COOKING** 20 MIN   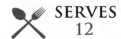 **SERVES** 12

DIRECTIONS

1. Preheat the oven to 350 °F.
2. Blend the cream cheese with a mixer until creamy.
3. Stir in the eggs, sweetener, vanilla, and xanthan gum. Blend well and fold in the almonds and blueberries.
4. Scoop into the molds and bake for 20 minutes.
5. Chill and serve.

Nutrition: Calories 155, Fat 14 g, Carb 2 g, Protein 3 g

79. BROWNIE MUFFINS

INGREDIENTS

- ½ tsp. salt
- 1 cup flaxseed meal
- ¼ cup cocoa powder
- 1 Tbsp. cinnamon
- ½ Tbsp. baking powder
- 2 Tbsp. coconut oil
- 1 egg
- ¼ cup sugar-free caramel syrup
- 1 tsp. vanilla extract

- ½ cup pumpkin puree
- ½ cup slivered almonds
- 1 tsp. apple cider vinegar

 PREPARATION
10 MIN

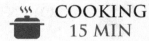 **COOKING**
15 MIN

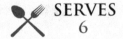 **SERVES**
6

DIRECTIONS

1. Preheat the oven to 350 °F.

2. Put all everything (except the almonds) in a bowl and mix well.

3. Place 6 paper liners in the muffin tin and add ¼-cup batter to each one.

4. Sprinkle almonds and press gently.

5. Bake for 15 minutes or until the top is set.

Nutrition: Calories 183, Fat 13 g, Carb 4.4 g, Protein 7 g

80. SAVORY CHEESE AND BACON MUFFINS

INGREDIENTS

- 1 ½ c. almond flour
- 2 tsps. baking powder
- ½ c. milk
- 2 eggs
- 1 tbsp. parsley, chopped
- 4 chopped bacon slices cooked
- onion, chopped
- ½ c. cheddar cheese, shredded
- ½ tsp. onion powder
- 1 tsp. salt
- 1 tsp. black pepper

 PREPARATION
15 MIN

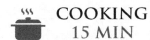 **COOKING**
15 MIN

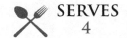 **SERVES**
4

DIRECTIONS

1. Preheat your air fryer to 360 °F.

2. Using a large bowl, add and stir all the ingredients until it mixes properly.

3. Then grease the muffin cups with a nonstick cooking spray or line it with a parchment paper. Pour the batter proportionally into each muffin cup.

4. Place it inside your air fryer and bake it for 15 minutes.

5. Thereafter, carefully remove it from your air fryer and allow it to chill.

6. Serve and enjoy!

Nutrition: Calories 240, Fat 18 g, Protein 17 g, Carb 4 g

81. PEPPER JACK AND CHEESE EGG MUFFINS

INGREDIENTS

- ¼ cup Shredded Pepper Jack Cheese
- 4 Bacon Slices
- 4 Eggs
- 1 Green Onion
- Garlic Powder
- Pepper
- ¼ tsp. Salt
- 1 ½ cup Water

 PREPARATION 15 MIN

 COOKING 15 MIN

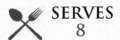 **SERVES** 8

DIRECTIONS

1. Set your Instant Pot to SAUTE.
2. Cook the bacon until crispy (for a few minutes).
3. Wipe off the bacon grease, pour the water inside, and lower the rack.
4. Beat the eggs along with the pepper, garlic powder, and salt.
5. Crumble the bacon and add to this mixture.
6. Stir in the onion and cheese.
7. Pour this mixture into 4 silicone muffin cups.
8. Arrange them on the rack and close the lid.
9. Cook on HIGH for 8 minutes.
10. Wait 2 minutes before releasing the pressure quickly.
11. Serve and enjoy!

Nutrition: Calories 282, Fat 12 g, Carbs 1 g, Protein 24 g

82. CARROT AND PECAN MUFFINS

INGREDIENTS

- ½ cup Chopped Pecans
- 1 cup Almond Flour
- 3 Eggs
- ¼ cup Coconut Oil
- 1 tsp. Baking Powder
- 1/3 cup. Truvia
- 1 c. Shredded Carrots
- 1 tsp. Apple Pie Spice
- ½ cup Heavy Cream
- 1 ½ cup Water

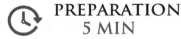 **PREPARATION**
5 MIN

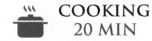 **COOKING**
20 MIN

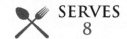 **SERVES**
8

DIRECTIONS

1. Pour the water into your Instant Pot and lower the rack.
2. Place all of the ingredients, except the carrots and pecans, in a mixing bowl.
3. Mix with an electric mixer until fluffy.
4. Fold in the pecans and carrots.
5. Divide the mixture between 8 silicone muffin cups.
6. Arrange on the rack and close the lid.
7. Cook on MANUAL for 15-20 minutes.
8. Do a quick pressure release.
9. Serve and enjoy!

NOTE: This recipe calls for the use of an Instant Pot or Pressure Cooker.

Nutrition: Calories 263, Fat 25 g, Carb 4 g, Protein 6 g

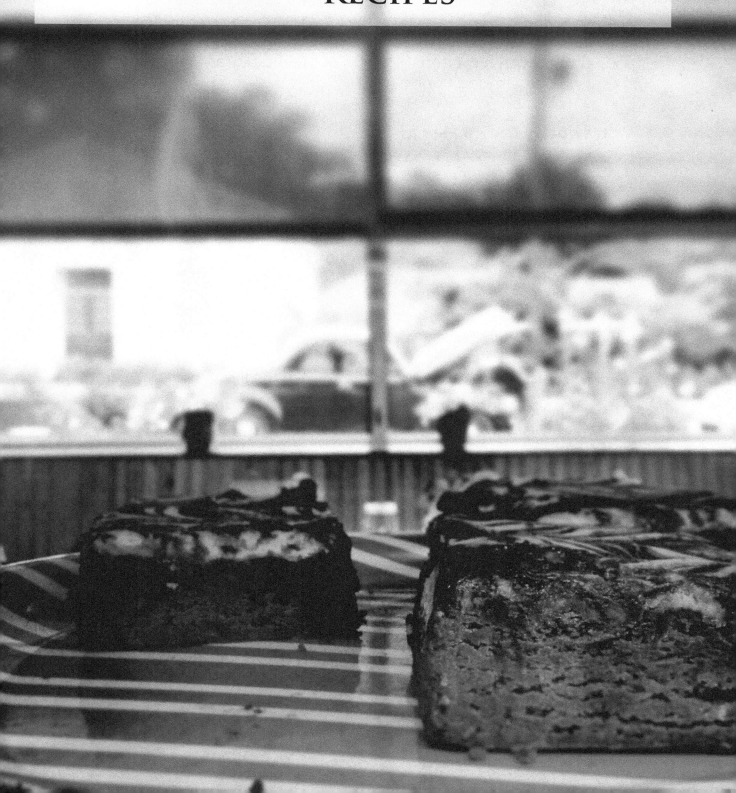

83. STRAWBERRY CREAM PIE

INGREDIENTS

Shortbread Crust:
- ¼ cup powdered swerve
- ¼ cup butter, melted
- 1 ½ cups almond flour
- ¼ tsp salt

Strawberry Cream Filling:
- ½ cup powdered swerve ¼ cup water
- ¾ tsp vanilla extract
- 1 ½ cups fresh strawberries, chopped

- 1 cup heavy whipping cream
- 2 ½ tsp grass-fed gelatin

 PREPARATION 20 MIN

 COOKING 10 MIN

 SERVES 10

DIRECTIONS

1. For the crust, take a mixing bowl of medium size, add almond flour, powdered swerve, salt and mix until combined.

2. Add melted butter to the mixture and mix well to prepare the dough.

3. Transfer the dough to a ceramic pie plate, pressing firmly with your fingers and place in the freezer in the meantime you are getting the filling ready.

4. For the filling, put strawberries and water in a food processer and puree the strawberries.

5. Put pureed strawberries in a saucepan of medium size and stir in the gelatin.

6. Keep at the medium low heat to allow simmering, until the gelatin gets dissolved. Remove from heat once ready and set aside to cool.

7. Mix the powdered swerve, vanilla extract and heavy whipping cream

in a large bowl. Keep mixing until you notice stiff peaks forming and add the cooled strawberry mixture into it to get the filling ready.

8. Take the prepared crust, spread the filling at the top and refrigerate for 3 hours.

9. Remove from the refrigerator once ready, top with cream, fresh berries and enjoy.

Nutrition: Calories 233, Fat 21.1 g, Protein 4.8 g, Carb 6.2 g

84. COCONUT PANNA COTTA

INGREDIENTS

Panna cotta:
- 1 cup canned coconut milk
- ¼ cup cold water
- ½ tsp vanilla extract
- 2 ½ tsp knox unflavored gelatin
- ¼ cup swerve
- 1 cup heavy whipping cream

Raspberry jam:
- 3 tbsp swerve
- 1 cup fresh raspberries
- 1 tbsp chia seeds
- 1 tbsp water

 PREPARATION
10 MIN

 COOKING
10 MIN

 SERVES
4

DIRECTIONS

1. Put together cold water and unflavored gelatin in a small bowl and leave it for 5 minutes or until it gets soft.

2. Put coconut milk, heavy whipping cream and sweetener in a saucepan and heat it over medium heat.

3. Take the hot cream mixture and add softened gelatin in that, stir well until combined, then add vanilla extract to the mixture and keep stirring until fully combined.

4. Take four custard cups, transfer the prepared mixture into them and place in the fridge for 2 hours.

5. Take a saucepan of medium size, add raspberries with 1 tablespoon water in that, keep at medium heat until boil and let simmer for 4-5 minutes.

6. Add chia seeds and sweetener after taking off the heat and place in the refrigerator for 2 hours.

7. Remove from the refrigerator once ready, put raspberry jam and panna cotta at the top and enjoy the delicious coconut panna cotta dessert.

Nutrition: Calories 352, Fat 35 g, Protein 3 g, Carb 8 g

85. RASPBERRY FOOL

INGREDIENTS

- 1 tsp sweet leaf (liquid stevia berry sweet drops)
- 18 oz fresh raspberries, divided
- 1 tsp sweet leaf (liquid stevia vanilla creme sweet drops)
- 1 pint heavy whipping cream
- 3 tbsp lemon juice
- Plain whipped cream for serving

 PREPARATION 20 MIN   **COOKING** 0 MIN   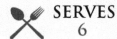 **SERVES** 6

DIRECTIONS

1. Take a mixing bowl, add liquid stevia berry sweet drops and lemon juice and mix together both the ingredients.

2. Add 12 oz raspberries to the mixture, coat well and set them aside for 8-10 minutes.

3. Mix the liquid stevia vanilla crème sweet drops with heavy whipping cream in stand mixer at high speed. Keep mixing until you see stiff peaks appearing at the top.

4. Fold in the coated raspberries gently and set aside.

5. Take 6 serving glasses and adjust some plain whipped cream at the bottom of each.

6. Transfer the prepared raspberry fool evenly to all the serving glasses.

7. Take the remaining 6 oz raspberries and use them for the topping with some plain whipped cream.

8. Refrigerate for some time if you prefer and enjoy the yummy raspberry fool.

Nutrition: Calories 317, Fat 29 g, Protein 4 g, Carb 9 g

86. FLOURLESS AVOCADO BROWNIES

INGREDIENTS

- 1/3 cup cacao powder
- ¼ cup melted ghee
- 1/3 cup lakanto
- 1 medium avocado
- 2 tbsp gelatin
- 3-4 tbsp unsweetened, unsalted almond butter
- 2 large eggs
- 1 tsp vanilla extract
- ½ tsp baking soda
- ½ cup low carb chocolate chips
- ¼ tsp salt

 PREPARATION
10 MIN

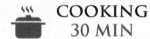 **COOKING**
30 MIN

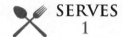 **SERVES**
1

DIRECTIONS

1. Preheat oven to 350°F and get the baking dish ready by lining it with parchment paper.

2. Put cacao powder, melted ghee, lakanto, avocado, gelatin and almond butter in the food processor and process to mix the ingredients.

3. Put eggs, vanilla extract, baking soda, chocolate chips and salt to the mixture in the food processor and blend to prepare the batter. Make sure that you don't over blend.

4. Transfer the batter to the baking dish with the help of a spatula and make it smooth from the top.

5. Place in the preheated oven after topping with chocolate chips if you prefer and bake for half an hour or until you notice the edges separating from the sides.

6. Remove from the oven once properly baked and allow to cool for some time.

7. Cut into pieces of square shape and serve the delicious flourless avocado brownies.

Nutrition: Calories 152, Fat 13.8 g, Protein 6.9 g, Carb 7 g

87. DARK CHERRY CRUNCH PIE

INGREDIENTS

- ½ cup pecan nuts, chopped
- 10 drops liquid stevia extract
- 1 cup desiccated coconut
- ¼ cup erythritol
- 3 tbsp extra virgin coconut oil, melted
- 1 cup almond flour

Topping:
- 1 tbsp Erythritol
- 1 cup almonds, flaked
- 5 drops liquid Stevia extract
- 1 ½ cup dark cherry chia jam
- 1 tbsp extra virgin coconut oil, melted
- 1 cup dried coconut,

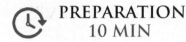 **PREPARATION** 10 MIN

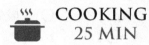 **COOKING** 25 MIN

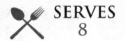 **SERVES** 8

DIRECTIONS

1. Preheat oven to 350°F and get a tart dish ready for baking.

2. Take a mixing bowl, add almond flour, coconut oil, desiccated coconut, chopped pecan nuts and mix until combined.

3. Add stevia and erythritol to the mixture and mix until fully combined.

4. Transfer the mixture to the baking dish and make edges with the help of your fingers.

5. Place in the preheated oven and bake for 15 minutes.

6. Remove from the oven once baked, transfer to a rack and spread the dark cherry chia jam at the top.

7. Mix coconut oil, coconut flakes, almond flakes, stevia, erythritol and salt in a small mixing bowl and sprinkle this mixture at the top of the baked pie.

8. Place in the oven again to bake for 10 minutes.

9. Remove from the oven and transfer to the rack to cool before you serve the delicious dark cherry crunch pie.

Nutrition: Calories 307, Fat 28.8 g, Protein 13.2 g, Carb 8.4 g

88. LEMON COCONUT CUSTARD PIE

INGREDIENTS

- ¼ cup coconut flour
- 1 tsp lemon zest
- 2 large eggs
- 1 tsp vanilla extract
- 1 cup coconut milk, canned
- ¾ tsp baking powder
- ¾ cup erythritol
- 4 ounces unsweetened shredded coconut
- 2 tbsp unsalted butter, melted
- ½ tsp lemon extract

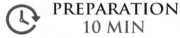 **PREPARATION** 10 MIN   **COOKING** 45 MIN   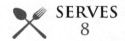 **SERVES** 8

DIRECTIONS

1. Preheat oven to 350°F and get a 9 inch pie dish ready by spraying it with cooking spray.

2. Take a large mixing bowl, add coconut flour, lemon zest, eggs, vanilla extract, coconut milk, baking powder and mix together all the ingredients.

3. Add lemon extract, butter and erythritol to the mixture and mix well until combined. Fold the unsweetened shredded coconut in the mixture.

4. Transfer the prepared mixture to the pie dish.

5. Place in the preheated oven and bake for 45 minutes or until you see that the top is golden brown and the edges are full brown.

6. Remove from the oven once baked properly and allow to cool.

7. Cut into triangular pieces and enjoy the amazing lemon coconut custard pie.

Nutrition: Calories 209, Fat 19 g, Protein 6 g, Carb 4 g

89. BERRY VANILLA JELLO RING

INGREDIENTS

Berry Jello:
- 1 cup water boiling
- 0.6 oz 2 x .3oz sugar free jello raspberry and strawberry
- 1 cup water cold

Creamy Vanilla Jello:
- 1 cup heavy cream
- 1 tsp vanilla extract

- 1 cup water boiling
- 3 tbsp erythritol
- 2 tbsp gelatin powder

 PREPARATION
10 MIN

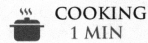 **COOKING**
1 MIN

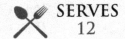 **SERVES**
12

DIRECTIONS

1. For the berry jello, take a heatproof jug and add the jello raspberry and strawberry in that.

2. Add the boiling water and keep stirring until the jello gets dissolved fully and then add the cold water.

3. Take a square container, line it with cling film and pour the dissolved jello into that.

4. Place in the fridge for 60 minutes.

5. Pull out of the fridge once the jello is set and cut into big cubes.

6. For the creamy vanilla jello, take a heatproof jug, add erythritol, gelatin and vanilla extract.

7. Add the boiling water and keep stirring until the ingredients are fully dissolved.

8. Stir in the heavy cream and set aside to cool.

9. Take a silicon ring mold, transfer half of the vanilla jello into that,

spread the cubes of berry jello over that, and then pour the remaining vanilla jello at the top. Place in the fridge for 2 hours.

10. Remove from the fridge once ready, unmold and enjoy the yummy berry vanilla jello ring.

Nutrition: Calories 76, Fat 7 g, Protein 3 g, Carb 1 g

90. NO BAKE COCONUT BARS

INGREDIENTS

- 4 tbsp coconut cream
- 10 tbsp shredded coconut
- 4 tbsp erythritol
- 2 oz chocolate chips

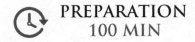 **PREPARATION**
100 MIN

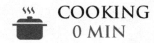 **COOKING**
0 MIN

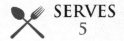 **SERVES**
5

DIRECTIONS

1. Take a small mixing bowl, add coconut cream, shredded coconut, erythritol, keep mixing until you get a crumbly and thick mixture.

2. Take a silicone mold in rectangular shape and transfer the prepared mixture into that, leaving a 0.2 inch space for the melted chocolate.

3. Place in the fridge to chill for half an hour.

4. Melt the chocolate with the help of double boiler and pour it at the top of chilled coconut filling in the silicone mold.

5. Place in the fridge to chill for another half hour.

6. Line a baking tray with parchment paper, get the bars released from the mold and transfer them into the baking tray.

7. Drop some melted chocolate at the top of each bar and place in the fridge once gain for half an hour.

8. Pull out of the fridge once ready and enjoy the delicious coconut bars.

Nutrition: Calories 187, Fat 18 g, Protein 4 g, Carb 3.2 g

91. PEANUT BUTTER BARS

INGREDIENTS

Peanut Butter Base:
- 5 tbsp almond flour
- 4 tbsp granulated erythritol
- ½ cup natural peanut butter
- 1 tsp vanilla extract
- 4 tbsp butter, melted

Topping:
- 2.50 oz sugar-free chocolate
- Chopped peanuts

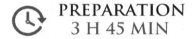 **PREPARATION** 3 H 45 MIN

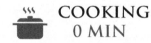 **COOKING** 0 MIN

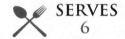 **SERVES** 6

DIRECTIONS

1. Take a large mixing bowl, add almond flour, erythritol, butter, peanut butter, vanilla extract and mix until smooth.

2. Transfer the mixture to the silicone mold, leaving 0.2 inch space for melted chocolate.

3. Place in the freezer to chill for 30 minutes.

4. Melt the chocolate with the help of double boiler and pour a part of it at the top of peanut butter filling in the silicone mold.

5. Place in the freezer again for 2 hours or until the bars get hard.

6. Remove from the freezer once hard, get the bars released from the silicone mold and transfer them to the baking rack lined with parchment paper.

7. Heat the remaining melted chocolate and pour it over the bars,

making sure that each bar is covered completely.

8. Spread chopped peanuts at the top and place in the freezer once again for 1 hour or until hard.

9. Remove from the freezer once ready and enjoy the delicious peanut butter bars.

Nutrition: Calories 315, Fat 27.3 g, Protein 9.7 g, Carb 6.5 g

92. CHOCOLATE MINT PUDDING

INGREDIENTS

- 2 tbsp coconut oil
- 1 tbsp unflavored unsweetened gelatin
- 3 ½ tbsp cocoa powder
- ¼ tsp gluten free mint extract
- ¼ tsp gluten free vanilla extract
- 1 egg yolk, beaten
- 3 tbsp cold water
- 1 ½ cups coconut milk, canned
- ½ cup erythritol
- 1 ½ tbsp Chocolate chips
- 2 tbsp whipped heavy cream

 PREPARATION 3 MIN   **COOKING** 4 MIN   **SERVES** 4

DIRECTIONS

1. Take the cold water in a small bowl, add gelatin, keep mixing using a fork until fully dissolved.
2. Be sure there are no lumps in it and set aside.
3. Add the coconut oil, coconut milk, cocoa powder, egg, mint extract, vanilla extract, erythritol in a saucepan at medium heat and keep whisking until smooth.
4. Add the gelatin mixture after reducing the heat to simmer.
5. Keep whisking until combined.
6. Remove from the heat once ready and set aside to cool.
7. Transfer into the containers once cooled and place in the refrigerator for 4 hours or until pudding is fully ready.
8. Remove from the refrigerator once ready, top with whipped heavy cream and chocolate chips and enjoy.

Nutrition: Calories 248, Fat 25 g, Protein 7 g, Carb 4 g

93. CAULIFLOWER CHOCOLATE PUDDING

INGREDIENTS

- 16 oz cauliflower florets
- ½ cup of water
- 5 tbsp raw cacao powder
- 3-5 tbsp maple syrup
- 2 tbsp MCT oil
- 10-15 drops liquid vanilla stevia
- ½ tsp vanilla extract
- ¼ - ½ tsp salt

 PREPARATION 10 MIN   **COOKING** 180 MIN   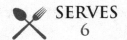 **SERVES** 6

DIRECTIONS

1. Start by adding water to an Instant Pot and seal its lid.
2. Cook the cauliflower for 2 minutes on Manual mode at High pressure.
3. Once soft, add cauliflower and water to a food processor.
4. Blend well then add the remaining ingredients.
5. Blend again until smooth then refrigerate for 3 hours.
6. Serve.

NOTE: This recipe calls for the use of an Instant Pot or Pressure Cooker.

Nutrition: Calories 214, Fat 19 g, Sodium 123 mg, Carb 6.5 g, Fiber 2.1 g, Protein 6.5 g

94. FLAVORED CHIA PUDDING

INGREDIENTS

- 1/3 cup chia seeds
- 1 ½ cups unsweetened almond milk
- ½ cup heavy whipping cream
- 2 tsp banana flavoring
- 1 tsp vanilla extract
- 1 tbsp erythritol

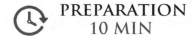 **PREPARATION**
10 MIN

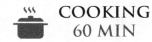 **COOKING**
60 MIN

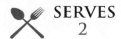 **SERVES**
2

DIRECTIONS

1. Add all the liquid into a jar adding the chia seeds last.

2. Mix well with a fork and cover it.

3. Refrigerate for 1 hour then garnish with coconut chips, chocolate chips, almonds, and berries.

4. Serve.

Nutrition: Calories 282, Fat 25.1 g, Sodium 117 mg, Carb 6.4 g, Fiber 3.2 g, Protein 9 g

95. MINT CHIA PUDDING

INGREDIENTS

- ¾ cup almond milk
- ¼ tsp vanilla extract
- ¼ tsp peppermint extract
- 2 tbsp chia seeds
- 2 tbsp dark chocolate chips

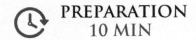 **PREPARATION**
10 MIN

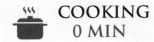 **COOKING**
0 MIN

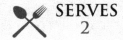 **SERVES**
2

DIRECTIONS

1. Add almond milk, peppermint extract, chia seeds, and vanilla extract to a bowl.
2. Mix and cover it with plastic wrap then refrigerate it overnight.
3. Garnish with chocolate chips.
4. Serve.

Nutrition: Calories 331, Fat 38.5 g, Sodium 283 mg, Carb 6.2 g, Fiber 1 g, Protein 5.1 g

96. DAIRY FREE COCONUT CHOCOLATE FUDGE

INGREDIENTS

- ¼ cup unsweetened almond milk
- ½ cup unsweetened cocoa powder
- ¼ cup powdered erythritol
- ½ cup coconut oil, softened
- 1 tsp vanilla extract
- 1/3 cup unsweetened flaked coconut

 PREPARATION 70 MIN

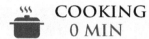 **COOKING** 0 MIN

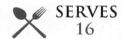 **SERVES** 16

DIRECTIONS

1. Add almond milk, cocoa powder, erythritol, coconut oil in a food processer and process until all the ingredients are combined.

2. Add the unsweetened flaked coconut, vanilla extract to the mixture in the food processer and process until well combined.

3. Take a rectangular shape container and get it ready by lining it with parchment paper.

4. Transfer the mixture to the container.

5. Place in the refrigerator for an hour or until the hardness is achieved.

6. Remove from the refrigerator once ready and get the fudge released from the container.

7. Cut into square shapes and enjoy the delicious dairy free coconut chocolate fudge.

Nutrition: Calories 77, Fat 8 g, Protein 10 g, Carb 2 g

97. CHOCOLATE COCONUT FUDGE POPS

INGREDIENTS

- 2 scoops of chocolate bone broth protein
- One 13 oz can of organic coconut milk
- 1 tsp of organic vanilla extract
- ¼ cup of raw cacao powder
- 10 drops of chocolate flavored stevia
- Dash of pink Himalayan salt

 PREPARATION
180 MIN

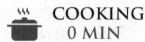 **COOKING**
0 MIN

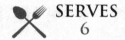 **SERVES**
6

DIRECTIONS

1. Put chocolate bone broth protein, coconut milk, cacao, chocolate flavored stevia in a food blender.

2. Blend on high for a minute or until all the ingredients are blended.

3. Check the taste. You can add little more stevia or salt if needed.

4. Add the vanilla extract and pink Himalayan salt to the mixture in the blender and blend until fully combined.

5. Take the popsicles mold and transfer the mixture evenly into the molds.

6. Place in the freezer for 3 hours or until you are satisfied with the hardness.

7. Remove from the freezer once the desired hardness is achieved.

8. Unmold by keeping in water for few minutes and enjoy the yummy chocolate coconut fudge pops.

Nutrition: Calories 160, Fat 12 g, Protein 8 g, Carb 5 g

98. COCONUT CHOCOLATE BARS

INGREDIENTS

- 1 large egg
- 2 ounces unsweetened desiccated coconut
- 4 ounces unsalted butter, melted
- 3 ounces almond flour
- 1 teaspoon vanilla extract
- 3 ounces surkin gold
- 1 tbsp unsweetened shredded coconut
- ½ tsp baking powder
- 2 tbsp unsweetened cocoa powder

Frosting:
- 1 tbsp unsalted butter, melted
- ½ cup surkin melis
- 2 tbsp hot water
- 2 tbsp unsweetened cocoa powder

 PREPARATION 10 MIN   **COOKING** 25 MIN   **SERVES** 16

DIRECTIONS

1. Preheat oven to 340°F and get a 7x11 baking tin ready by lining with parchment paper.

2. Take a mixing bowl, add cocoa powder, baking powder, desiccated coconut and mix until combined.

3. Add vanilla extract, egg and melted butter to the mixture and keep mixing until fully combined.

4. Transfer the mixture to the baking tin and make it even from the top using a spatula.

5. Place in the oven and bake for 25 minutes or until you feel springing back upon touching.

6. Frosting: add cocoa and surkin melis in a mixing bowl through a sifter.

7. Add melted butter and hot water to the mixture and keep stirring until it is ready to be spread.

8. Remove from the oven when properly baked, spread the frosting at the top and allow to cool.

9. Sprinkle the shredded coconut, cut into bars and enjoy.

Nutrition: Calories 121, Fat 12 g, Protein 2 g, Carb 2 g

99. ALMOND CINNAMON PANCAKES

INGREDIENTS

- 4 eggs
- 2 Tbsp heavy cream
- 3 Tbsp butter
- 3 tsp baking powder
- 3 Tbsp coconut flour
- ¼ cup almond flour
- ¼ tsp nutmeg
- ½ tsp cinnamon
- 2 tsp vanilla extract
- ¼ tsp salt

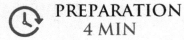 **PREPARATION**
4 MIN

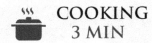 **COOKING**
3 MIN

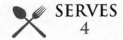 **SERVES**
4

DIRECTIONS

1. In a large bowl, add all ingredients and beat using a hand mixer until a smooth batter forms.
2. Spray the Instant Pot inside with cooking spray.
3. Set the Instant Pot on sauté mode.
4. Pour ¼ cup of batter into the pot and cook for 2–3 minutes.
5. Gently remove the pancake from the pot and make the remaining pancakes.
6. Serve and enjoy.

Nutrition: Calories 231, Fat 18.2 g, Carb 6.3 g, Protein 11.7 g

100. LOW-CARB COCONUT MACADAMIA BARS

INGREDIENTS

For crust:
- 2 ½ cups almond flour
- ½ teaspoon salt
- 2/3 cup Swerve sweetener
- 8 tablespoons unsalted butter, chilled, cut into small cubes

For filling:
- ½ cup butter
- 1 cup coconut cream
- 1 ½ cups chopped macadamia nuts
- 1 teaspoon vanilla extract
- 1 cup Swerve sweetener
- 2 2/3 cups flaked coconut
- 2 egg yolks

 PREPARATION
15 MIN

 COOKING
60 MIN

 SERVES
32

DIRECTIONS

1. To make crust: Add almond flour, salt and sweetener into the food processor bowl. Process until well incorporated.

2. Scatter the butter cubes and pulse until crumbly.

3. Line a large baking (13x9) dish with parchment paper.

4. Transfer the mixture into the baking dish. Press well on the bottom of the dish.

5. Bake in a preheated oven at 350° F for about 20-25 minutes or until light brown. Remove from the oven and set aside to cool for a while.

6. Meanwhile, make the filling as follows: Add butter into a saucepan. Place over medium heat.

7. When butter melts, add sweetener and coconut cream and whisk until well combined.

8. Add nuts, coconut, vanilla and yolks and whisk until well incorporated. Turn off the heat.

9. Spread the mixture over the crust.

10. Bake until golden brown on the edges. The center may look slightly undercooked but that's ok, it will harden when it cools. Cool completely.

11. Cut into 32 bars and serve.

NOTE: Leftovers can be stored in an airtight container in the refrigerator. These can keep for 4 – 5 days.

Nutrition: Calories 198, Fat 15.7 g, Carb 4.9 g, Protein 5.8 g

101. CHOCOLATE CHIP SCONES

INGREDIENTS

- 2 cups almond flour
- 1 tsp. baking soda
- ¼ tsp. sea salt
- 1 egg
- 2 tbsp. low-carb sweetener
- 2 tbsp. milk, cream or yogurt
- ½ cup sugar-free chocolate chips

 PREPARATION 10 MIN   **COOKING** 10 MIN   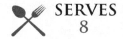 **SERVES** 8

DIRECTIONS

Preheat the oven to 350F.

1. In a bowl, add almond flour, baking soda, and salt and blend.

2. Then add the egg, sweetener, milk, and chocolate chips. Blend well.

3. Pour mixture in the bread machine loaf pan.

4. Place the bread pan in the machine, and select the cookies setting. If not available use pasta dough program.

5. Then press start once you have closed the lid of the machine.

6. Remove dough from bread machine when cycle is complete.

7. Pat the dough into a ball and place it on parchment paper.

8. Roll the dough with a rolling pin into a large circle. Slice it into 8 triangular pieces.

9. Place the scones and parchment paper on a baking sheet and

separate the scones about 1 inch or so apart.

10. Bake for 7 to 10 minutes or until lightly browned.

11. Cool and serve.

Nutrition: Calories 213, Fat 18 g, Carb 10 g, Protein 8 g

Conclusion

Perhaps it is now safe to say that we can enjoy some amazingly sweet recipe on a complete ketogenic diet without actually having any carbohydrates. With all these various recipes, your keto dessert menu will become full of colors and flavors.

With a good understanding of the low carb sweetener and keto substitutes, anyone can enjoy these delectable delights right at home. Just be more vigil while using certain ingredients like the chocolates, flours, and sweeteners, always read their labels to counter check the carb content, since not all companies ensure the standard carb quantity for low carb diet.

I hope that you found this one-of-a-kind cookbook to be valuable for creating a better version of yourself! There are many ways that you can make the best better in your physical life that spills into other aspects as well.

I hope that this book assisted you in gaining the confidence to purchase a pan and uses it regularly! If you wish to become more fit, you must be willing to give up fast food and junk food, for that is no way to fuel the one body you get in this life.

The next step is to put the information you have learned to the test in your life! Pick out a few recipes that caught your eye and make it a priority to take that first step to a better life by making and enjoying them!

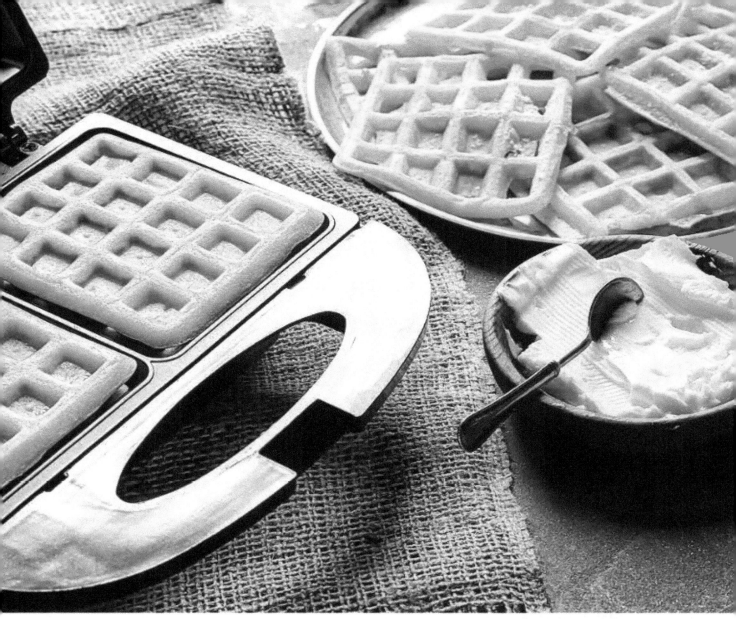

KETO CHAFFLES RECIPES

THE ULTIMATE COOKBOOK WITH 101 EASY RECIPES WHICH WILL
TEACH YOU HOW TO PREPARE DELICIOUS KETOGENIC WAFFLES FOR
YOUR LOW CARB AND GLUTEN-FREE DIET

Amanda White

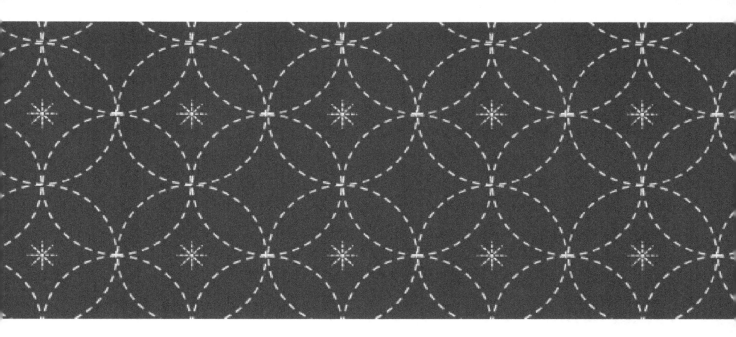

INTRODUCTION

Have you known about "Chaffles"? They've been overwhelming the keto world and, based on how famous they are, and they're digging in for the long haul! This cookbook will assist you in exploring and begin making the best Chaffles in your kitchen ASAP.

A chaffle is a keto dish made with eggs, melty cheddar and seasonings joined and prepared in a chaff producer, to make crunchy, low carb chaffles.

A chaffle can take somewhere in the range of 5-10 minutes to make contingent upon your chaff producer and what a number of you're making.

What sorts of cheddar would I be able to use in chaffles?

You need to be sure the cheddar you're utilizing can dissolve, but at the same time is tight. I prescribe cheeses like cheddar and mozzarella as a beginning stage.

Would you be able to make chaffles ahead?

Truly! You can make bunches early and freeze them for as long as seven days. Warmth them in your toaster, or by enveloping them by a soaked towel and microwaving for 20-30 seconds.

Note: sweet shuffle plans wind up tasting gooey again when re-warmed, so you may need to include a scramble of cinnamon, or some keto-accommodating sugar after it's warmed.

Here's the intriguing thing about this – although the chaff contains no grains, the base of this Keto chaff is cheddar.

- What's more, I realize you see this like, "did this lady extremely simply state cheddar?"
- Indeed – the most excellent stabilizer right now is mozzarella cheddar. Here's the reason?

I was a doubter about this strategy, too, when I saw it spring up on KetoMadMan's Instagram. Cheddar is the ideal base for these due to its adaptability. Mozzarella, specifically, has high fat and protein substance, and it's somewhat salty, so you get that astounding salty-sweet flavor. It's a gentle enough cheddar to use for a creamy formula, which is the thing that I did here. Cheddar additionally gets decent and firm when heated.

Is almond flour vital?

At the point when I tried plans, I attempted with some almond flour and without. What I saw was that chaffles without almond flour has a higher amount of an eggy taste, less structure, and will, in general, appear as though softened cheddar when you cut into them. They do get crunchy outwardly, yet you don't get that genuine "chaff" surface, and the cheddar gets somewhat stringy. Including a limited quantity of almond flour and blending your fixings well decreases the eggy taste, and gives it a higher amount of that "bready" chaff surface.

So, what does this keto chaff have an aftertaste like?

One thing I miss on a keto diet is a crunch. Stuff with a crunchy surface is alright on Keto, yet honestly, there's not at all like a good crunch. I'm happy to state that when you cut into this chaff, you will get that crunch you miss. Bryan said, "if you hadn't revealed to me this was made of cheddar, I wouldn't have known."

Concerning the taste, you can improve it up with your preferred glucose benevolent sugars like Swerve, erythritol, or Monk Fruit, or go flavorful with a smidgen of garlic powder and a more grounded cheddar like a sharp cheddar. It's adaptable.

What are Keto Chaffles without syrup? To me, ChocZero's Maple Pecan has genuinely been a lifeline for me. It's been energizing to, at present, have one of my preferred dishes without the stress.

Tips for Making Keto Chaffles

This is an exceptionally muddled procedure on the off chance that you don't slice the player down the middle before you make them. I had some victories in my chaff producer and cheddar all over the place. Be sure you divide it out to limit flood.

In case you're despite everything stressed over it, I prescribe a Silpat tangle for your ledge. You can put your chaff producer on top, and it makes for simple tidy up if your chaff overflows.

Appreciate the formula beneath and let me realize what you think about these keto chaffles/chaffles.

I got more than a couple of remarks about my syrup of decision. A couple of individuals asserted that Choczero contains maltodextrin. It doesn't. I got enough comments to alert me that something wasn't right, so I went to the source, and they addressed me openly. For me, the syrup had next with no impact on my glucose. I saw an expansion of 1-2 focuses (to analyze, I wake up 20-30 focuses higher doing only resting). Every individual has exceptional needs, so judge your needs and sensitivities cautiously. You can likewise include a sugar-like Swerve on the off chance that you truly need that additional sweetness.

I picked not to and instead utilized a low carb syrup that I feel is sufficiently sweet. This formula can be solidified and warmed in the microwave for 30 seconds – 1 moment. Let it cool for one moment, and the crunch returns right – it's crunchier than crisp, which appears to be a marvel to me! Be cautioned if you freeze it, and the mozzarella enhances more grounded in my tests. Include a scramble of cinnamon and teaspoon of spread on top before you eat it. They're best delighted in new. These can be solidified for as long as seven days in a ziplock sack without air. As indicated by clients, the formula makes four small scales chaffles in the DASH lower than usual chaff producer, or two chaffles in a standard measured chaffles creator. Eat what fits in your macros, yet the sustenance data recorded is for one colossal chaff, which is the serving size. Macros will shift by ingredients. Utilizing full fat, versus skim versus nonfat cheddar can increment or diminishing your nourishment data. This formula used nonfat cheddar, so make sure to recalculate your macros in case you're following intently.

Nourishment Facts

- Calories 150
- % Daily Value*
- Absolute Fat 9g
- Cholesterol 113mg

- Sodium 250.3mg
- Absolute Carbohydrate 6.5g
- Dietary Fiber 0.9g
- Sugars 0.5g
- Protein 10.7g
- Nutrient A 40.2μg

Chapter 1: Basic Of Ketogenic Diet And Its Benefits

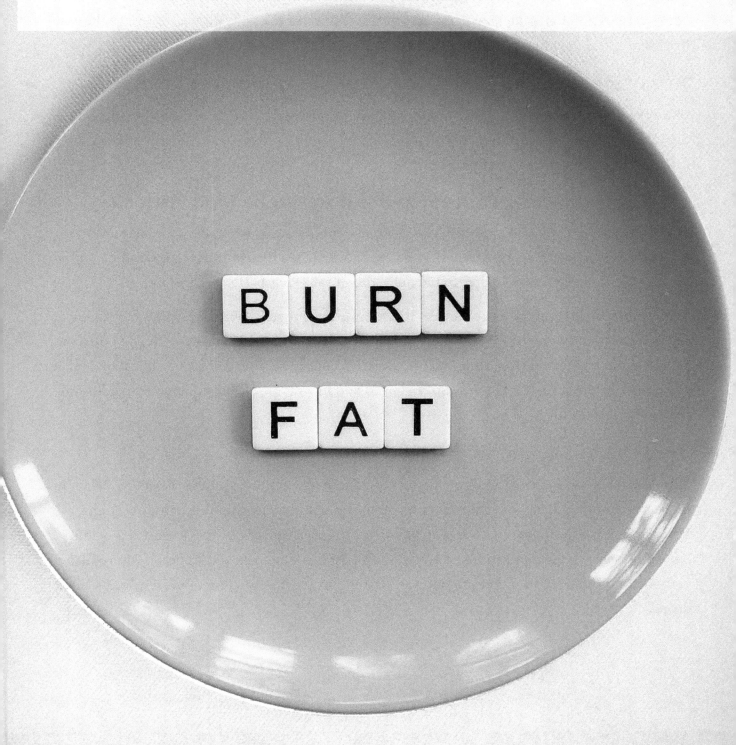

The ketogenic diet is a high-fat, moderate-protein, and low-carb diet. There's nothing very complicated about it. It's a little bit different than the standard low-carb dieting you've heard about because generally people on low-carb haven't worried about their protein intake. With keto, you eat proteins in adequate amounts but keep them in check. We'll see why that's the case in a bit.

But what about all that fat? Is it going to clog my arteries?

The answer for most people is a resounding no. The ketogenic diet is based on a diet of healthy fats. You probably already know the standard litany – omega-3's in fish, and olive oil are right for you, but animal fat, not so much.

Well, guess what. That turned out not to be true either.

Yes, it is true that olive oil is right for you. And so are fish. But what about animal fat? Well, about five years ago or so, researchers got a big shock. When the saturated fat found in animal meats was studied in detail – they found out it didn't raise heart attack risk at all.

So, it's safe to eat a fatty cut of steak. In fact, we encourage it. Basically, you can think of saturated fat as the neutral fat, and olive oil and fish oil are the best fats. It turned out that saturated fat only causes health problems when it's consumed in a diet heavy on carbs. When you're eating low carb, it's just fine. So, go ahead and have some steak and lamb, and add some butter if you want to.

Benefits of Ketogenic Diet

Low carb diets can reduce your appetite. Any diet increases hunger, and this is usually the main problem of dieting. It is the main reason why many people feel unhappy and eventually give up. Perhaps it is an accident that the word diet (nutrition) begins with the word (die) - to die. However, the use of low-carb foods leads to an automatic decrease in appetite. By reducing carbohydrate intake and increasing fat and protein intake, the total amount of calories eaten drops.

Low-carb diets lead to high weight loss. Reducing carbohydrate intake is one of the easiest and most effective ways to lose weight. Studies show that people on a low carbohydrate diet lose weight faster than people on a lean diet, even with substantial calorie restriction.

First of all, fat from the abdomen (abdominal fat) goes. Fat can be stored in different places. The location of fat accumulation determines how it affects our health.

Visceral fat envelops the internal organs and impairs their performance. Excess visceral fat is typically associated with increased inflammation and the development of type 2 diabetes. The Ketogenic Diet is very useful in getting rid of fat on the abdomen.

Significantly lowers triglycerides. Triglycerides are fat molecules that circulate in the blood. It is well known that fasting triglycerides are one of the signs of an increased risk of heart disease. The main reason for the high level of triglycerides in people living a sedentary lifestyle is the consumption of large amounts of carbohydrates, mainly pure sucrose and fructose. When people reduce carbohydrate intake, there is a very sharp decrease in the level of triglycerides in the blood. Also, keep in mind that low-fat diets often lead to an increase in triglyceride levels.

Increasing the level of "good" HDL cholesterol

High-density lipoprotein (HDL) is often called "good" cholesterol. The higher your HDL level compared to "bad" LDL, the lower the risk of heart disease. One of the best ways to increase "good" cholesterol is to eat healthy fat, and low-carb diets contain a lot of fat. It is therefore not surprising that HDL levels increase dramatically on healthy diets low in carbohydrates (for example, keto diets), while, on regular diets, the level of "good" cholesterol rises slightly.

Decreased blood sugar and insulin levels

Studies show that reducing carbohydrates dramatically reduces blood sugar and insulin levels. Some people with diabetes who are starting a keto diet may need to immediately reduce their insulin dose by 50%. In one study on people with type 2 diabetes, 95% reduced or stopped taking glucose-lowering drugs for six months. If you are taking blood sugar medications, talk with your doctor before making changes to carbohydrate intake, as your dosage may need to be adjusted to prevent hypoglycemia.

Normalization of blood pressure

High blood pressure, or hypertension, is a significant risk factor for many diseases, including heart disease, stroke, and renal failure. Low-carb diets are an effective way to lower blood pressure, which should reduce the risk of these diseases and help you live longer. Please note - if you start a keto diet and at the same time take pills to normalize blood pressure, you should consult with your doctor to adjust the dose of the medicine.

Keto diet leads to a reduction in LDL "bad" cholesterol

People who have high "bad" LDL (low-density lipoprotein) have an increased risk of worsening cardiovascular diseases due to vascular problems. However, particle size is important. Smaller particles are associated with a higher risk of cardiovascular disease, while larger particles are associated with a lower risk. Thus, reducing carbohydrate intake can significantly reduce the likelihood of heart and vessel problems.

The ketogenic (keto) diet is used in medicine to treat certain diseases of the brain

Your brain needs glucose, as some of its parts can only receive energy from it. That is why your liver produces glucose from protein if there is not enough carbohydrate (gluconeogenesis). However, most of your brain can also use ketones to generate energy. They are formed during fasting or significant restriction of carbohydrate intake. When the brain begins to receive energy from ketones, it greatly improves its condition and very beneficial effect on many processes. In one study, more than half of children on Ketogenic Diets experienced a reduction in the number of seizures by more than 50%, while 16% completely eliminated all symptoms. Very low-carb diets are currently being studied for the treatment of other brain diseases, such as Alzheimer's and Parkinson's. In the popular health food literature, very little is said about the benefits of low-carb diets, such as Keto Diets. These diets not only improve your cholesterol, blood pressure and blood sugar, but also reduce your appetite, help you lose weight, and lower triglyceride levels. If you are interested in improving your health, you should think about one of the options for such a diet.

Keto and Weight loss

The special form of diet encourages our body to adapt to a metabolic state; this is a unique state in which our body's energy supply derives from ketone bodies present in the blood. As your body begins utilizing fat instead of carbohydrates in the absence of glucose, our body goes into a physiological stage where it either burns fat supplied from food consumption or starts burning existing body fat.

Ketogenic diet pushes your body to maintain the level of carbohydrates as low as possible. By achieving such a low carbohydrate level, it inhibits the release of insulin after food consumption. Such inhibition is helpful in naturally achieving weight loss. In many ways, this unique diet form accelerates the speed at which our body loses weight and helps you in being total control over body weight.

Most ketogenic recipes are not high in protein; it is done on purpose. Fats do not affect on blood sugar and insulin levels in our body. Too much protein is converted to glucose and might increase your blood sugar and insulin level. The extra glucose from the protein can be a hindering factor for your body to go into the stage of ketosis.

Ketogenic Diet: Beyond Weight Loss

Ketogenic diet is not all about naturally losing weight as it promotes holistic health.

Improves Energy Level

When you are on the ketogenic diet, your body will increase the rate at which it oxidizes medium-chain fatty acids. Such physiological change improves your energy level and keeps you charged up to complete your routine tasks. Protein is also known to improve our energy levels. Most ketogenic foods are moderately rich in protein values to help you in being active all day long.

Keto diet promotes overall health by:

1. Promoting clearer thinking
2. Improving control over insulin

3. Facilitating better digestion

4. Promoting lower blood pressure

5. Decreasing stiffness and joint pain

6. Increasing satiety level through and minimizing overall food consumption

7. Improving body metabolism

8. Increasing the level of HDH cholesterol

9. Promoting a relaxed sleep cycle

CHAPTER 2: MAIN INGREDIENTS TO USE FOR KETO CHAFFLES PREPARATION

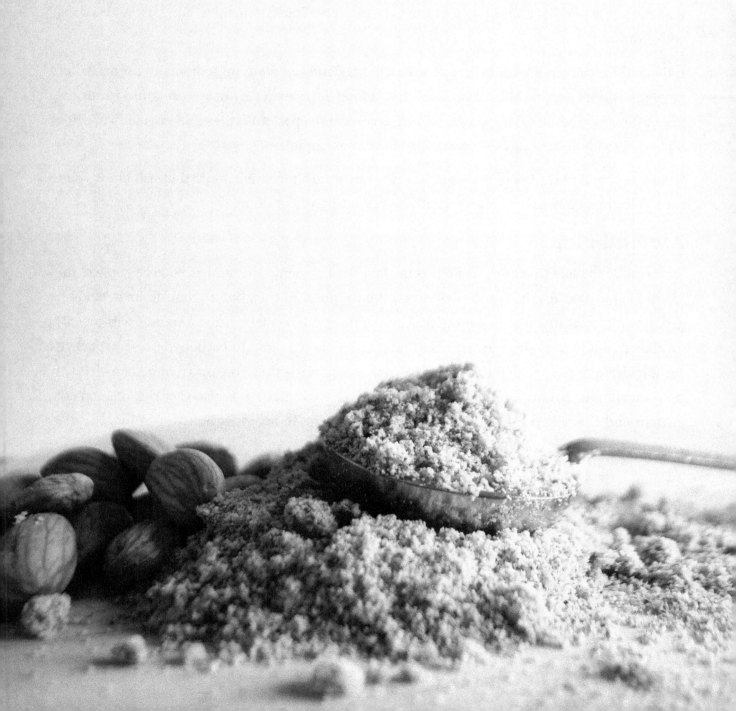

When you start cooking recipes for a ketogenic diet, one of the most difficult challenges is finding low-carbohydrate ingredients. The problem is even bigger when you have to bake bread, cakes, cookies, and similar foods.

Usually, for these purposes, we use wheat flour that gives baked goods the texture we love so much. But, unfortunately, wheat flour, in all its variations, has a very high carbohydrate content that can reach over 75 grams per 100 grams of product. You can imagine how this is absolutely keto-unfriendly!

Indeed, this recipe book deals mainly with Chaffles and the main ingredients to prepare them are eggs and cheese, so the problem of flour is not too severe. However, in some variations, wheat flour is used. Besides, you will also find several recipes of Waffles that normally use flour high in carbohydrates (such as wheat and rice, for example).

So below, you'll find a list of the main low carbohydrate alternative flours that will allow you to cook your own Chaffles and Waffles without regretting wheat flour.

Almond Flour

I won't hide the fact that almond flour is my favorite ketogenic alternative, so here you will find many recipes that use it. You probably could have guessed this, but almond flour is made by grinding almonds into a coarse powder. Almond flour can be made using almonds without skin or blanched almonds. It is an excellent alternative as it is low in carbohydrates. In fact, its carbohydrate content is about 10 grams per 100 grams and is therefore much more keto-friendly than wheat flour (which, I remind you, contains over 70% carbs). It is also very rich in good fats, protein and fiber. If you have diabetes or simply trying to avoid carbohydrates in your diet, almond flour is an excellent choice.

Almond flour is also gluten-free, which is very appreciated by those who have celiac disease or are intolerant. Of course, gluten is very important because it allows the dough to obtain that adorable soft consistency, and its lack is noticeable during baking.

But with some simple tricks, you can overcome the problem. For example:

- replace the wheat flour with the same amount of almond flour (so ratio 1:1)
- increase the amount of leavening agent since the specific weight of almond flour is higher than that of classic multipurpose flour.
- use less liquid in recipes to balance the greater volume.

Anyway, don't worry! The recipes that you will find here, already have all the exact dosages to be able to use almond flour safely.

Moreover, this recipe book concerns Chaffles and Waffles, whose dough does not need the same softness as bread or oven cakes.

Almond flour is best used in recipes such as cookies, quick bread, pancakes and waffles.

Almond Meal

It is a variant obtained using unpeeled almonds. Compared to almond flour, it will have a darker color and a coarser texture. It should be used in the same way as almond flour, and the same indications apply as in the paragraph above.

Coconut Flour

Coconut products are becoming more and more popular on the market; it is no surprise that coconut flour is becoming more popular as well. Coconut flour is created from the inside meat of the coconut being dried and ground into a fine powder. This specific type of flour has healthy fats, high in protein, and low in carbohydrates. If you have a nut allergy, wheat allergy, or diabetes, coconut flour will be an excellent alternative for your baking needs. The one thing you should know before purchasing coconut flour is that it is typically sweet from the coconut. It also has a strong scent of coconut and typically has a finer texture compared to other flours. If you do not like coconut, this taste can be hard to mask. However, this flour is excellent for bread, brownies, and cinnamon buns.

Nut Flours

Nut flours are derived from a variety of nuts (raw or dried) ground to a fine powder. Nut flours bring texture and moisture due to the oils inherent in the nuts themselves and bring about a rich taste. Notable nut flour variants, in addition to the already mentioned almond and coconut flour, are hazelnuts, chestnut, pecans, macadamias... but, as I said, I prefer almond flour.

Oat fibers

Is obtained by grinding the skin and shell of oatmeal grains. It should not be confused with oatmeal, which is derived from the grain itself (separated from the peel) and, due to its high carbs content, is not suitable for preparing ketogenic foods.

Practically oat fibers consist only of ground husks and are generally not used as the main ingredient for baking. The product obtained by grinding the hull is made up of over 90% insoluble fibers and is practically free of carbohydrates and calories.

This type of fiber is known to absorb water easily (up to 7 times its weight). This allows it to bind easily to fat and retain moisture, making bakery products more workable. They are, therefore, ideal in addition to the other alternative flours mentioned in this chapter to improve the consistency of the dough.

Oat fibers also help intestinal regularity and are gluten-free.

Xanthan Gum

Before we move onto the fun part of baking, you must learn that xanthan gum is going to be your new best friend. You may not realize this, but many of the gluten-free flour alternatives lack a binding agent. A binding agent is helpful to hold your food together, much like gluten does when used in baking and cooking. The moment you remove gluten, all mixtures will typically crumble and fall apart. Xanthan gum is made from lactose, sucrose, and glucose that have been fermented from a specific bacterium. When this is added to liquid, it creates a gum and is used with gluten-free baking. As a general guide, you will be using one teaspoon of xanthan gum for one cup of gluten-free flour that you use. For some mixes, this gum is already added, so when you are baking, you will always want to check the ingredient label. It should be noted that xanthan gum can be expensive, but it will last you a long time. If you have an allergy to xanthan gum, you can find ways around it.

Instead, you can try using psyllium husks, ground flaxseeds, or ground chia seeds. Psyllium can be sold in full husks or in powder. As you bake more, you will soon find what works for you and what doesn't! For a quick reference of flours, you can use while baking gluten-free, refer to the list below.

All-purpose Keto Flour

Cooking is nice, but sometimes you're in a hurry and don't have time to do the calculations to replace classic wheat flour with low-carb alternatives.

So, I came up with this mixture obtained with:

- 1 ½ cup almond flour
- ½ cup coconut flour
- ¼ cup oat fiber
- ¼ cup xanthan gum

This is what I like to call my multipurpose ketogenic flour. Just store it in a cool, dry place and use it instead of regular flour. If you don't like oat fibers, you can replace it with same amount of xanthan gum.

Low Carb Baking Mix

If you really don't have time and you don't have any alternative flours with you, the low carb baking mixes can be just right for you. Some of the most famous and easiest to buy online (also on Amazon) are:

- Keto and Co Pancake and Waffle Mix
- Julian Bakery Paleo Thin® Pancake & Waffle Mix
- Carbquik

There are many others, but between those that I have had the opportunity to try, the three indicated above are the ones that gave me the best results.

Since they are pre-packaged commercial mixes, I always recommend following the manufacturer's directions for use. However, I would like to point out that, even though they are quick solutions with more than satisfactory results, I personally prefer to use natural low carb flours.

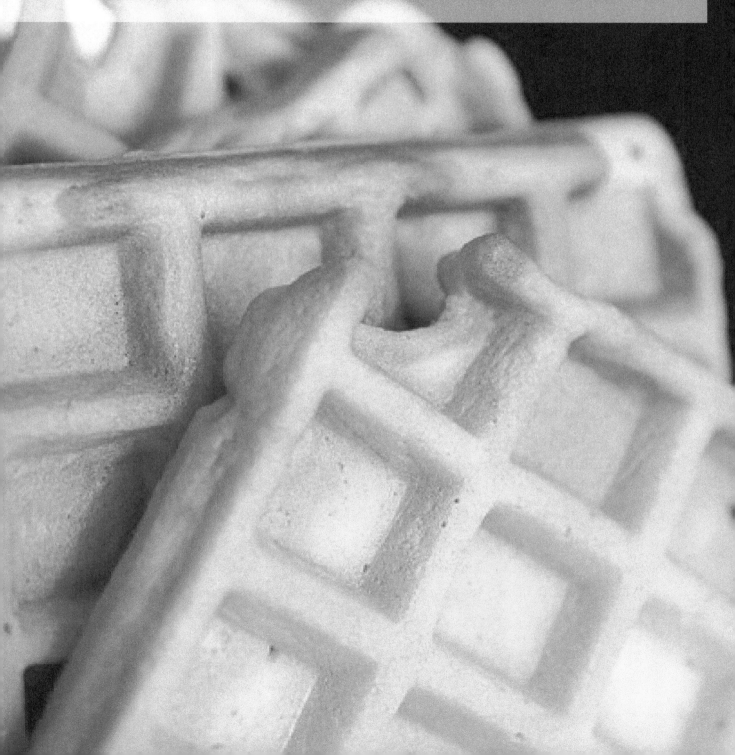

Chapter 3: Brief General Overview Of Main Types Of Keto Chaffles

Can I Replace the Chaffle Ingredients?

Sure! The basic ingredients for the chaffle are eggs and cheese, and everything else is fairly forgiving. You can play freely and exchange things you don't like.

If you are allergic or intolerant to the main ingredients, you have the following options:

Egg Substitution – If you can't eat eggs, you can substitute flax eggs in any chaffle recipe. Stir together 1 tablespoon of linseed with 3 tablespoons of water and leave for 15 minutes to thicken.

Cheese Replacement – I haven't tried it, but there is no doubt that vegan cheese substitutes will work for keto-chaffle shredded and cream cheeses. Check the label to make sure that the number of carbohydrates is still low.

What Are the Ingredients Typical Of a Chaffle?

Some of the usual ingredients you will use for a sweet chaffle are mozzarella cheese, milk, cocoa, cinnamon, almond flour, and low-carb sweeteners such as swerve or allulose. I love mine with a sugar-free salted caramel drizzle!

Mozzarella can be used in savory chaffles, but stronger, saltier cheeses such as cheddar or Colby jack are often combined with ingredients such as garlic powder, all bagel seasoning, tomato, jalapenos, etc.

Chaffle Variations

1. **Plain**. Chaffles are incredible, all alone as a morning meal nourishment. You can serve them up close by bacon, eggs, avocado, and other standard keto breakfast charge.
2. **Keto chaffle sandwich**. Make two chaffles and use them as bread for your preferred sandwich.
3. **Chaffle dessert**. Attempt one of the sweet chaffle varieties recorded beneath and present with keto maple syrup or your most loved keto frozen yogurt.
4. **Sweet chaffles:** Add cinnamon, vanilla extract and low carb sweetener of your choice. We like monk fruit sweetener but erythritol or SWERVE would work as well.

5. **Pumpkin chaffles**: Add pumpkin pie spice, maple extract and low carb sweetener.

6. **Chocolate chaffles**: Add cacao powder or unsweetened cocoa powder, vanilla extract, low carb sweetener and sugar free chocolate chips.

7. **Peanut butter chaffles**: Add peanut butter, vanill extract, low carb sweetener and top with chopped peanuts and a drizzle of peanut butter.

8. **Almond butter waffles**: Add almond butter, vanilla extract, low carb sweetener and top with strawberries, raspberries, blueberries and a drizzle of almond butter.

For Savory Chaffles

- **2 ingredient chaffles**: The original chaffle recipe uses 1/2 cup mozzarella cheese and 1 large egg.

- **Pizza chaffles**: Cook the chaffle batter until crispy then top with marinara sauce, shredded mozzarella, pepperoni, cherry tomatoes and basil. Bake at 375 F until cheese melts.

- **Chaffle sandwiches**: Cook the batter until crispy then stuff with any ingredients you like: Make ham and cheese chaffles, bacon and egg or turkey and cheese waffle sandwiches.

You can alter your chaffle in a wide range of ways. Here are a couple of alternatives.

Various Cheeses

Cheddar, mozzarella, parmesan, cream cheddar, Colby jack - any cheddar that melts well will work with a chaffle. Distinctive cheddar produces different flavors and somewhat various surfaces. Attempt a couple and locate your top choice.

Following some of the most used:

1. **Blue Cheese**: a small crumble of blue cheese contains (1/3 oz) has 32 calories, 0.2 g of carbs, 2 g of protein, and 2.5 g of fat. Blue cheese is produced from cow, goat or sheep's milk

2. **Feta Cheese:** is made of goat's milk, which can make it easier on the stomach even for people who are allergic to cow's milk cheese. ¼ cup of crumbled feta cheese gives 1.5 grams of carbs (none of that is fiber, so it's 1.5 grams net). It is a soft, salty, white cheese. It is made from sheep's or goat's milk. Feta gotten from sheep has it a tangy and sharp taste while the one from goat is milder. It can be used in making chaffles or crumpled over chaffles.

3. **Brie Cheese:** is very high in fat and also melty and delicious on almost everything. It contains 0.1 grams of carbs, 6 grams of protein, and 8 grams of fat per 1 ounce. It is a keto-friendly cheese that can be used in making chaffles.

4. **Cream Cheese:** this is a keto favorite mainly because the only thing it adds is mostly fat. One tablespoon contains 0.8 g of carbs, less than 1 g of protein, but 5 grams of fat, which shows that it is a great addition to a meal or snack when you need more fat. It can also be served with various keto-friendly vegetables.

5. **Paneer:** is a staple cheese, especially in Indian food. About 1-inch cube of Paneer contains 1 gram of carbs, along with 6 grams of protein and 7 grams of fat.

6. **Cheese Curds:** are tasty low-carb snacks in their own right but can also be used in making low-carb diets like chaffles. Apart from being used in making chaffles or as toppings for chaffles, cheese curds can be used in making a keto-friendly breading out of almond meal and some egg, coated and fried. It can also be used at the very end of the cooking period with any kind of roasted vegetables, like broccoli or cauliflower (use keto-friendly vegetables).

7. **Mozzarella Cheese:** is among the best cheese varieties for a keto diet. 1 serving of Mozzarella cheese contains 0.6g net carb, 7g protein, and 6g fat. It also contains bacteria that act as probiotics, which may improve gut health, promote immunity, and fight inflammation in the body. It is a traditionally southern Italian cheese made from Italian buffalo's milk. Mozzarella cheese has a milky sweetness, which makes it great for various cooking, including the chaffles. Mozzarella cheese has a mild enough flavor for sweet chaffles. It is a soft, white cheese with high moisture content.

8. **Cheddar cheese:** it is a relatively hard cheese with a hard texture. It can be sprinkled atop of chaffles or melted into a dip. 1oz of cheddar cheese contains 0.1g carb, 7g protein, and 9g of fat. Its taste depends on the variety, ranging from mild to extra sharp. It is a good source of vitamin K, which is important for heart and bone health.

9. **Swiss Cheese:** originated from Switzerland, it is a semi-hard cheese made from cow's milk and has a mild, nutty taste. 28g/1oz contains less than 1g carb, 8g of protein, and 9g fat. Its sodium content is more than in most cheeses and offers compounds that may help lower blood pressure.

10. **Mascarpone Cheese:** a quality achieved by its especially high percentage of saturated fat. 1oz of mascarpone cheese contains 0.5g carb, 13g fat, and 2g protein.

11. **Ricotta Cheese:** contains 13g fat, 11g protein, and 3g carbohydrate. It is technically made from milk of cows, sheep, goats, or water buffalo. The use of creamy ricotta cheese keeps the chaffles moist on the inside.

12. Other cheese suitable for making chaffles include Tilsit, Roquefort, Gouda.

TIPS

Caution is required in eating some higher-carb cheeses like:

1. Cottage cheese, which contains 5-6 grams of carbs per half a cup.

2. Labneh and any other similar yogurt cheeses which contain about 4-5 grams per serving, depending on the brand and exact style.

Go for full-fat versions of cheeses where possible, and always watch out for packaged shredded cheeses because some of them have anti-caking agents that add carbs to the total.

Exquisite Chaffles

Include exquisite fixings like herbs and flavors to your chaffle. For a pizza chaffle, include oregano, garlic powder, and diced pepperoni in the player, with tomato sauce and additional cheddar on top. Or then again, you could utilize cream cheddar and add everything bagel flavoring to the player for everything bagel chaffle. Present with more cream cheddar on top, tricks, onions, and smoked salmon.

Check out chaffles and concoct your preferred varieties. They're a fantastic expansion to a ketogenic diet and a great deal of enjoyable to try different things within the kitchen, and for motivation and progressively great keto food.

What else changes? Sugar yearnings become non-existent after the initial not many months, Lehner-Gulotta reports. Her patients disclose to her that they feel increasingly fulfilled after dinners, and they're not ravenous constantly. Peruse progressively about how the keto diet helped one lady shed 15 pounds in about a month and a half.

Do you need a claim to fame keto items to do this eating regimen?

If you invest any energy exploring the keto diet, you'll likely stumble into sites, internet-based life posts, and advertisements advancing an assortment of keto-consistent nourishments, from oils that you can add to your espresso to low-carb chocolate syrup. If that feels overpowering, disregard these items and set aside your cash, Lehner-Gulotta says. "You can get into ketosis by adjusting the manner in which you eat; you don't require exogenous ketones," she says.

The combinations for both sweet and savory versions are really endless. In the first 3 to 6 months, a ketogenic diet can help you lose more weight than some other diets. This may be because the transformation of Fat into energy requires more Calories than the transformation of carbohydrates into energy. A high-fat, high-Protein diet may also please you better, so you're eating less, but that's not yet confirmed. Typically, the more common ones are not serious: constipation, moderate low blood sugar, or indigestion. Low-carb diets can result in kidney stones or high acid levels in your bloodstream (acidosis) much less often. Other side effects may include headache, weakness, and irritability; bad breath; and fatigue.

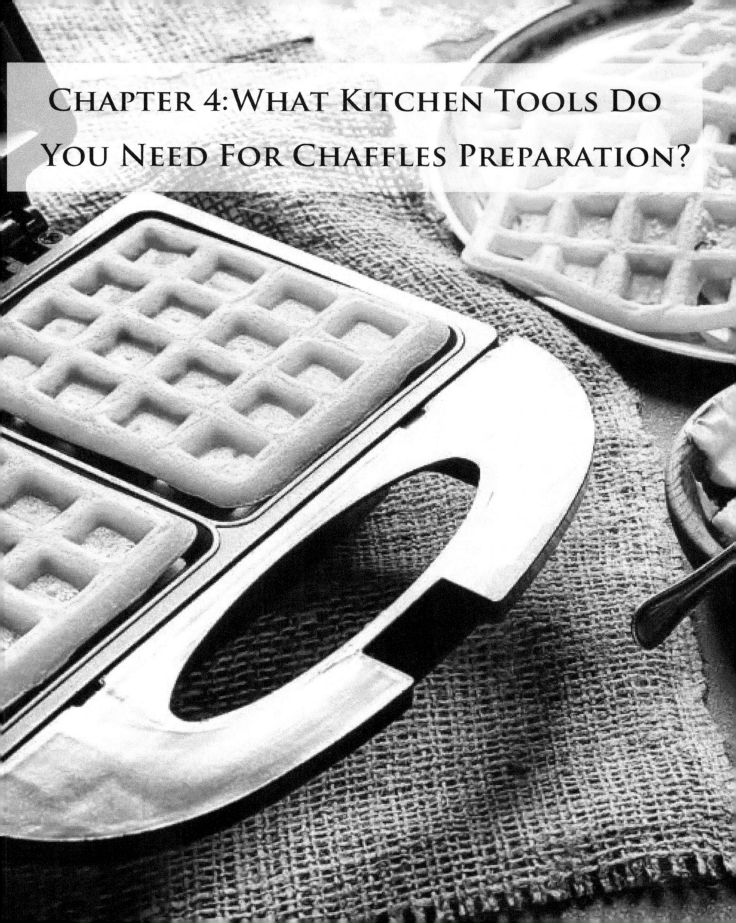

Chapter 4: What Kitchen Tools Do You Need For Chaffles Preparation?

In order to start preparing your Keto Chaffles or Waffles, you need to learn a few basic dough-making techniques and some simple tools. Some of these tools are probably already in your kitchen.

Waffle Maker

Obviously, this is the indispensable tool you can't do without. What Kind of Waffle Maker to Use for Chaffles? A mini waffle iron is perfect for making chaffles as it produces the ideal size (4 inches to be exact), cooks them fast, and crisp them up.

If you do not have one yet, choose the one that has a nonstick coating but chemical-free. The Dash mini waffle maker has recently been gaining popularity in the internet world.

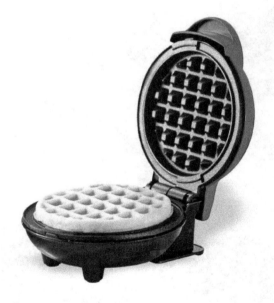

If it is your first time to use this kind of appliance, don't worry because it's user-friendly and will definitely not eat much space in your cupboard.

But if you think using a mini waffle maker is time-consuming because it makes 1 chaffle at a time, you can opt for a waffle maker that can make four chaffles at a time.

Like this one:

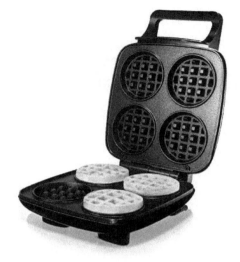

This is ideal for a big family or for someone who would like to cook in batch in order to be able to store ready-made food on the fridge. You can also use a Belgian waffle maker if you have this available at home. Since it is big, you need to adjust the recipe: 3 eggs are to 1.5 cup of cheese. You may also need to brush or spray oil onto the plate of this waffle maker, so chaffle won't stick.

Batter Cups

It is usually supplied together with the waffle maker, the batter cup, is a simple graduated plastic container which, when filled to the indicated level, avoids pouring too much dough into the waffle maker making it overflow.

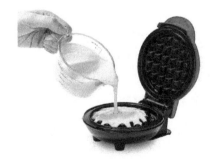

It will help you not to dirty the kitchen. Each batter cup is specific to its waffle maker model.

Batter Dispensers

Similar to batter cups, batter dispensers are just another way to cleanly pour batter onto the grids of your waffle maker. These help to cut down on waste by reducing dripping and splattering during pouring, and they also help you provide consistent results.

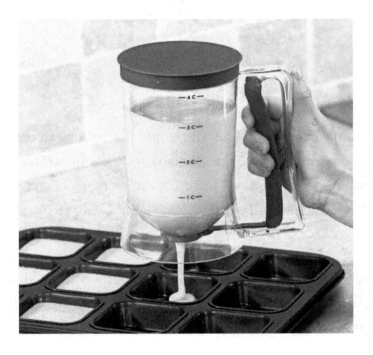

Bowls

I love using the large metal mixing bowl that I found at a restaurant supply store, but any bowl will do. Make sure you have a variety of sizes so you can measure out different quantities of ingredients. Whenever I shop at thrift stores, I like finding small bowls for a few cents here and there to add to my collection. Having little bowls for ingredients in smaller amounts, like salt, yeast, chopped herbs, and so on, is nice, but it's not absolutely necessary—any vessel will do.

Dough Scraper

I recommend getting a metal and a plastic dough scraper. They cost just a few dollars at kitchen stores, at restaurant supply stores, or on Amazon, and they are so useful. A metal scraper is helpful for cutting and scraping dough off your work area, and a plastic scraper is flexible enough to help scrape the dough out of the bowl after rinsing.

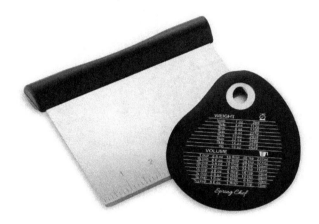

Kitchen Scale

Almost all of the ingredients in the recipes are measured in grams, so you will need a kitchen scale that weighs in metrics. Weighing your ingredients is the best way to get the most consistent results in your baking, and once you get used to weighing your ingredients, I promise you won't want to go back.

It is so much simpler and makes a huge difference in the final loaf of bread.

Kitchen scales are relatively inexpensive these days; small ones can be found for around $20. They typically have a "mode" button that will easily switch them from ounces to grams.

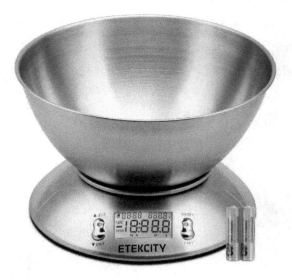

Notebook and Pen

I can't say enough that when you are starting out, different baking results will occur, and you will want to know why you got those results. The only way to find out is to record what you did. Think of it like running a series of scientific experiments. Everything being equal, knowing what variables have changed and what haven't can lead you to where you went right or wrong.

Other items you may need that are usually part of any kitchen:

- Teaspoon
- Tablespoon
- Kitchen towels
- Nonstick cooking spray
- Parchment paper
- Plastic wrap
- Scissors
- Spray bottle

Chapter 5: Keto Chaffles Tips And FAQS For Beginners

Ready to jump at the bar? Basic Chaffles only require a few daily ingredients: eggs and a handful of grated cheese with a little baking soda, if desired, to make it very light. Then you are only limited by your imagination and personal taste.

I personally prefer recipes for chaffles that contain coconut or almond flour for a less moist taste (you can only use protein to get the same effect). Extraordinary breads are even less spicy, use mayonnaise as a binder, and really taste like soft white bread and like a pillow. Sweet spots are seasoned with cream cheese. Optional additions give special notes - for example, cocoa powder, vanilla, chocolate chips and/or cinnamon as a dessert of turkey or meat slices, jalapeno slices, herbal spices or more seasoned garlic spices.

You can double the recipe below to make super tasty waffles (waffles are waffles, right?). But when you use it for sandwiches, the size of a mini waffle maker is perfect. Here are some tips for making perfect recipes:

- Preheat the waffle iron for a few minutes before using it and bring it to temperature.
- Even if your waffle iron is brand new and has a whole Teflon coating, spray the iron lightly with cooking spray or melt melted butter in all angles before adding the dough. If not, the stones can jam.
- Fill the hot iron with a light hand. The dough will come off after you close the lid, and if you mix it with the waffles, the dough will come out, leaving a terrible mess.
- Be patient. Resist the urge to open the waffle iron while still steaming.
- If you are serving more than one serving, keep the grill warm and crispy in the oven at 200 degrees.

- Don't be afraid to be creative. Try different types of cheese, herbs, food supplements, and side dishes.
- Don't check the dirt by opening the waffle iron too fast! You want it to cook until it's ripe and crispy. If nothing else, make the cooking side a little longer than you think.
- You can certainly experiment with other cheeses that are good for keto - goat cheese and halloumi work well - but mozzarella is usually recommended because it's mild and not as high as other choices.
- If you want more protein and flavor, you can also add 1 slice of ham when you mix eggs and cheese. Bacon can also work (enough if you follow a strict keto diet.)
- If you prefer sweet cubes, substitute mozzarella cream cheese. I like this tip! I can't imagine mozzarella on my cakes.
- Sprinkle a little extra cheese on waffle iron before adding the egg and cheese mixture to get a warm, crispy crust. My husband and I love this shrimp and cheese trick.
- It might be difficult to make it super crispy on the plate because the steam from the stew softens them like all waves. They are best eaten or frozen immediately, although I have found that a little almond flour helps the texture.
- Make loot: The mini-wafer maker in the dashboard is available in many good colors at prices under $ 15! You really can't go wrong with a waffle maker. If you don't already have a lot of keto bloggers, you're obsessed with Dash Mini Waffle Maker for Rifles. It is not only inexpensive but also multi-functional and available in many pleasant colors. Plus, it works really well; My best friend has been using it for years to make eggs for her children and swear by it. I personally use my Cuisinart classic waffle maker smoothly - it's only a few dollars more.
- Do more than you need - stains can be stored in the refrigerator for several days. I'm hot using my toaster, but you can also heat it in a pan on your stove.
- There are different variations! After reducing the basics, try some alternative recipes for a nasty touch on your own favorite recipe blog or magazine.

Learn from my mistakes…and successes. These tips should help.

Chaffle making: the most common questions

Who invented the original chaffle recipe?

Sometimes new word variations like 'chaffle' just seem to arrive out of the blue. Therefore it is very difficult to determine the origin of new words. So who really can appreciate disgust is dealing with a serious argument. There are many credit trackers who claim the honor of creating a basic recipe. After all, there are lots of praise and appreciation for baking. Yet it's still pretty ambiguous where the term first manifested.

How many eggs do I need to make chaffle?

One free egg is usually enough for two mini waffles. After adding the mixture to your keto iron, you can prepare one egg sandwich. We recommend native chicken eggs because chickens have a better life. Waffle irons are available in a variety of kitchen-friendly colors, and waffles come out perfectly every time. I pressed the blue model. For clarity, there is no difference between a glass and a waffle maker for making husks. The last recipe is different, and both work with your device. Several derived terms are united in occasional conversation. Then get involved in social media, which quickly becomes fashionable and viral. Bloggers and influencers, hoping to gain additional excellence, popularized the word and snowball. This can happen flexibly, and only time will tell who really gets the loan.

Why does everyone use Storebound Dash Maker?

Many people do this because they have seen many creators on YouTube, and bloggers use it. Dash is not the only waffle maker on the planet. They are, of course, a great product, but you can use any waffle maker. I have seen many people pull some good devices from their garage and pursue themselves as professionals. Don't you have a waffle iron that you haven't touched since you received it from your aunt as a wedding gift more than ten years ago?

Can you freeze the chaffle? Can you warm the barrier?

Of course! Whatever plastic you think is good in the freezer will work. Even freezer bags. If this is a basic grill, allow it to cool before putting it in the freezer. The heat and condensation make them sticky. For other stones coated with crazy materials, you might want to split them with parchment paper. If you heat up, you might want to avoid microwaves unless you don't care. You will become pliers! The best way is to use a toaster, hot air container, deep frying pan, or frying pan in the oven. So in many cases, you can. I have no problem with freezing it. But the truth is they are so simple that they don't need time to defeat them! I think the air fryer is the best for warming up and makes your shrimp feel fresher when you get home.

Looking for other storage ideas or tools?

If it's more than an egg and cheese, is it still disgusting? That seems to be a V-Sauce question. Okay, it's not my fault that people scream like that, but I can't create new groups and websites for every new version of this. People take ideas and improve them. That's why the internet is used. Exchange ideas and help each other. For organizational purposes, we will call them all chaffles if it is relative enough, and we will throw them on the waffle iron.

When do you eat chaffle?

Most often, fruits are a recipe for breakfast. However, there are no hard and fast rules unless you fast. Prepare soup for lunch or dinner if you suddenly feel like it.

Like chaffle tastes like eggs?

It all depends on how many eggs you want in your breakfast recipe. I find that most grills taste crisp, light, and crispy. The best advice is to experiment with different combinations and numbers of eggs.

Pro tip - If you sprinkle cheese on your waffle iron before you put the mixture in it, the tip of your grill will be fresher and fresher.

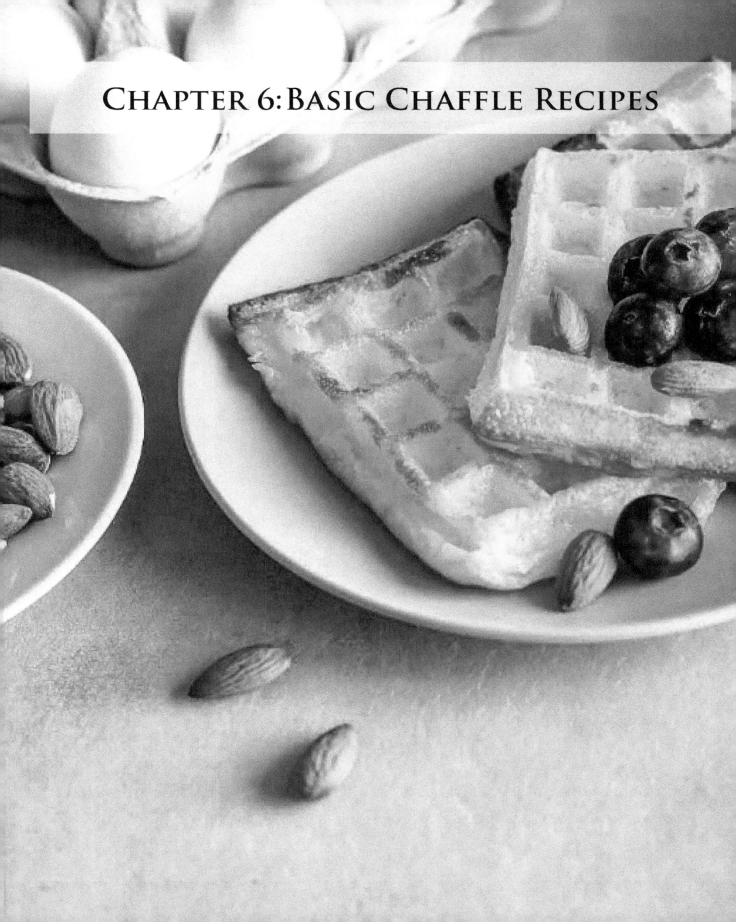

CHAPTER 6: BASIC CHAFFLE RECIPES

1. BUTTER & CREAM CHEESE CHAFFLES

INGREDIENTS

- 2 tablespoons butter, melted and cooled
- 2 large organic eggs
- 2 ounces cream cheese, softened
- ¼ cup powdered erythritol
- 1½ teaspoons organic vanilla extract
- Pinch of salt
- ¼ cup almond flour
- 2 tablespoons coconut flour
- 1 teaspoon organic baking

 PREPARATION 10 MIN

 COOKING 16 MIN

 SERVES 4

DIRECTIONS

1. Preheat a mini waffle iron and then grease it.

2. In a bowl, add the butter and eggs and beat until creamy.

3. Add the cream cheese, erythritol, vanilla extract, and salt, and beat until well combined.

4. Add the flours and baking powder and beat until well combined.

5. Place ¼ of the mixture into preheated waffle iron and cook for about 4 minutes.

6. Repeat with the remaining mixture.

7. Serve warm.

Nutrition: Calories 217, Net Carbs 3.3 g, Total Fat 18 g, Saturated Fat 8.8 g, Cholesterol 124 mg, Sodium 173 mg, Total Carbs 6.6 g, Fiber 3.3 g, Sugar 1.2 g, Protein 5.3 g

2. PEANUT BUTTER CHAFFLES

INGREDIENTS

- 1 organic egg, beaten
- ½ cup mozzarella cheese, shredded
- 3 tablespoons granulated erythritol
- 2 tablespoons peanut butter

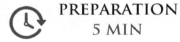 **PREPARATION**
5 MIN

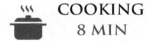 **COOKING**
8 MIN

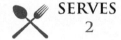 **SERVES**
2

DIRECTIONS

1. Preheat a mini waffle iron and then grease it.
2. In a medium bowl, put all ingredients and with a fork, mix until well combined.
3. Place half of the mixture into preheated waffle iron and cook for about 4 minutes.
4. Repeat with the remaining mixture.
5. Serve warm.

Nutrition: Calories 145, Net Carbs 2.6 g, Total Fat 11.5 g, Saturated Fat 3.1 g, Cholesterol 86 mg, Sodium 147 mg, Total Carbs 3.6 g, Fiber 1 g, Sugar 1.7 g, Protein 8.8 g

3. ALMOND BUTTER CHAFFLES

INGREDIENTS

- 1 large organic egg, beaten
- 1/3 cup mozzarella cheese, shredded
- 1 tablespoon erythritol
- 2 tablespoons almond butter
- 1 teaspoon organic vanilla extract

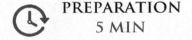 **PREPARATION**
5 MIN

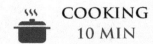 **COOKING**
10 MIN

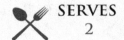 **SERVES**
2

DIRECTIONS

9. Preheat a mini waffle iron and then grease it.
10. In a medium bowl, put all ingredients and with a fork, mix until well combined.
11. Place half of the mixture into preheated waffle iron and cook for about 3–5 minutes.
12. Repeat with the remaining mixture.
13. Serve warm.

Nutrition: Calories 153, Net Carbs 2 g, Total Fat 12.3 g, Saturated Fat 2 g, Cholesterol 96 mg, Sodium 65 mg, Total Carbs 3.6 g, Fiber 1.6 g, Sugar 1.2 g, Protein 7.9 g

4. CINNAMON CHAFFLES

INGREDIENTS

For Chaffles:
- 1 large organic egg, beaten
- ¾ cup mozzarella cheese, shredded
- ½ tablespoon unsalted butter, melted
- 2 tablespoons blanched almond flour
- 2 tablespoons erythritol
- ½ teaspoon ground cinnamon
- ½ teaspoon Psyllium husk powder

- ¼ teaspoon organic baking powder
- ½ teaspoon organic vanilla extract

For Topping:
- 1 teaspoon powdered Erythritol
- ¾ teaspoon ground cinnamon ¾ cup mozzarella cheese, shredded

 PREPARATION
10 MIN

 COOKING
8 MIN

 SERVES
2

DIRECTIONS

1. Preheat a waffle iron and then grease it.

2. For chaffles: In a medium bowl, put all ingredients and with a fork, mix until well combined.

3. Place half of the mixture into preheated waffle iron and cook for about 3–5 minutes.

4. Repeat with the remaining mixture.

5. Meanwhile, for topping: in a small bowl, mix together the erythritol and cinnamon.

6. Place the chaffles onto serving plates and set aside to cool slightly.

7. Sprinkle with the cinnamon mixture and serve immediately.

Nutrition: Calories 142, Net Carbs 2.1 g, Total Fat 10.6 g, Saturated Fat 4 g, Cholesterol 106 mg, Sodium 122 mg, Total Carbs 4.1 g, Fiber 2 g, Sugar 0.3 g, Protein 7.7 g

5. LAYERED CHAFFLES

INGREDIENTS

- 1 organic egg, beaten and divided
- ½ cup cheddar cheese, shredded and divided
- Pinch of salt

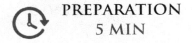 **PREPARATION** 5 MIN

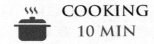 **COOKING** 10 MIN

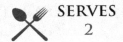 **SERVES** 2

DIRECTIONS

13. Preheat a mini waffle iron and then grease it.

14. Place about 1/8 cup of cheese in the bottom of the waffle iron and top with half of the beaten egg.

15. Now, place 1/8 cup of cheese on top and cook for about 4–5 minutes.

16. Repeat with the remaining cheese and egg.

17. Serve warm.

Nutrition: Calories 145, Net Carbs 0.5 g, Total Fat 11.6 g, Saturated Fat 6.6 g, Cholesterol 112 mg, Sodium 284 g, Total Carbs 0.5 g, Fiber 0 g, Sugar 0.3 g, Protein 9.8 g

6. BLUEBERRY CREAM CHEESE CHAFFLES

INGREDIENTS

- 1 organic egg, beaten
- 1/3 cup mozzarella cheese, shredded
- 1 teaspoon cream cheese, softened
- 1 teaspoon coconut flour
- ¼ teaspoon organic baking powder
- ¾ teaspoon powdered erythritol
- ¼ teaspoon ground cinnamon
- ¼ teaspoon organic vanilla
- Pinch of salt
- 1 tablespoon fresh blueberries

 PREPARATION
10 MIN

 COOKING
8 MIN

 SERVES
2

DIRECTIONS

3. Preheat a mini waffle iron and then grease it.

4. In a bowl, place all ingredients except for blueberries and beat until well combined.

5. Fold in the blueberries.

6. Place half of the mixture into preheated waffle iron and cook for about 4 minutes.

7. Repeat with the remaining mixture.

8. Serve warm.

Nutrition: Calories 90, Net Carbs 2.9 g, Total Fat 5 g, Saturated Fat 2.7 g, Cholesterol 97 mg, Sodium 161 mg, Total Carbs 5.7 g, Fiber 2.8 g, Sugar 1.2 g, Protein 5.7 g

7. RASPBERRY CHAFFLES

INGREDIENTS

- 1 organic egg, beaten
- 1 tablespoon cream cheese, softened
- ½ cup mozzarella cheese, shredded
- 1 tablespoon powdered erythritol
- ¼ teaspoon organic raspberry extract
- ¼ teaspoon organic vanilla extract

 PREPARATION
10 MIN

 COOKING
8 MIN

 SERVES
2

DIRECTIONS

1. Preheat a mini waffle iron and then grease it.

2. In a medium bowl, put all ingredients and with a fork, mix until well combined.

3. Place half of the mixture into preheated waffle iron and cook for about 4 minutes.

4. Repeat with the remaining mixture.

5. Serve warm.

Nutrition: Calories 69, Net Carbs 0.6 g, Total Fat 5.2 g, Cholesterol 91 mg, Sodium 88 mg, Total Carbs 0.6 g, Fiber 0 g, Sugar 0.2 g, Protein 5.2 g

8. RED VELVET CHAFFLES

INGREDIENTS

- 2 tablespoons cacao powder
- 2 tablespoons erythritol
- 1 organic egg, beaten
- 2 drops super red food coloring
- ¼ teaspoon organic baking powder
- 1 tablespoon heavy whipping cream

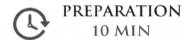 **PREPARATION** 10 MIN

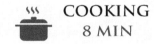 **COOKING** 8 MIN

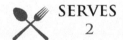 **SERVES** 2

DIRECTIONS

10. Preheat a mini waffle iron and then grease it.

11. In a medium bowl, put all ingredients and with a fork, mix until well combined.

12. Place half of the mixture into preheated waffle iron and cook for about 4 minutes.

13. Repeat with the remaining mixture.

14. Serve warm.

Nutrition: Calories 70, Net Carbs 1.7 g, Total Fat 6 g, Saturated Fat 3 g, Cholesterol 92 mg, Sodium 34 mg, Total Carbs 3.2 g, Fiber 1.5 g, Sugar 0.2 g, Protein 3.9 g

9. WALNUT PUMPKIN CHAFFLES

INGREDIENTS

- 1 organic egg, beaten
- ½ cup mozzarella cheese, shredded
- 2 tablespoons almond flour
- 1 tablespoon sugar-free pumpkin puree
- 1 teaspoon erythritol
- ¼ teaspoon ground cinnamon
- 2 tablespoons walnuts, toasted and chopped

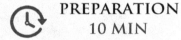 **PREPARATION** 10 MIN   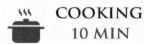 **COOKING** 10 MIN   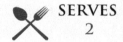 **SERVES** 2

DIRECTIONS

1. Preheat a mini waffle iron and then grease it.

2. In a bowl, add all ingredients except pecans and beat until well combined.

3. Fold in the walnuts.

4. Place half of the mixture into preheated waffle iron and cook for about 5 minutes.

5. Repeat with the remaining mixture. Serve warm.

Nutrition: Calories 148, Net Carbs 1.6 g, Total Fat 11.8 g, Cholesterol 86 mg, Sodium 74 mg, Total Carbs 3.3 g, Fiber 1.7 g, Sugar 0.8 g, Protein 6.7 g

10. PUMPKIN CREAM CHEESE CHAFFLES

INGREDIENTS

- 1 organic egg, beaten
- ½ cup mozzarella cheese, shredded
- 1½ tablespoon sugar-free pumpkin puree
- 2 teaspoons heavy cream
- 1 teaspoon cream cheese, softened
- 1 tablespoon almond flour
- 1 tablespoon erythritol
- ½ teaspoon pumpkin pie spice
- ½ teaspoon organic baking powder
- 1 teaspoon organic vanilla extract

 PREPARATION 10 MIN

 COOKING 10 MIN

 SERVES 2

DIRECTIONS

1. Preheat a mini waffle iron and then grease it.
2. In a medium bowl, put all ingredients and, with a fork, mix until well combined.
3. Place half of the mixture into preheated waffle iron and cook for about 3–5 minutes.
4. Repeat with the remaining mixture.
5. Serve warm.

Nutrition: Calories 110, Net Carbs 2.5 g, Total Fat 7.8 g, Saturated Fat 3.1 g, Cholesterol 94 mg, Sodium 82 mg, Total Carbs 3.3 g, Fiber 0.8 g, Sugar 1 g, Protein 5.2 g

11. BASIC CHAFFLES RECIPE

INGREDIENTS

- 1 large egg
- 1/2 cup mozzarella cheese finely chopped

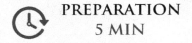 **PREPARATION**
5 MIN

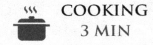 **COOKING**
3 MIN

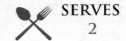 **SERVES**
2

DIRECTIONS

1. Connect a waffle maker and heat.

2. Break the eggs into small bowls and beat with a fork. Add mozzarella cheese and mix.

3. Spray the non-stick spray on the waffle iron.

4. Pour half of the egg mixture into a heated waffle iron and cook for 2-3 minutes.

5. Carefully remove the waffle and cook the remaining dough.

6. Serve warm with butter and sugar-free syrup.

Note: Try adding a little vanilla or cinnamon for the next level of breakfast chaffle!

Nutrition: Calories 202, Total Fat 13 g, Saturated Fat 6 g, Trans Fat 0 g, Unsaturated Fat 5 g, Cholesterol 214 mg, Sodium 364 mg, Carbohydrates 3 g, Net Carbohydrates 3 g, Fiber 0 g, Sugar 1 g, Sugar Alcohols 0 g, Protein 16 g

12. PUMPKIN CHAFFLES

INGREDIENTS

- 1/2 oz cream cheese
- One large egg
- 1/2 cup mozzarella cheese (shredded)
- 2 tablespoons pumpkin puree
- 2 1/2 tablespoons erythritol
- 3 tsp coconut flour
- 1/2 tbsp pumpkin pie spice
- 1/2 teaspoon of vanilla essence (optional)
- 1/4 teaspoon baking powder (optional)

 PREPARATION 5 MIN

 COOKING 5 MIN

 SERVES 2

DIRECTIONS

1. Preheat the waffle iron for about 5 minutes until hot.

2. If your recipe includes cream cheese, put it in a bowl first. Gently heat in a microwave (15-30 seconds) or double boiler until soft and stir.

3. Stir all remaining ingredients (except toppings, if any).

4. Pour a sufficient amount of chaffle dough into the waffle maker and cover the surface firmly. (For a normal waffle maker, about 1/2 cup, for a mini waffle maker, about 1/4 cup.)

5. Cook for about 3-4 minutes until brown and crisp.

6. Carefully remove the chaffle from the waffle maker and set aside for a crisp noise. (Cooling is important for the texture!) If there is any dough, repeat with the remaining dough.

Nutrition: Calories 208, Fat 16 g, Protein 11 g, Total carbs 4 g, Pure carbohydrates 2 g, Fiber 2 g, Sugar 0 g

13. KETO BELGIAN CHAFFLE

INGREDIENTS

- 2 large eggs
- 1.5 C shred cheddar/jack cheese (other cheeses can be substituted)

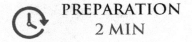 **PREPARATION** 2 MIN

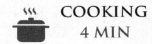 **COOKING** 4 MIN

 **SERVES** 2

DIRECTIONS

1. Preheat by inserting a waffle iron. While heating, break the eggs into small bowls, whisk and mix.

2. Next, add the shredded cheese and mix.

3. Pour the chaffle dough evenly into the preheated waffle iron. Each waffle cavity can be completely filled. This fabric expands, but not as much as regular waffle fabric.

4. Close the waffle iron lid and cook for 4 minutes.

5. When ready, lift the lid and pierce the end of the chaffle and remove it. This creates two Belgian-sized chaffles.

Nutrition: Calories 87, Total Fat 5.7 g, Cholesterol 104 mg, Sodium 136.9 mg, Total Carbohydrate 2.8 g, Dietary Fiber 0.2 g, Sugars 1.1 g, Protein 6.3g

14.GRILLED CHEESE CHAFFLE

INGREDIENTS

- 1 egg
- ¼ teaspoon garlic powder
- ½ cup shred cheddar
- 2 American cheese or ¼ cup shredded cheese
- 1 tablespoon butter

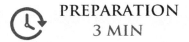
PREPARATION
3 MIN

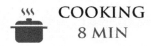
COOKING
8 MIN

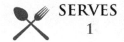
SERVES
1

DIRECTIONS

1. In a small bowl, mix bacon, garlic powder and shredded cheddar cheese.

2. After heating the dash waffle maker, add half the mixture of the scramble. Cook and cook for 4 minutes.

3. Add the remainder of the scramble mixture and cook for 4 minutes.

4. Steam the stove pan over moderate heat when both chaffles are finished.

5. Attach 1 spoonful of butter and dissolve.

6. Place one chaffle in the pan once the butter has melted.

7. Place your favorite cheese on top of the chaffle and finish with a second chaffle.

8. Cook the chaffle for 1 minute on the first side, turn it over and cook for another 1-2 minutes on the other side to finish the cheese melting.

9. Cut it from the bread when the cheese melts and eat it!

Nutrition: Calories 549 kcal, Carbohydrates 3 g, Protein 27 g, Fats 48 g, Saturated Fats 28 g, Cholesterol 295mg, Sodium 1216 mg, Potassium 172 mg, Sugar 1 g

15. GARLIC PARMESAN CHAFFLE

INGREDIENTS

- 1/2 cup mozzarella cheese (shredded)
- 1/3 cup grated parmesan cheese
- 1 large egg
- 1 piece of garlic (chopped or used 1/2 to reduce the flavor of garlic)
- 1/2 tsp Italian seasoning
- 1/4 teaspoon baking powder (optional)

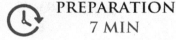 **PREPARATION** 7 MIN   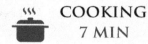 **COOKING** 7 MIN   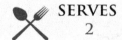 **SERVES** 2

DIRECTIONS

1. Preheat the waffle iron for about 5 minutes until hot.

2. If your recipe includes cream cheese, put it in a bowl first. Gently heat in a microwave (15-30 seconds) or double boiler until soft and stir.

3. Stir all remaining ingredients.

4. Pour a sufficient amount of chaffle dough into the waffle maker and cover the surface firmly. (For a normal waffle maker, about 1/2 cup, for a mini waffle maker, about 1/4 cup.)

5. Cook for about 3-4 minutes until brown and crisp.

6. Carefully remove the chaffle from the waffle maker and set aside for a crisp noise. (Cooling is important for the texture!) If there is any dough, repeat.

Nutrition: Calories 208, Fat 16 g, Protein 11 g, Total carbs 4 g, Pure carbohydrates 2 g, Fiber 2 g, Sugar 0 g

16. TRADITIONAL KETO LOW CARB CHAFFLE

INGREDIENTS

- 1 egg
- 1/2 cup shredded cheddar cheese

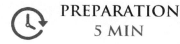 **PREPARATION**
5 MIN

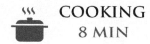 **COOKING**
8 MIN

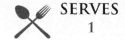 **SERVES**
1

DIRECTIONS

7. Turn on or plug in the waffle maker, heat and grease both sides.

8. After breaking the eggs in a small bowl, add 1/2 cup of cheddar cheese and mix.

9. Pour half of the dough into the waffle maker and close the top.

10. Cook for 3-4 minutes or until the desired degree of baking is achieved.

11. Carefully remove from the waffle maker and leave for 2-3 minutes to give time to crisp.

Follow the Directions again to make a second chaffle.

This recipe of traditional chaffle makes a great sandwich.

Nutrition: Calories 291 kcal, Carbohydrates 1 g, Protein 20 g, Fat 23 g, Saturated Fat 13 g, Cholesterol 223 mg, Sodium 413 mg, Potassium 116 mg, Sugar 1 g, Iron 1 mg

17. CHAFFLE BREAKFAST SANDWICH

INGREDIENTS

For chaffle:
- 1 egg
- 1/2 cup of mozzarella cheese
- 2 tablespoons almond flour

For sandwiches:
- 1 egg
- One slice of cheese
- Two slices of bacon

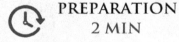 **PREPARATION**
2 MIN

 COOKING
7 MIN

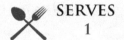 **SERVES**
1

DIRECTIONS

1. Preheat the iron of your waffle.

2. When preheating the waffle iron, bring together in a bowl the milk, egg, and almond flour.

3. Using Cooking Spray, spray the waffle iron and pour the batter over the waffle iron.

4. Open it and let it steam for the waffle.

5. Fry the bacon in a pan while the waffle is frying. Make any kind of egg you want. Cook the microwave bacon.

6. Bring your breakfast sandwich together and eat it!

Nutrition: Calories 493, Sugar 2g, Fat 32 g, Saturated Fat 11 g, Carbohydrate 6 g, Fiber 3 g, Protein 46 g

18. SPICY JALAPENO POPPER CHAFFLE

INGREDIENTS

- 1 oz cream cheese
- One large egg
- 1 cup cheddar cheese (shredded)
- 2 tablespoons bacon bit
- 1/2 tbsp jalapeno
- 1/4 teaspoon baking powder (optional)
- Healthy yam keto sweetener

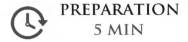 **PREPARATION** 5 MIN

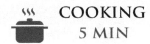 **COOKING** 5 MIN

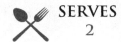 **SERVES** 2

DIRECTIONS

- Preheat the waffle iron for about 5 minutes until hot.
- If your recipe includes cream cheese, put it in a bowl first. Gently heat in a microwave (15-30 seconds) or double boiler until soft and stir.
- Stir all remaining ingredients (except toppings, if any).
- Pour a sufficient amount of chaffle dough into the waffle maker and cover the surface firmly. (For a normal waffle maker, about 1/2 cup, for a mini waffle maker, about 1/4 cup.)
- Cook for about 3-4 minutes until brown and crisp.
- Carefully remove the chaffle from the waffle maker and set aside for a crisp noise. (Cooling is important for the texture!) If there is any dough, repeat.

Nutrition: Calories 243, Fat 19 g, Protein 11 g, Total carbs 5 g, Pure carbohydrates 2 g, Fiber 2 g, Sugar 0 g

19. BACON CHAFFLE OMELETS

INGREDIENTS

- 2 slices bacon, raw
- 1 egg
- 1 tsp maple extract, optional
- 1 tsp all spices

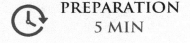 **PREPARATION** 5 MIN

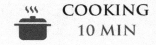 **COOKING** 10 MIN

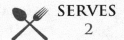 **SERVES** 2

DIRECTIONS

1. Put the bacon slices in a blender and turn it on.
2. Once ground up, add in the egg and all spices.
3. Go on blending until liquefied.
4. Heat your waffle maker on the highest setting and spray with non-stick cooking spray.
5. Pour half the omelet into the waffle maker and cook for 5 minutes max.
6. Remove the crispy omelet and repeat the same steps with rest batter.
7. Enjoy warm.

Nutrition: Calories per Serving 59 Kcal, Fats 4.4 g, Carbs 1 g, Protein 5 g,

20. ZUCCHINI CHAFFLES

INGREDIENTS

- 1/2 cup mozzarella cheese, finely shredded
- 1 egg
- 4 tbsp parmesan cheese, finely shredded
- 1 cup zucchini, grated
- ¼ tsp garlic powder
- ¼ tsp black pepper, ground
- ½ tsp Italian seasoning
- ¼ tsp salt

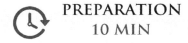 **PREPARATION**
10 MIN

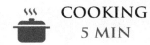 **COOKING**
5 MIN

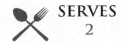 **SERVES**
2

DIRECTIONS

1. Sprinkle the zucchini with a pinch of salt and set it aside for a few minutes.
2. Squeeze out the excess water.
3. Warm up your mini waffle maker.
4. Mix all the ingredients in a small bowl.
5. For a crispy crust, add a teaspoon of shredded cheese to the waffle maker and cook for 30 seconds.
6. Then, pour the mixture into the waffle maker and cook for 5 minutes or until crispy.
7. Carefully remove.
8. Enjoy!

Nutrition: Calories per Serving 190 Kcal, Fats 13 g, Carbs 4 g, Protein 16 g

21. AVOCADO CHAFFLE TOAST

INGREDIENTS

- ½ avocado
- 1 egg
- ½ cup cheddar cheese, finely shredded
- 1 tbsp almond flour
- 1 tsp lemon juice, fresh
- Salt, ground pepper to taste
- Parmesan cheese, finely shredded for garnishing

 PREPARATION 4 MIN   **COOKING** 8 MIN   **SERVES** 2

DIRECTIONS

1. Warm up your mini waffle maker.

2. Mix the egg, almond flour with cheese in a small bowl.

3. For a crispy crust, add a teaspoon of shredded cheese to the waffle maker and cook for 30 seconds.

4. Then, pour the mixture into the waffle maker and cook for 5 minutes or until crispy.

5. Repeat with remaining batter.

6. Mash avocado with a fork until well combined and add lemon juice, salt, pepper

7. Top each chaffle with avocado mixture. Sprinkle with parmesan and enjoy!

Nutrition: Calories per Serving 250 Kcal, Fats 23 g, Carbs 9 g, Protein 14 g

22. BROCCOLI CHAFFLES

INGREDIENTS

- ½ cup cheddar cheese, finely shredded
- 1 egg
- 1/3 cup broccoli, fresh chopped
- 1 tbsp almond flour
- 1/3 tsp garlic powder

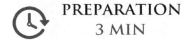 **PREPARATION**
3 MIN

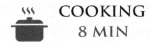 **COOKING**
8 MIN

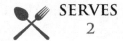 **SERVES**
2

DIRECTIONS

1. Warm up your mini waffle maker.
2. Mix the egg, almond flour, garlic powder with cheese in a small bowl.
3. Add half broccoli to the cheese mixture.
4. For a crispy crust, add a teaspoon of shredded cheese to the waffle maker and cook for 30 seconds.
5. Then, pour the mixture into the waffle maker and cook for 5 minutes or until crispy.
6. Repeat with remaining batter. Serve with fried slice of bacon and enjoy!

Nutrition: Calories per Serving 180 Kcal, Fats 13 g, Carbs 2 g, Protein: 11 g

23. CHICKEN CHAFFLES

INGREDIENTS

- 2 oz chicken breasts, cooked, shredded
- 1/2 cup mozzarella cheese, finely shredded
- 2 eggs
- 6 tbsp parmesan cheese, finely shredded
- 1 cup zucchini, grated
- ½ cup almond flour
- 1 tsp baking powder
- ¼ tsp garlic powder
- ¼ tsp black pepper, ground
- ½ tsp Italian seasoning
- ¼ tsp salt

 PREPARATION 5 MIN

 COOKING 15 MIN

 SERVES 4

DIRECTIONS

1. Sprinkle the zucchini with a pinch of salt and set it aside for a few minutes.

2. Squeeze out the excess water and warm up your mini waffle maker.

3. Mix chicken, almond flour, baking powder, cheeses, garlic powder, salt, pepper and seasonings in a bowl.

4. Use another small bow for beating eggs. Add them to squeezed zucchini, mix well.

5. Combine the chicken and egg mixture, and mix.

6. For a crispy crust, add a teaspoon of shredded cheese to the waffle maker and cook for 30 seconds.

7. Then, pour the mixture into the waffle maker and cook for 5 minutes or until crispy.

8. Carefully remove. Repeat with remaining batter the same steps. Enjoy!

Nutrition: Calories per Serving 135 Kcal, Fats 10 g, Carbs 3 g, Protein 11 g

24. CRUB CHAFFLES

INGREDIENTS

- 1 lb crab meat
- 1/3 cup Panko breadcrumbs
- 1 egg
- 2 tbsp fat Greek yogurt
- 1 tsp Dijon mustard
- 2 tbsp parsley and chives, fresh
- 1 tsp Italian seasoning
- 1 lemon, juiced
- Salt, pepper to taste

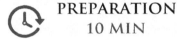 **PREPARATION** 10 MIN

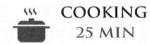 **COOKING** 25 MIN

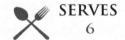 **SERVES** 6

DIRECTIONS

1. Preheat the waffle maker
2. Mix all the ingredients in a small mixing bowl, except crab meat.
3. Add the meat. Mix well.
4. Form the mixture into round patties.
5. Cook 1 patty for 3 minutes.
6. Remove it and repeat the process with the remaining crab chaffle mixture.
7. Once ready, remove and enjoy warm.

Nutrition: Calories per Serving 99 Kcal, Fats 8 g, Carbs 4 g, Protein 16 g

25. PROTEIN CHAFFLES

INGREDIENTS

- ¼ cup almond milk
- ¼ cup plant-based protein powder
- 2 tbsp almond butter
- 1 tbsp psyllium husk

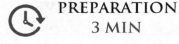 **PREPARATION**
3 MIN

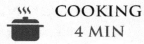 **COOKING**
4 MIN

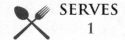 **SERVES**
1

DIRECTIONS

1. Preheat the waffle maker.
2. Combine almond milk, protein powder, psyllium husk and mix thoroughly until the mixture gets the form of a paste.
3. Add in butter, combine well and form round balls.
4. Place the ball in the center of preheated waffle maker.
5. Cook for 4 minutes.
6. Remove, top as prefer and enjoy.

Nutrition: Calories per Serving 310 Kcal, Fats 19 g, Carbs 5 g, Protein 25 g

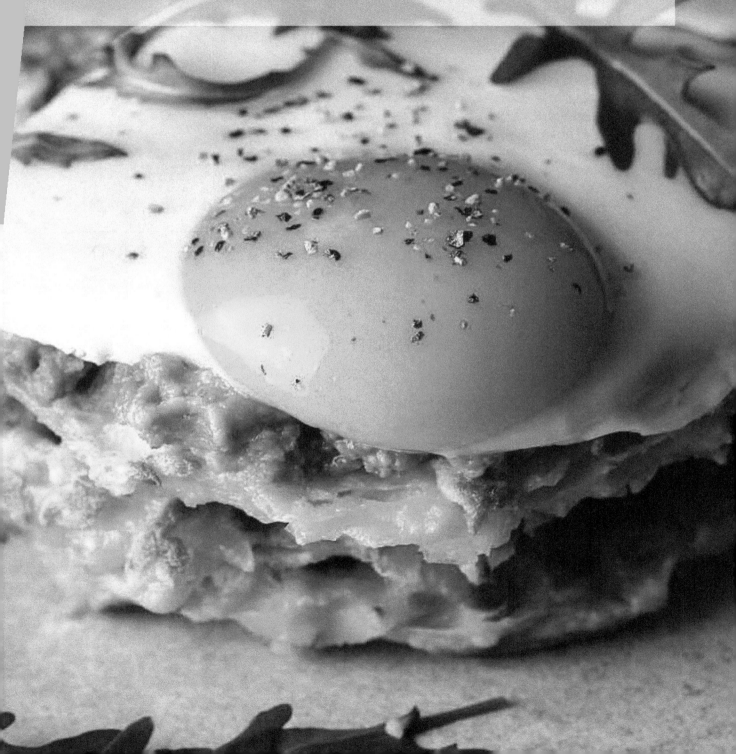

Chapter 7: Medium Difficulty Chaffle Recipes

26. HOT BROWN SANDWICH CHAFFLE

INGREDIENTS

- 1 egg, beaten
- 1/4 cup cheddar cheese, shredded and divided
- 2 slices fresh tomato
- 1/2 lb. roasted turkey breast
- 1/2 tsp parmesan cheese, grated
- 2 bacon, cooked
- 2 oz cream cheese, cubed
- 1/3 cup heavy cream
- 1/4 cup swiss cheese, shredded
- 1/4 tsp ground nutmeg
- White pepper

 PREPARATION
16 MIN

 COOKING
10 MIN

 SERVES
2

DIRECTIONS

1. Preheat the waffle maker.

2. Start by making the chaffle, once heated up, sprinkle 1 tbsp cheddar cheese onto the iron.

3. After 30 seconds, top the cheese with beaten egg.

4. Once the egg starts to cook, top the mixture with another layer of cheese.

5. Close the waffle maker lid and allow to cook for 3-5 minutes until the chaffle is crispy and golden brown.

6. Take out the cooked chaffle and repeat the steps until you've used up all the batter.

7. Make the sauce by combining heavy cream and cream cheese in a small saucepan.

8. Place saucepan over medium heat and whisk until the cheese completely dissolves.
9. Add in Swiss cheese and parmesan, then continue whisking to melt the cheese.
10. Add in the white pepper and nutmeg.
11. Continue whisking until you achieve a smooth consistency.
12. Remove the saucepan from heat.
13. Prepare the sandwich by setting the oven for broiling.
14. Cover a cookie sheet with aluminum foil.
15. Lightly grease the foil with butter, and place two chaffles on it.
16. Top the chaffles with 4 oz of turkey and a slice of tomato each. Add some sauce and grated parmesan on top.
17. Broil the chaffle sandwiches for 2-3 minutes until you see the sauce bubble and brown spots appear on top.
18. Remove from the oven. Put them on a heatproof plate.
19. Arrange bacon slices in a crisscross manner on top of the sandwich before serving.

Nutrition: Calories 572, Carbohydrates 3 g, Fat 41 g, Protein 41 g

27. BRULEED FRENCH TOAST CHAFFLE MONTE CRISTO

INGREDIENTS

- 1 egg
- 1/8 tsp baking powder
- 1/4 tsp cinnamon
- 1/2 tsp monk fruit
- 1 tbsp cream cheese
- 2 tsp brown sugar substitute
- 2 oz deli ham
- 2 oz deli turkey
- 1 slice provolone cheese
- 1/2 tsp sugar-free jelly

 PREPARATION 10 MIN

 COOKING 5 MIN

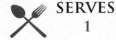 **SERVES** 1

DIRECTIONS

1. Preheat the waffle maker.

2. Place all the chaffle ingredients, except the sugar substitute, inside a blender. Make sure to place the cream cheese closest to the blades. Blend the ingredients until you achieve a smooth consistency.

3. Sprinkle the waffle maker with 1/2 tsp of brown sugar substitute.

4. Onto the waffle maker, pour 1/2 of the batter. Sprinkle another 1/2 teaspoon of the brown sugar substitute.

5. Close the lid and allow the batter to cook for 3-5 minutes.

6. Remove the chaffle. Repeat the steps until you used up all the batter.

7. Prepare the chaffle by spreading jelly on one surface of the chaffle.

8. Following this order, place the ham, turkey, and cheese in a small, microwaveable bowl. Place inside the microwave. Heat until the cheese is melted.

9. Invert the bowl onto the chaffle so that the contents transfer onto the chaffle. The cheese should be under the ham and turkey, directly sitting on top of the chaffle.

10. Top with the other chaffle and flip it over before serving.

Nutrition: Calories 368, Carbohydrate 7 g, Fat 22 g, Protein 34 g

28. LEMON CHAFFLE DOME CAKE

INGREDIENTS

- 2 eggs
- 2 oz cream cheese, softened
- 1 tbsp coconut flour
- 2 tsp heavy cream
- 2 tsp lemon juice
- 1/2 tsp vanilla extract
- 1/4 tsp stevia powder
- 1/4 tsp baking soda
- 8 oz cream cheese, softened
- 2 oz unsalted butter, softened
- 1 tbsp stevia powder
- 1 tbsp lemon zest

 PREPARATION
10 MIN

 COOKING
30 MIN

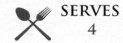 **SERVES**
4

DIRECTIONS

1. Preheat the mini waffle maker.

2. Combine all the chaffle ingredients using a blender.

3. Onto the preheated waffle maker, pour 1/4 of the batter.

4. Close the lid. Let the batter cook for 4-5 minutes. Remove the cooked chaffle using a pair of silicone tongs.

5. Repeat the steps to use up the remaining batter.

6. Let the chaffles cool completely.

7. Make the lemon frosting by combining the ingredients in a bowl.

8. Assemble by cutting two of the chaffles in half.

9. Use cling wrap to line a small bowl.

10. Place a whole chaffle in the bowl, carefully molding it to the shape of the bowl.

11. Line each side with the four chaffle halves.
12. Add half the amount of lemon frosting.
13. Cover the frosting with the last whole chaffle.
14. Cover the bowl with cling wrap. Put in the fridge for 30 minutes. You don't need to chill the remaining lemon frosting.
15. Invert the chaffle dome onto a plate.
16. Spread the remaining lemon frosting over it. Add decorations if desired.
17. Chill the cake for another 30 minutes. Serve.

Nutrition: Calories 405, Carbohydrates 3 g, Fat 38 g, Protein 9 g

29. KEEMA CURRY CHAFFLE

INGREDIENTS

- 2 eggs
- 3 oz mozzarella cheese, shredded
- 3 tbsp almond flour
- 1/2 tsp baking powder
- 1/4 tsp garlic powder
- 10.5 oz ground beef
- 1 tbsp avocado oil
- 1/4 tsp salt
- 1/2 tsp garlic powder
- 1/4 tsp ginger powder
- 1/2 cup tomato puree
- 2 tbsp curry powder

- 2 tbsp Worcestershire sauce
- 4 tsp parmesan cheese, finely grated

 PREPARATION
10 MIN

 COOKING
10 MIN

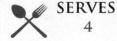 **SERVES**
4

DIRECTIONS

1. Start by making the curry, over medium heat, heat avocado oil in a frying pan.

2. Add in the ground meat and cook until it turns brown.

3. Add the ginger powder, garlic powder, and salt. Stir well.

4. Stir in the Worcestershire sauce and the tomato puree.

5. Finally, add the curry powder and stir it in.

6. Allow to simmer for about 6-10 minutes over low heat.

7. Preheat the mini waffle maker.

8. Combine all chaffle ingredients, except cheese, in a small mixing bowl.

9. Sprinkle some cheese onto the heated waffle maker and let it melt.

10. When the cheese melts, immediately pour 1/4 of the batter on top of it. Spread 2 tsp of keema curry then sprinkle some more cheese.

11. Close the lid. Cook for 4 minutes.

12. Remove the cooked chaffle and repeat the steps until you've used up all the batter.

13. Once all chaffles are cooked, use the remaining keema curry on top.

14. Top all the chaffles with parmesan cheese.

Nutrition: Calories 374, Carbohydrate 8 g, Fat 25 g, Protein 27 g

30. BROCCOLI AND CHEESE CHAFFLES

INGREDIENTS

- 1 egg
- 1/2 cup cheddar cheese
- 1/4 cup broccoli, freshly chopped
- 1/4 tsp garlic powder
- 1 tbsp almond flour

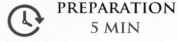 **PREPARATION** 5 MIN

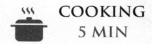 **COOKING** 5 MIN

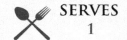 **SERVES** 1

DIRECTIONS

1. Preheat the waffle maker.

2. In a mixing bowl, combine cheddar cheese, almond flour, garlic powder, and egg. If you don't have a whisk, you can use a fork.

3. Pour in the cheese batter and half the chopped broccoli in the waffle maker. Allow to cook for 4 minutes.

4. Let the chaffle cool for 1-2 minutes before serving.

Nutrition: Calories 170, Carbohydrates 2 g, Fat 13 g, Protein 11 g

31. CHEESE AND HOT HAM CHAFFLES

INGREDIENTS

- 1 egg
- 1/2 cup Swiss cheese, shredded
- 1/4 cup Deli ham, chopped
- 1/4 tsp garlic salt
- 1 tbsp mayonnaise
- 2 tsp Dijon mustard

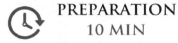 **PREPARATION**
10 MIN

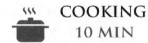 **COOKING**
10 MIN

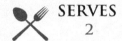 **SERVES**
2

DIRECTIONS

1. Preheat the waffle maker.

2. In a small bowl, start whisking the egg. Then add the ham, cheese, and garlic salt. Mix all the ingredients well.

3. Scoop up half of the batter and place in the hot waffle maker. Allow this to cook for 3-4 minutes.

4. Remove the cooked chaffle and repeat the prior step for the remaining batter.

5. For the dip, stir the Dijon mustard and mayonnaise together until full mixed.

Optional: You may slice the chaffles in halves, or just tear them up and dip them in the sauce.

Nutrition: Calories 435, Carbohydrate 4 g, Fat 32 g, Protein 31 g

32. TACO CHAFFLES

INGREDIENTS

- 1 egg white
- 1/4 cup Monterey Jack cheese, shredded
- 1/4 cup cheddar cheese, shredded
- 3/4 tsp water
- 1 tsp coconut flour
- 1/4 tsp baking powder
- 1/8 tsp chili powder
- Pinch of salt

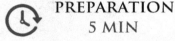 **PREPARATION** 5 MIN

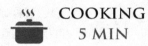 **COOKING** 5 MIN

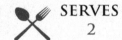 **SERVES** 2

DIRECTIONS

1. Preheat the waffle maker.
2. Mix all the ingredients into a mixing bowl.
3. Divide the batter into two. Spoon the first half into the waffle maker and close the lid.
4. Allow the batter to cook for up to 4 minutes.
5. Remove the taco chaffle once cooked and set aside. Cook the remaining batter.
6. Using a muffin pan, set the taco chaffles between the cups, carefully molding it to form a shape similar to a taco shell.

Nutrition: Calories 258, Carbohydrates 4 g, Fat 19 g, Protein 18 g

33. CRUNCH CEREAL CAKE CHAFFLE

INGREDIENTS

- 1 egg
- 2 tbsp almond flour
- 1/2 tsp coconut flour
- 1 tbsp butter, melted
- 1 tbsp cream cheese, softened
- 1/4 tsp vanilla extract
- 1/4 tsp baking powder
- 1 tbsp confectioners' sweetener
- 1/8 tsp xanthan gum
- 20 drops captain cereal flavoring
- Whipped cream

 PREPARATION 15 MIN

 COOKING 10 MIN

 SERVES 1

DIRECTIONS

1. Preheat the mini waffle maker.
2. Blend or mix all the chaffles ingredients until the consistency is creamy and smooth. Allow to rest for a few minutes so that the flour absorbs the liquid ingredients.
3. Scoop out 2-3 tbsp of batter and put it into the waffle maker. Allow to cook for 2-3 minutes.
4. Top the cooked chaffles with freshly whipped cream.
5. Add syrup and drops of Captain Cereal flavoring for a great flavor.

Nutrition: Calories 154, Carbohydrate 5.6 g, Fat 11.2 g, Protein 4.6 g

34. BAKED POTATO CHAFFLE USING JICAMA

INGREDIENTS

- 1 jicama root
- 1/2 onion, medium, minced
- 2 cloves garlic, pressed
- 1 cup cheese
- 1 eggs, whisked
- Salt and pepper

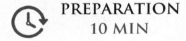 **PREPARATION** 10 MIN

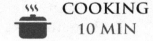 **COOKING** 10 MIN

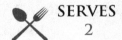 **SERVES** 2

DIRECTIONS

1. Peel the jicama root and shred it using a food processor.

2. Place the shredded jicama root in a colander to allow the water to drain. Mix in 2 tsp of salt as well.

3. Squeeze out the remaining liquid.

4. Microwave the shredded jicama for 5-8 minutes. This step pre-cooks it.

5. Mix all the remaining ingredients together with the jicama.

6. Start preheating the waffle maker.

7. Once preheated, sprinkle a bit of cheese on the waffle maker, allowing it to toast for a few seconds.

8. Place 3 tbsp of the jicama mixture onto the waffle maker. Sprinkle more cheese on top before closing the lid.

9. Cook for 5 minutes. Flip the chaffle and let it cook for 2 more minutes.

10. Serve your baked jicama by topping it with sour cream, cheese, bacon pieces, and chives.

Nutrition: Calories 168, Carbohydrates 5.1 g, Fat 11.8 g, Protein 10 g

35. FRIED PICKLE CHAFFLE STICKS

INGREDIENTS

- 1 egg
- 1/2 cup mozzarella cheese
- 1/4 cup pork panko
- 6-8 pickle slices, thinly sliced
- 1 tbsp pickle juice

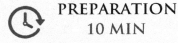 **PREPARATION**
10 MIN

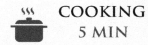 **COOKING**
5 MIN

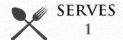 **SERVES**
1

DIRECTIONS

1. Mix all the ingredients, except the pickle slices, in a small bowl.

2. Use a paper towel to blot out excess liquid from the pickle slices.

3. Add a thin layer of the mixture to a preheated waffle iron.

4. Add some pickle slices before adding another thin layer of the mixture.

5. Close the waffle maker's lid and allow the mixture to cook for 4 minutes.

6. Optional: Combine hot sauce with ranch to create a great-tasting dip.

Nutrition: Calories 465, Carbohydrate 3.3 g, Fat 22.7 g, Protein 59.2 g

36. CHOCOLATE CHIP CHAFFLES

INGREDIENTS

- 1 egg
- 1 tsp coconut flour
- 1 tsp sweetener
- ½ tsp vanilla extract
- ¼ cup heavy whipping cream, for serving
- ½ cup almond milk ricotta, finely shredded
- 2 tbsp sugar-free chocolate chips

 PREPARATION 4 MIN

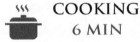 **COOKING** 6 MIN

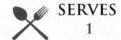 **SERVES** 1

DIRECTIONS

1. Preheat your mini waffle iron.
2. Mix the egg, coconut flour, vanilla, and sweetener. Whisk together with a fork.
3. Stir in the almond milk ricotta.
4. Pour half of the batter into the waffle iron and dot with a pinch of chocolate chips.
5. Close the waffle iron and cook for 5 minutes.
6. Repeat with remaining batter.
7. Serve hot with the whipped cream.

Nutrition: Calories 304 Kcal, Fats 16 g, Carbs 7 g, Protein 3 g

37. PUMPKIN CHAFFLES

INGREDIENTS

- 2 eggs
- ½ cup mozzarella cheese, shredded
- 1 tsp coconut flour
- ¾ tsp baking powder
- 2 tsp pumpkin puree
- ¾ tsp pumpkin pie spice
- 4 tsp heavy whipping cream
- 2 tsp Sugar-free maple syrup
- ½ tsp vanilla
- A pinch of salt

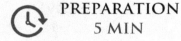 **PREPARATION** 5 MIN

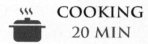 **COOKING** 20 MIN

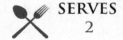 **SERVES** 2

DIRECTIONS

1. Preheat your chaffle maker.
2. In a small mixing bowl, combine all the ingredients and mix.
3. Pour the batter into the waffle maker and cook for 5 minutes.
4. Repeat this process until you have 4 chaffles.
5. Once ready, allow to cool and serve with sugar-free maple syrup.

Nutrition: Calories 200 Kcal, Fats 17 g, Carbs 4 g, Protein 12 g

38. OREO CHAFFLES

INGREDIENTS

Chocolate Chaffle:
- 2 eggs
- 2 tbsp cocoa, unsweetened
- 2 tbsp sweetener
- 2 tbsp heavy cream
- 2 tsp coconut flour
- 1/2 tsp baking powder
- 1 tsp vanilla

Filling:
- Whipped cream

 PREPARATION 2 MIN

 COOKING 5 MIN

 SERVES 2

DIRECTIONS

1. Preheat the mini waffle maker.
2. In a small bowl, add all chaffle Ingredients and mix well.
3. Pour half of the mixture into the waffle iron. Cook for 5 minutes.
4. Once ready, carefully remove and repeat with the remaining chaffle mixture.
5. Allow the cooked chaffles to sit for 3 minutes.
6. Once they have cooled, spread the whipped cream on the chaffles and stack them cream side facing down to form a sandwich.
7. Slice into halves and enjoy.

Nutrition: Calories 390 Kcal, Fats 40 g, Carbs 3 g, Protein 10 g

39. PEANUT BUTTER CHAFFLES

INGREDIENTS

For the chaffle:
- 3 eggs
- 3 tbsp cocoa powder, unsweetened
- 1 ½ tbsp sweetener
- 3 tbsp chocolate chips, sugar free
- 1 tsp espresso powder
- ½ cup finely shredded almond milk ricotta

For peanut butter filling:
- 4 tbsp creamy peanut butter
- 3 tbsp powdered sweetener
- 1 tbsp butter, softened

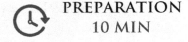 **PREPARATION**
10 MIN

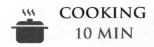 **COOKING**
10 MIN

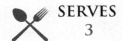 **SERVES**
3

DIRECTIONS

Chaffles:

1. Preheat the waffle iron.
2. Whisk together the eggs, sweetener, chocolate chops, cocoa powder, and espresso powder in a mixing bowl.
3. Pour in the almond milk ricotta. Mix thoroughly.
4. Pour half of the batter to the waffle pan and cook for 5 minutes.
5. Repeat with the remaining batter.
6. Set aside.

Peanut butter filling:

7. Add all the filling Ingredients to small bowl and mix using a fork until you have a smooth and creamy batter.

Assembling:

8. Spread the chaffles with the peanut butter and close to form a sandwich.
9. Slice into 3 quarters and enjoy.

Nutrition: Calories 215, Kcal Fats 15 g, Carbs 3 g, Protein 9 g

40. CHOCOLATE CHAFFLE

INGREDIENTS

- 1 egg
- 1 oz almond milk ricotta
- 1/8 tsp Monk fruit extract
- 1/8 tsp almond flavor extract
- 1 tbsp coconut oil
- 1.5 tsp cocoa powder

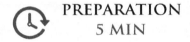 **PREPARATION** 5 MIN

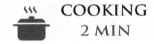 **COOKING** 2 MIN

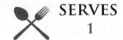 **SERVES** 1

DIRECTIONS

1. Melt the coconut oil and mix with the ricotta.
2. Whisk the egg and add to the coconut oil mixture.
3. Pour in the remaining Ingredients and continue whisking.
4. Once you have a thick batter, pour it into your waffle maker and cook for 5 minutes.
5. Remove, set aside to cool, and enjoy.

Nutrition: Calories 166, Kcal Fats 25 g, Carbs 4 g, Protein 10 g

41. PUMPKIN CHAFFLES

INGREDIENTS

- 1 egg
- 1/3 cup almond milk Ricotta, finely shredded
- 1 tbsp pureed pumpkin
- ¼ tsp cinnamon

 PREPARATION
3 MIN

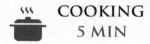 **COOKING**
5 MIN

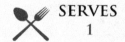 **SERVES**
1

DIRECTIONS

1. Pre-heat the waffle maker.
2. Mix the eggs, pumpkin puree, cheese, cinnamon and cloves in a small bowl.
3. Spray the waffle maker with non stick cooking spray.
4. Evenly pour the egg mixture into the waffle maker and cook for 5 minutes.
5. Carefully remove the chaffle from the pan and enjoy!

Nutrition: Calories 117 Kcal, Fats 13 g, Carbs 3 g, Protein 14 g

42. CHURRO CHAFFLES

INGREDIENTS

- 2 eggs
- 1 cup mozzarella cheese, shredded
- 4 tbsp swerve sweetener
- 1 tsp cinnamon

 PREPARATION
4 MIN

 COOKING
5 MIN

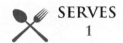 **SERVES**
1

DIRECTIONS

1. Preheat your waffle iron.
2. Whisk the eggs with a fork in a bowl. Add in the shredded cheese.
3. Pour half of the egg and cheese mixture into the waffle maker. Cook for 5 minutes or until golden brown.
4. In the meantime, add the cinnamon and the sweetener in a separate bowl.
5. By now, the chaffle is ready. Cut into slices and dip them into the cinnamon mixture while.
6. Serve and enjoy!

Nutrition: Calories 76 Kcal, Fats 4.4 g, Carbs 4 g, Protein 5.5 g

43. CHURRO CHAFFLES (VERSION 2)

INGREDIENTS

- 1 tbsp coconut cream
- 1 egg
- 6 tbsp almond flour
- ¼ tsp xanthan gum
- ½ tsp cinnamon
- 2 tbsp keto brown sugar

Coating:
- 2 tbsp butter, melt
- 1 tbsp keto brown sugar

 PREPARATION
5 MIN

 COOKING
10 MIN

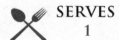 **SERVES**
1

DIRECTIONS

1. Add all the waffle Ingredients in a small bowl and mix until thick and sticky.
2. Warm up your waffle maker.
3. Pour half of the batter to the waffle pan and cook for 5 minutes.
4. Carefully remove the cooked waffle and repeat the steps with the remaining batter.
5. Allow the chaffles to cool and spread with the melted butter and top with the brown sugar.
6. Enjoy.

Nutrition: Calories 178 Kcal, Fat 15.7 g, Carb 3.9 g, Protein 2 g

44. CHOCOLATE BROWNIE CHAFFLES

INGREDIENTS

- 1 large egg
- ½ tsp baking powder
- 1 tbsp heavy cream
- 2 tbsp almond flour
- 1 tbsp cacao powder
- 1 ½ tbsp swerve sweetener
- 1 tsp vanilla extract
- ¼ cup dark chocolate chips

 PREPARATION
4 MIN

 COOKING
5 MIN

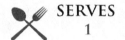 **SERVES**
1

DIRECTIONS

1. Mix well all the Ingredients.
2. Place 2 tablespoons of the batter onto the waffle maker.
3. Cook for 5 minutes.
4. Once ready, remove from the chaffle maker and allow to cool.
5. Enjoy.

Nutrition: Calories 358 Kcal, Fat 16 g, Carb 7 g, Protein 3 g

45. UBE CHAFFLES WITH ICE CREAM

INGREDIENTS

- 1/3 cup mozzarella cheese, shredded
- 1 tbsp whipped cream cheese
- 2 tbsp sweetener
- 1 egg
- 2-3 drops ube or pandan extract
- 1/2 tsp baking powder
- Keto ice cream

 PREPARATION 4 MIN

 COOKING 10 MIN

 SERVES 2

DIRECTIONS

1. Preheat your mini waffle maker.
2. Combine together all the Ingredients in a small bowl, except ube extract. Mix well.
3. Add in 2 or 3 drops of ube extract, mix until creamy and smooth.
4. Pour half of the batter mixture in the mini waffle maker and cook for about 5 minutes.
5. Repeat the same steps with the remaining batter mixture.
6. Top with keto ice cream and enjoy.

Nutrition: Calories 265 Kcal, Fat 16 g, Carb 7 g, Protein 22 g

46. STRAWBERRY SHORTCAKE CHAFFLE

INGREDIENTS

Sweet Chaffle:
- 1 tbsp almond flour
- ½ cup mozzarella cheese
- 1 egg
- 1 tbsp granulated swerve
- ¼ tsp vanilla extract
- Keto whipped cream

Strawberry Topping:
- 3 fresh strawberries
- ½ tbsp granulated swerve

 PREPARATION
5 MIN

 COOKING
12 MIN

 SERVES
2

DIRECTIONS

1. Heat up your mini waffle maker.

1. Clean and chop up your fresh strawberries.

2. Place them in a small mixing bowl, add ½ the granulated swerve and set aside.

3. In a separate mixing bowl, add the egg, almond flour, mozzarella cheese, vanilla extract, and the remaining granulated swerve.

4. Pour 1/3 of your batter mixture into the mini waffle maker. Cook for 4 minutes.

5. Repeat the process until you have 3 chaffles.

6. While your third chaffle is cooking, prepare your whipped cream.

Assembling:

7. Start by placing the whipped cream and chopped strawberries on top of the chaffles.

8. Next, drizzle all the juices that remain in the bowl and top with the strawberries.

Nutrition: Calories 112 Kcal, Fat 9 g, Carbs 2 g, Protein 7 g

47. CHAFFLE BIRTHDAY CAKE

INGREDIENTS

- Butter cream icing
- 3 tbsp cream cheese
- 1 tbsp almond flour
- 5 tbsp coconut flour
- 1 tsp baking powder
- 6 eggs
- 2 tbsp birthday cake syrup

 PREPARATION
10 MIN

 COOKING
16 MIN

 **SERVES**
4

DIRECTIONS

1. Thoroughly mix all the chaffle Ingredients until you have a thick texture.

2. Scoop 3 tbsp of the mixture into your waffle maker. Cook for 4 minutes and set aside.

3. Repeat the process until you have 4 cake chaffles.

4. Just like a normal cake, start assembling your cake by placing one chaffle at the bottom as the base and add a butter cream icing layer. Repeat the same process.

5. Pipe your cake edges with the icing and pile colorful shredded coconut at the center.

6. Once all the layers are completed, top with more icing and shredded coconut sprinkles. Enjoy!

Nutrition: Calories 390 Kcal, Fat 35 g, Carb 18.9 g, Protein 11 g

48. CREAM CAKE CHAFFLE

INGREDIENTS

For Chaffle:
- 4 oz cream cheese, softened
- 4 eggs
- 4 tbsp coconut flour
- 1 tbsp almond flour
- 1 ½ tsp baking powder
- 1 tbsp butter, softened
- 1 tsp vanilla extract
- ½ tsp cinnamon
- 1 tbsp sweetener
- 1 tbsp shredded coconut, colored and unsweetened
- 1 tbsp walnuts, chopped

For Italian Cream Frosting:
- 2 oz cream cheese, softened
- 2 tbsp butter, room temperature
- 2 tbsp sweetener
- ½ tsp vanilla

 PREPARATION 7 MIN

 COOKING 12 MIN

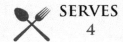 **SERVES** 4

DIRECTIONS

1. Add the almond flour, coconut flour, eggs, cream cheese, softened butter, vanilla, sweetener, and baking powder in a blender and blend until smooth.

2. Add the walnuts and shredded coconut to the mixture.

3. Blend the Ingredients on the high setting until you have a creamy mixture.

4. Preheat your waffle maker and add ¼ of the Ingredients.

5. Cook for 3 minutes and repeat the process until you have 4 chaffles.

6. Remove and set aside.

7. In the meantime, start making your frosting by mixing all the Ingredients together.

8. Stir until you have a smooth and creamy mixture.

9. Cool, frost the cake and enjoy.

Nutrition: Calories 127 Kcal, Fat 10 g, Carb 5.5 g, Protein 7 g

49. CHAFFLE GLAZED WITH RASPBERRY

INGREDIENTS

Donut Chaffle Ingredients:
- 1 egg
- ¼ cup mozzarella cheese, shredded
- 2 tsp cream cheese, softened
- 1 tsp sweetener
- 1tsp almond flour
- ½ tsp baking powder
- 20 drops glazed donut flavoring

Raspberry Jelly Filling:
- ¼ cup raspberries
- 1 tsp chia seeds
- 1 tsp confectioners sweetener
- Donut Glaze:
- 1 tsp powdered sweetener
- Heavy whipping cream

 PREPARATION 7 MIN

 COOKING 5 MIN

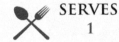 **SERVES** 1

DIRECTIONS

Chaffles:

1. Preheat your waffle maker.

2. Mix all the chaffle Ingredients.

3. Spray your waffle maker with cooking oil and add the batter mixture into the waffle maker.

4. Cook for 3 minutes and set aside.

Raspberry Jelly Filling:

5. Mix all the Ingredients under the filling portion.

6. Place in a pot and heat on medium.

7. Gently mash the raspberries and set aside to cool.

Donut Glaze:

8. Stir together the Ingredients in a small dish.

Assembling:

9. Lay your chaffles on a plate and add the fillings mixture between the layers.

10. Drizzle the glaze on top and enjoy.

Nutrition: Calories 188 Kcal, Fat 23 g, Carb 12 g, Protein 17 g

50. VANILLA CHAFFLES

INGREDIENTS

- 2 tbsp butter, softened
- 2 oz cream cheese, softened
- 2 eggs
- ¼ cup almond flour
- 2 tbsp coconut flour
- 1 tsp baking powder
- 1 tsp vanilla extract
- ¼ cup confectioners
- Pinch of pink salt

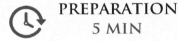 **PREPARATION** 5 MIN

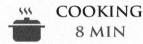 **COOKING** 8 MIN

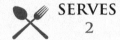 **SERVES** 2

DIRECTIONS

1. Preheat the waffle maker and spray with non-stick cooking spray.
2. Melt the butter and set aside for a minute to cool.
3. Add the eggs into the melted butter and whisk until creamy.
4. Pour in the sweetener, vanilla, extract, and salt. Blend properly.
5. Next add the coconut flour, almond flour, and baking powder. Mix well.
6. Pour into the waffle maker and cook for 4 minutes.
7. Repeat the process with the remaining batter.
8. Remove and set aside to cool.
9. Enjoy.

Nutrition: Calories 202 Kcal, Fat 27 g, Carb 9 g, Protein 23 g

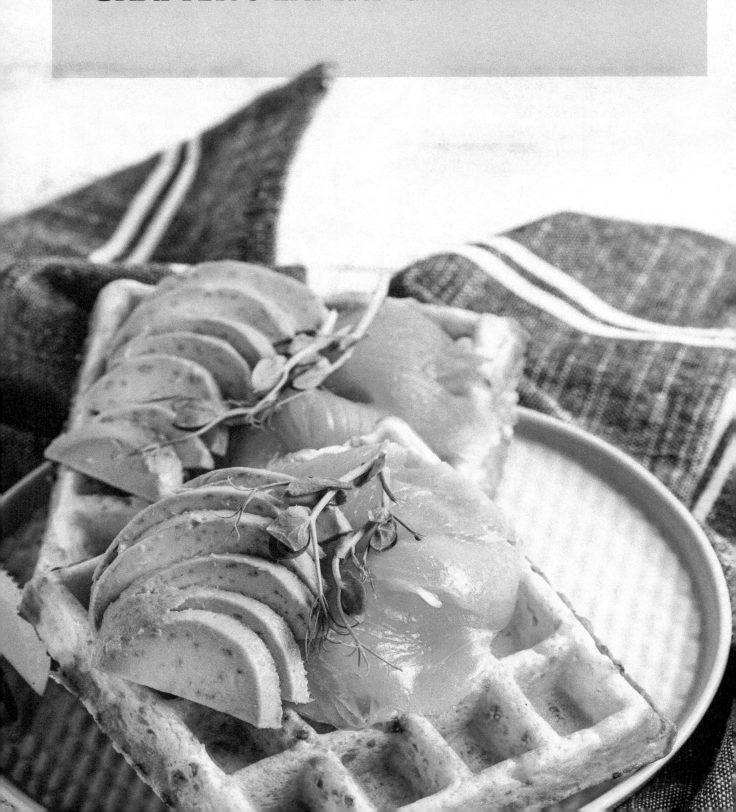

51. KETO STRAWBERRY SHORTCAKE CHAFFLE

INGREDIENTS

- 1 egg
- 1 tablespoon heavy whipped cream
- 1 tsp coconut flour
- 2 tablespoons of Lacanto Golden Sweetener (use 20% off wine)
- 1/2 teaspoon cake batter extract
- 1/4 teaspoon baking powder

 PREPARATION 2 MIN

 COOKING 4 MIN

 SERVES 2

DIRECTIONS

1. Preheat the maker of mini waffles.

2. Combine all the ingredients of the chaffle in a small bowl.

3. Pour half of the mixture of the chaffle into the waffle iron center. Allow 3-5 minutes to cook. If the chaffle rises, lift the lid slightly for a couple of seconds until it begins to go back down and restore the lid as it finishes.

4. Carefully remove the second chaffle and repeat it. Let the chaffles sit for a couple of minutes to crisp up.

5. Add your desired and enjoyed amount of whipped cream and strawberries!

NOTES: Recipe is perfect in a standard waffle maker for either two mini chaffles or one chaffle.

Nutrition (before the amount of strawberries and whipped cream you want): Calories 268, Total Fat 11.8 g, Cholesterol 121 mg, Sodium 221.8 mg, Total Carbohydrate 5.1 g, Dietary Fiber 1.7 g, Sugars 1.2 g, Protein 10 g, Vitamin A 133.5 µg, Vitamin C 7.3 mg

52. SLOPPY JOE CHAFFLE

INGREDIENTS

- 1 lb. ground beef
- 1 tsp onion powder
- 1 teaspoon of garlic
- 3 tbsp tomato paste
- 1/2 teaspoon
- 1/4 teaspoon pepper
- Chili powder 1 tbs
- 1 teaspoon of cocoa powder (optional but recommended)
- Usually 1/2 cup bone soup beef flavor
- 1 teaspoon coconut amino or soy sauce as you like

- 1 teaspoon mustard powder
- 1 teaspoon of brown or screen golden
- 1/2 teaspoon paprika

For corn bread chaffle:
- Make two chaffles
- 1 egg
- 1/2 cup cheddar cheese
- 5-slice jalapeno, very small diced (pickled or fresh)
- 1 tsp Frank Red hot sauce
- 1/4 teaspoon corn extract is optional but tastes like real

 PREPARATION 10 MIN

 COOKING 5 MIN

 SERVES 4

DIRECTIONS

1. First, cook the minced meat with salt and pepper.
2. Add all remaining ingredients.
3. Cook the mixture while making the chaffle.
4. Preheating waffle maker.
5. Put the eggs in a small bowl.
6. Add the remaining ingredients.
7. Spray to the waffle maker with a non-stick cooking spray.
8. Divide the mixture in half.
9. Simmer half of the mixture for about 4 minutes or until golden.
10. For a chaffled crispy rind, add 1 teaspoon cheese to the waffle maker for 30 seconds before adding the mixture.
11. Pour the warm stubby Joe Mix into the hot chaffle and finish! Dinner is ready!

Nutrition: Calories 156, Total Fat 3.9 g, Cholesterol 67.8 mg, Sodium 392.6 mg, Total Carbohydrate 3.9 g, Dietary Fiber 1.2 g, Sugars 1.6 g, Protein 25.8 g, Vitamin A 33.1 µg, Vitamin C 3.1 mg

53. BACON EGG & CHEESE CHAFFLE

INGREDIENTS

- ¾ of a chopped chess cup (I used a blend of sharp cheddar and mozzarella cheese)
- 2 eggs (scrambled)
- 3 slices of thin bacon.
- a pinch of salt
- ¼ teaspoon pepper

 PREPARATION
3 MIN

 COOKING
7 MIN

 SERVES
2

DIRECTIONS

1. Cut small pieces of bacon.

2. Scramble the egg in a medium-sized bowl and mix salt and pepper in the cheese, then add the pieces of bacon and mix them all together.

3. Preheat your waffle iron when it is open at the proper cooking temperature and pour the mixture into the center of the iron to ensure that it is distributed evenly.

4. Close your waffle iron and set the timer for 4 minutes and do not open too quickly. No matter how good it begins to smell, let it cook. A good rule to follow is that if the waffle machine stops steaming, the chaffle will be done.

5. When the time is up, gently open the waffle iron and make sure not all of it sticks to the top.

6. If so, use a Teflon or other non-metallic spatula to pry the Chaffle softly away from the top and then gently pull the Chaffle from the bottom and onto the plate after you have fully opened the unit.

Nutrition: Calories 490, Fat 15.7 g, Sodium 209 mg, Carbohydrates 9.9 g, Potassium 128 mg, Fiber 2.9 g, Sugar 0.9 g, Protein 11.5 g, Vitamin A 345 IU, Calcium 175 mg, Iron 1.8 mg

54. CRUNCHY KETO CINNAMON CHAFFLE

INGREDIENTS

- 1 tablespoon almond flour
- 1 egg
- 1 teaspoon of vanilla
- Cinnamon 1 shake
- 1 teaspoon baking powder
- 1 cup mozzarella cheese

 PREPARATION 5 MIN   **COOKING** 10 MIN   **SERVES** 2

DIRECTIONS

1. Mix the egg and vanilla extract in a bowl.
2. Mix powder, almond flour and cinnamon with baking.
3. Finally, add the cheese in the mozzarella and coat with the mixture evenly.
4. Spray oil on your waffle maker and let it heat up to its maximum setting.
5. Cook the waffle, test it every 5 minutes until it becomes golden and crunchy. A tip: make sure you put half of the batter in it. It can overflow the waffle maker, rendering it a sloppy operation. I suggest you put down a silpat mat to make it easy to clean.
6. With butter and your favorite low-carb syrup, take it out carefully.

Nutrition: Calories 450, Fat 15.7 g, Sodium 209 mg, Carbohydrates 9 g, Potassium 128 mg, Fiber 2.9 g, Sugar 1.5 g, Protein 14.5 g, Vitamin A 345 IU, Calcium 175 mg, Iron 1.8 mg

55. CRISPY BURGER BUN CHAFFLE

INGREDIENTS

- 1 egg
- 1/2 cup mozzarella cheese shredded
- 1/4 teaspoon baking powder
- 1/4 teaspoon glucomannan powder
- 1/4 teaspoon allulose or other sweetener
- 1/4 teaspoon caraway seed or other seasoning

 PREPARATION 5 MIN   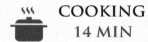 **COOKING** 14 MIN   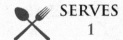 **SERVES** 1

DIRECTIONS

1. In a pot, add all the ingredients and blend together with a fork.

2. Spoon part of the mixture into the waffle maker, depending on whether you want them soft or crispy, cook for 5 to 7 minutes.

3. Prepare as you usually do your burger. Usually I cook a bacon strip in a cast iron pan and then fry a burger over medium low heat with salt and pepper in the bacon fat. I add the cheese a couple of minutes after frying, pour in a 1/4 cup of water and place a metal bowl over the burger to steam the cheese. I like my burgers with lettuce, tomato, onion, a bit of ranch dressing, salt, and pepper. But, that's me. You're doing it.

4. Pop it in the toaster oven when the first chaffle comes out to keep it warm while the second chaffle is being made, again for 5 to 7 minutes.

Nutrition: Calories 258, Fat 18.5 g, Carbohydrates 11 g, Sugar 1.3 g, Protein 16.5g

56. VEGAN KETO CHAFFLE WAFFLE

INGREDIENTS

- 1 tablespoon flax seed
- 2 glasses of water
- ¼ cup low carb vegan cheese
- 2 tablespoons coconut powder
- 1 tbsp low carb vegan cream cheese
- A pinch of salt

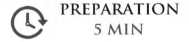 **PREPARATION** 5 MIN

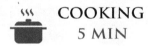 **COOKING** 5 MIN

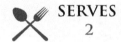 **SERVES** 2

DIRECTIONS

1. Preheat the waffle maker to medium high heat.
2. In a small bowl, mix flax seed meal and water. Leave for 5 minutes until thick and sticky.
3. Make flax eggs
4. Whisk all vegan chaffle ingredients together.
5. Meat vegan keto waffle
6. Pour vegan waffle dough into the center of the waffle iron. Close the waffle maker and cook for 3-5 minutes or until the waffles are golden and firm. If using a mini waffle maker, pour only half the dough.
7. Pour the waffle mixture into the waffle maker
8. Remove the vegan chaffle from the waffle maker and serve.

Nutrition: Calories 168, Fat 11.8 g, Cholesterol 121 mg, Sodium 221.8 mg, Total Carbohydrate 5.1 g, Dietary Fiber 1.7 g, Sugars 1.2 g, Protein 10g, Vitamin A 133.5 µg, Vitamin C 7.3 mg

57. GLUTEN-FREE CHAFFLES RANCHEROS

INGREDIENTS

- 2 tbsp. olive oil
- 1 onion and garlic.
- 1 cup of chopped tomato juice and black beans
- Cumin and eggs
- 1 cup almond milk
- 1 tbsp. jalapeno and butter.

 PREPARATION 10 MIN   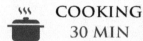 **COOKING** 30 MIN   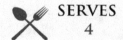 **SERVES** 4

DIRECTIONS

1. Take a pan and put some oil in it. Heat it for 4 minutes and add garlic and onions chopped.

2. Add tomato juice and sauce in it. Stir the mixture for 3 minutes.

3. Put cumin, beans, and salt in the mix. Cook it for 4 minutes

4. In a bowl, combine egg, jalapeno, butter, onion, salt, garlic, and milk.

5. Pour this batter in the waffle maker and heat it for 3 minutes.

6. Cook the egg and move it to the waffle and beans.

Nutrition: Calories 460, Carbohydrates 11 g, Proteins 17 g, Fats 24 g, Saturated Fat 1 g, Fiber 2 g

58. PUMPERNICKEL CHAFFLES

INGREDIENTS

- 3 cups of almond milk
- ¼ cup of sugar-free maple extract
- 3 eggs
- 3/4 cup almond flour
- Butter and sweetener.
- Salt and zero carb chocolate

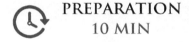 **PREPARATION** 10 MIN   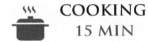 **COOKING** 15 MIN   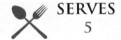 **SERVES** 5

DIRECTIONS

1. Heat the pan and add almond milk in it. Cook it until it boils.
2. Add maple extract, salt, and chocolate in it. Stir it for 4 minutes.
3. Add eggs and yeast in the mixture. Pour flour in the batter and cool it.
4. Beat eggs, butter, and sweetener together.
5. Pour it in the waffle maker and cook it for 3 minutes.
6. Serve waffles with butter.

Nutrition: Calories 950, Carbohydrates 16 g, Proteins 25 g, Fats 65 g, Saturated Fat 16 g, Fiber 5 g

59. LOADED "LIKE-POTATO" CHAFFLES

INGREDIENTS

- 2 jicama root (like potatoes replacement)
- 3 tbsp. butter and almond flour.
- 1 cup of cream
- 1/2 cup of cooked bacon
- 1 cup cheddar cheese, shredded.
- 1 tsp. salt and baking powder.

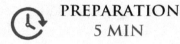 **PREPARATION** 5 MIN

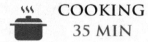 **COOKING** 35 MIN

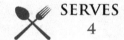 **SERVES** 4

DIRECTIONS

1. Peel the jicama root and shred it using a food processor.
2. Place the shredded jicama root in a colander to allow the water to drain. Mix in 2 tsp of salt as well.
3. Squeeze out the remaining liquid.
4. Microwave the shredded jicama for 5-8 minutes. This step pre-cooks it.
5. Mix all the remaining ingredients together with the jicama.Heat the oven on 200 F and waffle maker also.
6. Add butter on the maker and pour the mixture into it. Cook it 7 minutes.
7. Put waffle in the oven for 2 min and serve it with cream.

Nutrition: Calories 1392, Carbohydrates 19 g, Proteins 28 g, Fats 86 g, Saturated Fat 16 g, Fiber 15 g, Sugar 6 g

60. KIMCHI-CHEDDAR CHAFFLES

INGREDIENTS

- 2 cups of almond flour and cheddar cheese.
- 1 cup cabbage Kimchi and buttermilk.
- 1 tsp. baking powder and soda.
- Salt and 1 tsp. butter.
- 3 eggs
- 1 tbsp. chili peppers and scallion.

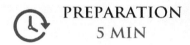 **PREPARATION** 5 MIN

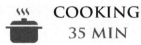 **COOKING** 35 MIN

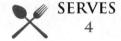 **SERVES** 4

DIRECTIONS

1. Heat the waffle maker and turn it on.
2. Combine baking powder, salt, and almond flour in a bowl.
3. In the next bowl, add Kimchi, cheese, eggs, buttermilk, butter, and scallion.
4. Pour the egg mix with the flour mix and place it on the waffle maker.
5. Cook it for 4 minutes and serve it with cream.

Nutrition: Calories 676, Carbohydrates 12 g, Proteins 32 g, Fats 56 g, Saturated Fat 31 g, Fiber 6 g, Sugar 8 g

61. RAISIN BELGIAN WAFFLE BREAD

INGREDIENTS

- 1 cup almond flour
- 1 tbsp. baking powder and caraway seeds.
- 1 cup of butter and almond milk.
- 1 tbsp. raisins, honey, sugar-free maple syrup, and oil.
- 1 tsp. baking powder and cinnamon.
- 2 eggs.

 PREPARATION
10 MIN

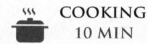 **COOKING**
10 MIN

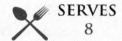 **SERVES**
8

DIRECTIONS

1. Take one bowl and add almond flour in it. Stir it with few seeds, baking powder.
2. Add salt, cinnamon, and raisins in it. Take another bowl, add almond milk and eggs in it.
3. Put some butter and honey in it. Place it into the flour mix.
4. Pour the mixture in the maker and cook it for 4 minutes.
5. Serve it with sugar-free maple syrup.

Nutrition: Calories 1291, Carbohydrates 60 g, Proteins 34 g, Fats 79 g, Saturated Fat 12.4 g, Fiber 30 g, Sugar 11 g

62. SAVORY CHAFFLES WITH CREMINI MUSHROOMS AND POACHED EGGS

INGREDIENTS

- 1 cup almond flour
- 1 tsp. baking powder
- 1 tbsp. Swerve and butter.
- 1 cup onion
- 1 tbsp. rosemary and salt
- 2 eggs
- 2 tbsp. oil

 PREPARATION
10 MIN

 COOKING
30 MIN

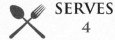 **SERVES**
4

DIRECTIONS

1. Heat the waffle maker with olive oil.
2. Take a bowl and add almond flour, egg, salts, and baking powder in it.
3. Use another bowl and mix rosemary and butter properly.
4. Take a pan and cook mushrooms and parsleys.
5. Serve with eggs on waffles and mushroom sauce.

Nutrition: Calories 501, Carbohydrates 13 g, Proteins 18 g, Fats 31 g, Saturated Fat 6 g, Fiber 9 g, Sugar 2 g

63. WAFFLED "LIKE-POTATO" BLINI WITH SMOKED SALMON

INGREDIENTS

- 2 jicama root (like potatoes substitute)
- Salmon
- 2 eggs
- 2 tbsp. dill and onion, chopped
- 3 tbsp. butter and almond flour
- Salt.
- Cream

 PREPARATION 5 MIN

 COOKING 40 MIN

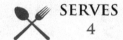 **SERVES** 4

DIRECTIONS

1. Peel the jicama root and shred it using a food processor.
2. Place the shredded jicama root in a colander to allow the water to drain. Mix in 2 tsp of salt as well.
3. Squeeze out the remaining liquid.
4. Microwave the shredded jicama for 5-8 minutes. This step pre-cooks it.
5. Heat the oven on 200 F and turn on the waffle maker on heat.
6. Take a bowl and mix onion, eggs, baking powder, and salt properly.
7. Add butter, dill, jicama, and almond flour in the mixture.
8. Pour this on waffle maker and cook it for 5 minutes.
9. Serve it with cream and salmon.

Nutrition: Calories 336, Carbohydrates 9 g, Proteins 29 g, Fats 20 g, Saturated Fat 4 g, Fiber 20 g, Sugar 3 g

64. CALZONE CHAFFLES

INGREDIENTS

- 2 cups of almond flour and buttermilk
- 2 tbsp. sweetener and baking powder.
- 1 cup mozzarella cheese
- 1 lb. salami
- 2 eggs
- 1 tbsp. butter
- Salt

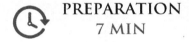 **PREPARATION** 7 MIN

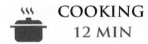 **COOKING** 12 MIN

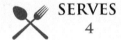 **SERVES** 4

DIRECTIONS

1. Combine buttermilk, eggs, and butter in one bowl and stir it properly.

2. Take another bowl and mix cheese, sweetener, salt, baking powder, and almond flour.

3. Heat the waffle maker and pour the batter in it. Place salami and mozzarella cheese on it.

4. Cook it for 10 minutes and serve it with sauce.

Nutrition: Calories 390, Carbohydrates 18 g, Proteins 25 g, Fats 27 g, Saturated Fat 0 g, Fiber 21 g, Sugar 2 g

65. VEGGIE CHAFFLE FRITTATA

INGREDIENTS

- 4 onions, chopped.
- ½ cup of parmesan, feta cheese.
- ½ cup almond flour and mushrooms.
- 2 tbsp. parsley and baking powder.
- 2 cups spinach
- 1 bell pepper

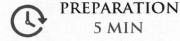 **PREPARATION** 5 MIN

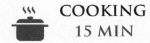 **COOKING** 15 MIN

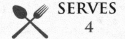 **SERVES** 4

DIRECTIONS

1. Take a pan and heat onion and pepper properly. Add mushrooms in it.
2. Cook it for 4 minutes. In a bowl, mix eggs and add almond flour and baking powder in it.
3. Now, place parmesan, cheese, parsley, and spinach.
4. Put it in the maker and heat it for 3 minutes. Serve it with sauce.

Nutrition: Calories 747, Carbohydrates 15 g, Proteins 57 g, Fats 51 g, Saturated Fat 21 g, Fiber 34 g, Sugar: 3 g

66. HOT PESTO CHAFFLES

INGREDIENTS

- 1 cup almond milk
- 1 cup mozzarella, shredded
- 1 cup coconut flour
- 3 tablespoons basil pesto
- 1 teaspoon hot paprika
- 1 teaspoon chili powder
- 2 eggs, whisked
- 1 tablespoon ghee, melted
- 1 teaspoon baking soda

 PREPARATION 10 MIN

 COOKING 7 MIN

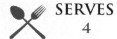 **SERVES** 4

DIRECTIONS

1. In a bowl, mix the almond milk with the cheese, pesto and the other ingredients and whisk.

2. Heat up the waffle maker.

3. Pour ¼ of the mix, cook for 7 minutes and transfer to a plate.

4. Repeat with the rest of the mix

5. Enjoy!

Nutrition: Calories 250, Fat 13 g, Fiber 4 g, Carbs 7.2 g, Protein 15 g

67. MONTE CRISTO CHAFFLES

INGREDIENTS

- 2 cups of almond flour and buttermilk
- 2 tbsp. sweetener and butter
- 4 eggs
- 1 cup cheese
- 1 lb. of ham
- 1 tbsp. baking powder and salt.

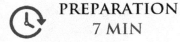 **PREPARATION**
7 MIN

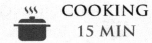 **COOKING**
15 MIN

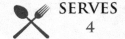 **SERVES**
4

DIRECTIONS

1. Combine buttermilk, eggs, and butter in one separate bowl.
2. Turn on the waffle maker for heating.
3. In another bowl, mix salt, sweetener, cheese, and baking powder.
4. Add almond flour into the mixture.
5. In a pan cook an egg with butter and place it on the waffles.
6. Serve it with maple and ham.

Nutrition: Calories 440, Carbohydrates 11 g, Proteins 29 g, Fats 21 g, Saturated Fat 7 g, Fiber 1 g, Sugar 3 g

68. CRISPY CHICKEN CHAFFLE WRAP

INGREDIENTS

- 3 chicken pieces
- Salt and pepper
- 1 tbsp. buttermilk
- 1 cup of almond flour
- 2 tsp. garlic powder and paprika
- 1 cup shredded cheese and milk
- Egg and olive oil

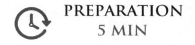 **PREPARATION** 5 MIN

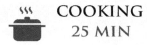 **COOKING** 25 MIN

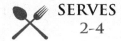 **SERVES** 2-4

DIRECTIONS

1. Marinate the chicken with buttermilk and salt.
2. Take a bowl and add paprika, garlic powder, salt, pepper, and almond flour.
3. Place chicken in this mixture. Fry chicken for 4 times.
4. Take a bowl and mix cheese, salt, pepper, milk, and oil together.
5. Add egg in it and stir it properly.
6. Cook it in the waffle maker and place it over chicken pieces.

Nutrition: Calories 170, Carbohydrates 6 g, Proteins 16 g, Fats 10 g, Saturated Fat 2 g, Fiber 2 g, Sugar 1 g

69. PULLED PORK CHAFFLE TOASTS

INGREDIENTS

- 2 cups of almond milk
- 2 tbsp. butter
- 2 tbsp. sugar-free maple syrup
- 2 cups Carbquik
- 1 egg
- 1 large pork

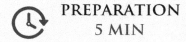 **PREPARATION**
5 MIN

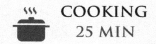 **COOKING**
25 MIN

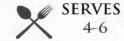 **SERVES**
4-6

DIRECTIONS

1. Preheat the waffle maker and turn it on.

2. Take a bowl and add butter, Carbquik, and egg in it. Stir it with the ladle and mix it properly.

3. Add almond milk in the bowl and make a smooth blend.

4. Place pork on the waffle maker and pour the batter around it. Cook it for 5 minutes.

5. Serve it with sugar-free maple syrup.

Nutrition: Calories 534, Carbohydrates 6 g, Proteins 23 g, Fats 30 g, Saturated Fat 9 g, Fiber 1 g, Sugar 3 g

70. ELOTE-STYLE CORNBREAD CHAFFLES

INGREDIENTS

- 2 cups of buttermilk
- 2 eggs
- 5 tbsp. butter and Swerve
- 1 cup of almond flour
- 1 tbsp. baking powder and salt
- 1 tbsp. baking soda

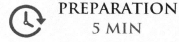 **PREPARATION** 5 MIN

 COOKING 25 MIN

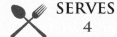 **SERVES** 4

DIRECTIONS

1. In a bowl, mix buttermilk, egg, butter, and oil.

2. Take another bowl and blend almond flour and ingredients and mix together.

3. Mix mayo, garlic, and lemon. Add paprika, pepper, and sauce in it.

4. Pour it on the waffle maker and place cheese and cream on it.

5. Heat it for 5 minutes and serve it.

Nutrition: Calories 240, Carbohydrates 16 g, Proteins 13 g, Fats 18 g, Saturated Fat 9 g, Fiber 1 g, Sugar 4 g

71. CHIVE WAFFLE TARTINE WITH OYSTER MUSHROOMS AND LEEKS

INGREDIENTS

- 1 cup almond flour
- 1 tsp. baking powder
- 2 tbsp. butter.
- 1 cup olives
- 1 tbsp. mushrooms and salt
- 2 eggs
- 2 tbsp. oil

 PREPARATION
10 MIN

 COOKING
30 MIN

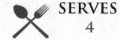 **SERVES**
4

DIRECTIONS

1. Heat the waffle maker with olive oil.
2. Take a bowl and add flour, egg, salts, and baking powder in it.
3. Use another bowl and mix mushrooms and butter properly.
4. Pour this batter in the waffle maker and cook it 6 minutes.
5. Take a pan and cook olives and parsleys.
6. Serve with eggs on waffles and mushroom sauce.

Nutrition: Calories 490, Carbohydrates 18 g, Proteins 26 g, Fats 48 g, Saturated Fat 7.6 g, Fiber 15 g, Sugar 4 g

72. SPICED SWEET POTATO WAFFLE TOSTADA

INGREDIENTS

- 2 jicama root (like potatoes substitute)
- 1 cup of almond flour and almond milk
- 1 cup cheddar cheese
- 1/2 diced onion, garlic, and bell pepper
- 2 eggs
- 2 tbsp. chili powder, pepper, and salt
- 1 tsp. cumin and coconut oil

 PREPARATION 10 MIN   **COOKING** 30 MIN   **SERVES** 4

DIRECTIONS

1. Peel the jicama root and shred it using a food processor.
2. Place the shredded jicama root in a colander to allow the water to drain. Mix in 2 tsp of salt as well.
3. Squeeze out the remaining liquid.
4. Microwave the shredded jicama for 5-8 minutes. This step pre-cooks it.
5. Heat the oven on 200 F and turn on the waffle maker on heat.
6. Add almond flour, cheese, eggs, garlic, almond milk, oil, and onion in a bowl.
7. Put salt and pepper in it.
8. Pour the batter in the waffle maker for 4 minutes.
9. Serve the waffles.

Nutrition: Calories 1800, Carbohydrates 18 g, Proteins 64 g, Fats 138.7 g, Saturated Fat 44.3 g, Fiber 12.7 g, Sugar 3 g

73. NEW YEAR KETO CHAFFLE CAKE

INGREDIENTS

- 4 oz. almond flour
- 2 cup cheddar cheese
- 5 eggs
- 1 tsp. stevia
- 2 tsp baking powder
- 2 tsp vanilla extract
- 1/4 cup almond butter, melted
- 3 tbsp. almond milk
- 1 cup cranberries
- 1 cup coconut cream

 PREPARATION 5 MIN   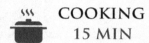 **COOKING** 15 MIN   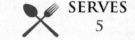 **SERVES** 5

DIRECTIONS

1. Crack eggs in a small mixing bowl, mix the eggs, almond flour, stevia, and baking powder.

2. Add the melted butter slowly to the flour mixture, mix well to ensure a smooth consistency.

3. Add the cheese, almond milk, cranberries and vanilla to the flour and butter mixture be sure to mix well.

4. Preheat waffles maker according to manufacturer instruction and grease it with avocado oil.

5. Pour mixture into waffle maker and cook until golden brown.

6. Make 5 chaffles

7. Stag chaffles in a plate. Spread the cream all around.

8. Cut in slice and serve.

Nutrition (Amount per serving 112 g): Calories 243, Fats 44,72 g, Protein 7.87 g, Net Carbs 1.67 g, Fiber 10 g, Starch 0 g

74. THANKSGIVING KETO CHAFFLES

INGREDIENTS

- 4 oz. cheese, shredded
- 5 eggs
- 1 tsp. stevia
- 1 tsp baking powder
- 2 tsp vanilla extract
- 1/4 cup almond butter, melted
- 3 tbsps. almond milk
- 1 tsp avocado oil for greasing

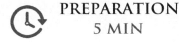 **PREPARATION**
5 MIN

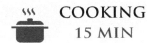 **COOKING**
15 MIN

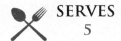 **SERVES**
5

DIRECTIONS

1. Crack eggs in a small mixing bowl; mix the eggs, almond flour, stevia, and baking powder.

2. Add the melted butter slowly to the flour mixture, mix well to ensure a smooth consistency.

3. Add the almond milk and vanilla to the flour and butter mixture, be sure to mix well.

4. Preheat waffles maker according to the manufacturer's instruction and grease it with avocado oil.

5. Pour the mixture into the waffle maker and cook until golden brown.

6. Dust coconut flour on chaffles and serve with coconut cream on the top.

Nutrition (Amount per serving 134 g): Calories 273, Fats 47 g, Protein 11 g, Net Carbs 4 g, Fiber 10 g, Starch 0 g

75. NEW YEAR CINNAMON CHAFFLE WITH COCONUT CREAM

INGREDIENTS

For Chaffles:
- 2 large eggs
- 1/8 cup almond flour
- 1 tsp. cinnamon powder
- 1 tsp. sea salt
- 1/2 tsp. baking soda
- 1 cup shredded mozzarella

For Topping:
- 2 tbsps. coconut cream
- 1 tbsp. unsweetened chocolate sauce

 PREPARATION 5 MIN

 COOKING 5 MIN

 SERVES 2

DIRECTIONS

1. Preheat waffle maker according to the manufacturer's directions.
2. Mix together recipe ingredients in a mixing bowl.
3. Add cheese and mix well.
4. Pour about ½ cup mixture into the center of the waffle maker and cook for about 2-3 minutes until golden and crispy.
5. Repeat with the remaining batter.
6. For serving, coat coconut cream over chaffles. Drizzle chocolate sauce over chaffle.
7. Freeze chaffle in the freezer for about10 minutes.
8. Serve on Christmas morning and enjoy!

Nutrition: (Amount per serving 122 g): Total Calories 260 kcal, Fats 16.11 g, Protein 24.5 g, Net Carbs 2.38 g, Fiber 0.7 g, Starch 0 g

76. THANKSGIVING PUMPKIN SPICE CHAFFLE

INGREDIENTS

- 1 cup egg whites
- ¼ cup pumpkin puree
- 2 tsps. pumpkin pie spice
- 2 tsps. coconut flour
- ½ tsp. vanilla
- 1 tsp. baking powder
- 1 tsp. baking soda
- 1/8 tsp cinnamon powder
- 1 cup mozzarella cheese, grated
- 1/2 tsp. garlic powder

 PREPARATION 5 MIN

 COOKING 5 MIN

 SERVES 4

DIRECTIONS

1. Switch on your square waffle maker. Spray with non-stick spray.

2. Beat egg whites with beater, until fluffy and white.

3. Add pumpkin puree, pumpkin pie spice, coconut flour in egg whites and beat again.

4. Stir in the cheese, cinnamon powder, garlic powder, baking soda, and powder.

5. Pour ½ of the batter in the waffle maker.

6. Close the maker and cook for about 3 minutes.

7. Repeat with the remaining batter.

8. Remove chaffles from the maker.

9. Serve hot and enjoy!

Nutrition: (Amount per serving 105 g): Total Calories 132 kcal, Fats 5.93 g, Protein 15.86 g, Net Carbs 1.61 g, Fiber 0.2 g, Starch 0 g

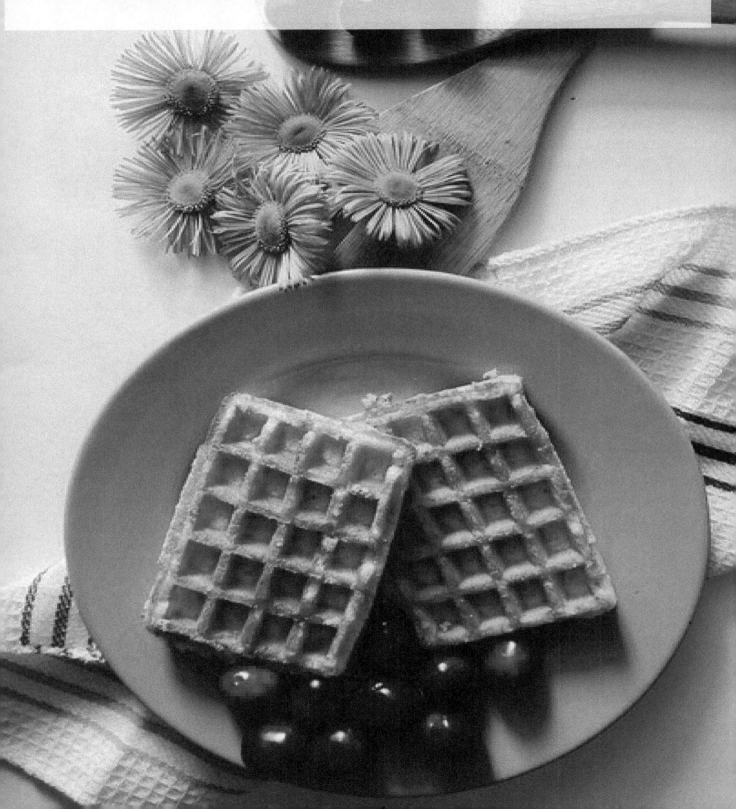

77. TOFU AND ESPRESSO CHAFFLES

INGREDIENTS

- 2 cups almond flour
- 2 teaspoons cinnamon powder
- 1 tablespoon baking soda
- ½ teaspoon vanilla extract
- 11 ounces soft tofu, non GMO, crumbled
- ½ cup butter, melted
- 4 tablespoons stevia
- 1 tablespoon espresso

 PREPARATION
10 MIN

 COOKING
20 MIN

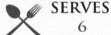 **SERVES**
6

DIRECTIONS

1. In a bowl, mix the flour with baking soda and cinnamon and stir.

2. In your blender, mix tofu with espresso and the other ingredients, pulse well, add to the flour mix and stir until you obtain a batter.

3. Heat up the waffle iron, pour 1/6 of the batter and cook for 6 minutes.

4. Repeat with the rest of the batter and serve the chaffles cold.

Nutrition: Calories 220, Fat 27 g, Fiber 2 g, Carbs 11 g, Protein 16 g

78. CRANBERRY CHAFFLES

INGREDIENTS

- 1 and ¾ cup almond flour
- 2 teaspoons baking powder
- ¼ cup swerve
- ¼ cup fat free Greek yogurt
- ¼ cup coconut butter
- 2 eggs, whisked
- 2 tablespoons cream cheese, soft
- ½ cup cranberries
- 1 teaspoon vanilla extract

 PREPARATION
10 MIN

 COOKING
10 MIN

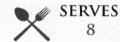 **SERVES**
8

DIRECTIONS

1. In a bowl, combine the flour with the baking powder and the other ingredients and whisk.
2. Heat up the waffle iron, pour 1/8 of the batter.
3. Cook for 5 minutes.
4. Repeat with the rest of the batter and serve the chaffles cold.

Nutrition: Calories 200, Fat 20 g, Fiber 0 g, Carbs 8 g, Protein 17 g

79. ALMOND BUTTER CHAFFLES

INGREDIENTS

- 2 eggs, whisked
- 2 tablespoons cream cheese, soft
- 1 cup almond butter
- 1 teaspoon almond extract
- ¼ cup almond flour
- 2 tablespoons stevia
- ½ teaspoon baking soda

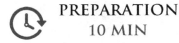 **PREPARATION** 10 MIN

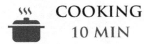 **COOKING** 10 MIN

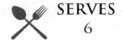 **SERVES** 6

DIRECTIONS

1. In a bowl, combine the cream cheese with the almond butter and the other ingredients and whisk.

2. Heat up the waffle iron, pour 1/6 of the batter and cook for 7 minutes.

3. Repeat with the rest of the batter, divide the chaffles between plates and serve.

Nutrition: Calories 140, Fat 12 g, Fiber 3 g, Carbs 2 g, Protein 8 g

80. AVOCADO AND YOGURT CHAFFLES

INGREDIENTS

- 2 cups coconut flour
- ½ cup cream cheese, soft
- ½ cup yogurt
- ½ teaspoon baking soda
- 1 teaspoon baking powder
- 2 tablespoons stevia
- 2 eggs, whisked
- 3 tablespoons coconut oil, melted

 PREPARATION
5 MIN

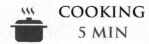 **COOKING**
5 MIN

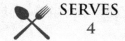 **SERVES**
4

DIRECTIONS

1. In a bowl, mix the flour with the yogurt and the other ingredients and whisk well.
2. Pour ¼ of the batter in your waffle iron, close.
3. Cook for 5 minutes.
4. Repeat this with the rest of the batter and serve your chaffles right away.

Nutrition: Calories 200, Fat 18 g, Fiber 2 g, Carbs 3 g, Protein 8 g

81. CHAFFLES AND RASPBERRY SYRUP

INGREDIENTS

For Chaffles:
- 2 tablespoons stevia
- 1 and ¼ cup coconut milk
- ¼ cup coconut oil, melted
- ½ teaspoon almond extract
- 1 cup almond flour
- ½ cup coconut flour
- 1 and ½ teaspoons baking powder
- ¼ teaspoon cinnamon powder

For the Syrup:
- 1 and 1/3 cup raspberries
- 4 tablespoons lemon juice
- ½ cup water

 PREPARATION 10 MIN

 COOKING 20 MIN

 SERVES 4

DIRECTIONS

1. In a bowl, mix the stevia with the coconut oil, milk and the other ingredients except the ones for the syrup and whisk.

2. Pour ¼ of the batter in your waffle iron, cover and cook for about 5 minutes.

3. Transfer to a plate and repeat with the rest of the batter.

4. Meanwhile, combine the raspberries with the lemon juice and the water, whisk heat up over medium heat for 10 minutes.

5. Drizzle the raspberry mix over your chaffles and serve.

Nutrition: Calories 230, Fat 16 g, Fiber 5 g, Carbs 3 g, Protein 10 g

82. PUMPKIN SEEDS CHAFFLES

INGREDIENTS

- 1 tablespoon coconut oil, melted
- 1 cup almond flour
- 1 egg, whisked
- 3 tablespoons cream cheese, soft
- 1 and ½ cups almond milk
- 3 tablespoons stevia
- 2 tablespoons pumpkin seeds
- 1 teaspoon vanilla extract
- 1 teaspoon baking soda

 PREPARATION
6 MIN

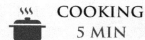 **COOKING**
5 MIN

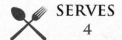 **SERVES**
4

DIRECTIONS

1. In a bowl, mix the melted coconut oil with the flour and the other ingredients and whisk well.

2. Heat up the waffle iron, pour ¼ of the batter and cook for 5 minutes.

3. Repeat with the rest of the batter.

4. Serve the chaffles cold.

Nutrition: Calories 220, Fat 14 g, Fiber 3 g, Carbs 3 g, Protein 9 g

83. ALMOND AND NUTMEG CHAFFLES

INGREDIENTS

- 1 cup coconut flour
- ½ cup cream cheese, soft
- ½ teaspoon nutmeg, ground
- 1 cup almond flour
- 3 eggs, whisked
- ¼ cup almond butter, melted

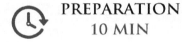 **PREPARATION** 10 MIN

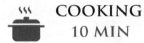 **COOKING** 10 MIN

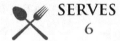 **SERVES** 6

DIRECTIONS

1. In a bowl, combine the flour with the cream cheese and the other ingredients and whisk.

2. Heat up the waffle iron, pour 1/6 of the batter and cook for 7 minutes.

3. Repeat with the rest of the batter and serve.

Nutrition: Calories 200, Fat 18 g, Fiber 3 g, Carbs 4 g, Protein 8 g

84. LEMON CHAFFLES

INGREDIENTS

- 1 cup almond flour
- 1 teaspoon baking powder
- ½ cup heavy cream
- 3 tablespoons cream cheese, soft
- 1 teaspoon baking soda
- 3 tablespoons coconut oil, melted
- 1 cup almond milk
- 3 tablespoons stevia
- ¼ cup lemon juice

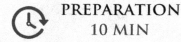 **PREPARATION**
10 MIN

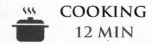 **COOKING**
12 MIN

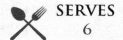 **SERVES**
6

DIRECTIONS

1. In a bowl, combine the flour with the cream and the other ingredients and whisk well.

2. Heat up the waffle iron, pour 1/6 of the batter and cook for 7 minutes.

3. Repeat with the rest of the batter and serve cold.

Nutrition: Calories 346, Fat 20 g, Fiber 1 g, Carbs 6 g, Protein 9

85. PEPPERMINT CHAFFLES

INGREDIENTS

- ¼ cup cream cheese, soft
- 2 eggs, whisked
- 1 cup coconut flour
- ½ cup coconut milk
- 3 tablespoons ghee, melted
- ¼ teaspoon vanilla extract
- ¼ teaspoon peppermint extract

 PREPARATION
10 MIN

 COOKING
10 MIN

 SERVES
8

DIRECTIONS

1. In a bowl, mix the cream cheese with the eggs and the other ingredients and whisk well.

2. Heat up the waffle iron, pour 1/8 of the batter and cook for 6 minutes.

3. Repeat with the rest of the batter and serve the peppermint chaffles cold.

Nutrition: Calories 170, Fat 16 g, Fiber 4 g, Carbs 4 g, Protein 8.4 g

86. LIME CHAFFLES

INGREDIENTS

- 1/3 cup almond butter, melted
- Juice and zest of 1 lime
- 1 cup almond flour
- ½ cup almond milk
- 3 tablespoons cream cheese, soft
- 1 egg, whisked
- 1 tablespoon stevia
- 1 and ½ tablespoons coconut oil

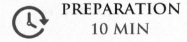 **PREPARATION**
10 MIN

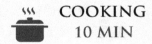 **COOKING**
10 MIN

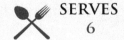 **SERVES**
6

DIRECTIONS

1. In a bowl, combine the almond butter with the lime juice, zest and the other ingredients and whisk well.

2. Heat up the waffle iron, pour 1/6 of the batter inside and cook for 7 minutes.

3. Repeat with the rest of the batter and serve the chaffles cold.

Nutrition: Calories 182, Fat 14 g, Fiber 2.3 g, Carbs 3 g, Protein 8.4 g

87. BLACKBERRY AND CRANBERRY CHAFFLES

INGREDIENTS

- 1 and ¾ cup coconut flour
- Zest from 1 lime, grated
- ¼ cup blackberries
- ¼ cup cranberries
- 2 teaspoons baking powder
- ¼ cup swerve
- ¼ cup heavy cream
- ¼ cup cream cheese, warm
- 2 eggs, whisked
- 1 teaspoon vanilla extract

 PREPARATION
10 MIN

 COOKING
10 MIN

 SERVES
6

DIRECTIONS

1. In a bowl, mix the flour with the berries, lime zest and the other ingredients and whisk well.

2. Heat up the waffle iron, pour 1/6 of the batter and cook for 8 minutes.

3. Repeat with the rest of the batter and serve.

Nutrition: Calories 200, Fat 16 g, Fiber 4 g, Carbs 5.4 g, Protein 8 g

88. FRUITY CHAFFLES

INGREDIENTS

- ½ cup almond flour
- ½ cup almond milk
- ½ cup coconut flour
- ½ cup cream cheese, soft
- 2 eggs, whisked
- 1 plum, pitted and chopped
- 1 avocado, peeled, pitted and chopped
- 1 mango, peeled, pitted and chopped
- ¼ teaspoon cinnamon, ground
- ½ teaspoon baking powder

 PREPARATION
10 MIN

 COOKING
10 MIN

 **SERVES**
6

DIRECTIONS

1. In your food processor, combine the flour with the milk, cream cheese and the other ingredients and pulse well.

2. Heat up the waffle iron over medium-high heat, pour 1/6 of the batter and cook for 8 minutes.

3. Repeat with the rest of the batter and serve the chaffles cold.

Nutrition: Calories 240, Fat 22 g, Fiber 5 g, Carbs 7 g, Protein 6.5

89. CHIA CHAFFLES

INGREDIENTS

- 1 cup almond flour
- 1 cup coconut cream
- 2 tablespoons chia seeds
- ¼ cup cream cheese, soft
- ¼ teaspoon almond extract
- ½ teaspoon baking soda
- 1 and ½ teaspoon baking powder
- 2 tablespoons swerve
- 2 eggs
- 3 tablespoons coconut oil, melted

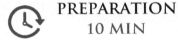 **PREPARATION** 10 MIN

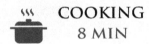 **COOKING** 8 MIN

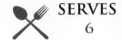 **SERVES** 6

DIRECTIONS

1. In a bowl, combine the flour with the cream, cream cheese and the other ingredients and whisk well.

2. Pour 1/6 of the batter in your waffle iron, close and cook for 6 minutes.

3. Repeat this with the rest of the batter and serve.

Nutrition: Calories 200, Fat 10 g, Fiber 2.3 g, Carbs 7, Protein 6 g

90. SWEET TOMATO CHAFFLES

INGREDIENTS

- 1 cup almond flour
- 3 tablespoons tomato passata
- 1 cup cream cheese, soft
- 2 eggs, whisked
- 1 tablespoon stevia
- 1 teaspoon avocado oil
- ½ cup coconut cream
- 1 tablespoon coconut butter, melted

 PREPARATION 5 MIN   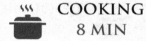 **COOKING** 8 MIN   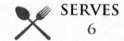 **SERVES** 6

DIRECTIONS

1. In a bowl, combine the flour with the passata and the other ingredients and whisk well.

2. Pour 1/6 of the batter into the heated waffle maker and cook for 8 minutes.

3. Repeat with the rest of the batter and serve.

Nutrition: Calories 220, Fat 14 g, Fiber 3 g, Carbs 4.5 g, Protein 7.5 g

91. SWEET CAULIFLOWER CHAFFLES

INGREDIENTS

- 1 tablespoon coconut oil, melted
- 1 and ½ cups almond milk
- 1 cup cauliflower rice
- 3 tablespoons stevia
- ½ cup almond flour
- ½ cup cream cheese, soft
- 1 egg, whisked
- 1 teaspoon vanilla extract
- 1 teaspoon baking soda

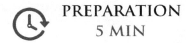 **PREPARATION**
5 MIN

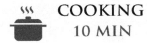 **COOKING**
10 MIN

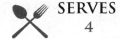 **SERVES**
4

DIRECTIONS

1. In a bowl, mix the almond milk with the cauliflower rice and the other ingredients and whisk well.

2. Pour ¼ of the batter in the waffle iron, cook for 8 minutes and transfer to a plate.

3. Repeat with the rest of the batter and serve the chaffles warm.

Nutrition: Calories 220, Fat 13 g, Fiber 3 g, Carbs 6 g, Protein 6.6 g

92. CHAFFLES WITH BLACKBERRY SAUCE

INGREDIENTS

Batter:
- cooking spray (such as Pam®)
- 2 cups almond flour
- 2 cups almond milk
- 2 eggs
- 1/3 cup vegetable oil
- 1 tablespoon baking powder
- 1/2 teaspoon salt
- 1/2 cup mozzarella cheese, shredded

Blackberry Sauce:
- 2 cups fresh blackberries
- 1/3 cup white Swerve
- 1 tablespoon lemon juice

 PREPARATION 15 MIN

 COOKING 15 MIN

 SERVES 4

DIRECTIONS

1. Preheat a waffle iron according to manufacturer's instructions.

2. Prepare the cooking surface with cooking spray.

3. Beat flour, milk, eggs, vegetable oil, baking powder, and salt together in a bowl using an electric mixer until batter is thoroughly mixed.

4. Add mozzarella cheese and stir well.

5. Pour about 1/4 cup batter per waffle into the preheated waffle iron and cook according to manufacturers' instructions.

6. Stir blackberries together in a saucepan over high heat until heated through, 3 to 4 minutes.

7. Decrease heat to medium and add sugar, cornstarch, and lemon juice to blackberries; cook and stir until sauce is thickened, about 5 minutes.

Nutrition: Calories 575, Total Fat 44.6 g, Cholesterol 103 mg, Sodium 746 mg, Total Carbohydrate 18 g, Protein 26.4 g

93. COCONUT OIL CHAFFLES

INGREDIENTS

- 1 ½ cups almond flour
- 2 tablespoons Swerve
- 2 teaspoons baking powder
- ½ cup mozzarella cheese, shredded
- ½ teaspoon salt
- 1 ½ cups almond milk, room temperature
- 1/3 cup virgin coconut oil, melted
- 1 large egg, beaten
- ½ teaspoon vanilla extract

 PREPARATION
10 MIN

 COOKING
5 MIN

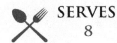 **SERVES**
8

DIRECTIONS

1. Preheat a waffle iron according to the manufacturer's instructions.
2. Whisk flour, sugar, baking powder, and salt together in a bowl
3. Make a well in the center of the flour mixture.
4. Beat milk, coconut oil, egg, and vanilla extract together in another bowl, add mozzarella cheese and stir well.
5. Pour into well in the flour mixture and stir until batter is just combined.
6. Ladle batter into preheated waffle iron and cook until golden and crisp, 2 to 5 minutes.

Nutrition: Calories 220, Total Fat 18.1 g, Cholesterol 27 mg, Sodium 295 mg, Total Carbohydrate 11.7 g, Protein 7.6 g

94. PECAN CHAFFLES

INGREDIENTS

- 2 cups almond flour
- 2 tablespoons Swerve
- 3 teaspoons baking powder
- 1/2 teaspoon salt
- 1/2 cup mozzarella cheese, shredded
- 2 large eggs, separated
- 1-3/4 cups fat-free milk
- 1/4 cup canola oil
- 1/2 cup chopped pecans

 PREPARATION
10 MIN

 COOKING
20 MIN

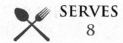 **SERVES**
8

DIRECTIONS

1. Preheat waffle maker.
2. Whisk together first four ingredients.
3. In another bowl, whisk together egg yolks, milk and oil.
4. Add to flour mixture, stirring just until moistened.
5. In a clean bowl, beat egg whites on medium speed until stiff but not dry.
6. Add mozzarella cheese and stir well.
7. Fold into batter. Bake chaffles according to manufacturer's directions until golden brown, sprinkling batter with pecans after pouring.

Freeze option: Cool chaffles on wire racks. Freeze between layers of waxed paper in a resealable plastic freezer bag. Reheat chaffles in a toaster or toaster oven on medium setting.

Nutrition: Calories 241, Total Fat 17 g, Cholesterol 48 mg, Sodium 338 mg, Total Carbohydrate 9 g, Protein 14 g, Fiber 3 g

95. CARBQUIK CHAFFLES

INGREDIENTS

- ½ cup egg substitute
- 1-3/4 cups almond milk
- ½ cup fat-free plain yogurt
- 1 tablespoon vanilla extract
- 2 cup Carbquik
- Sugar substitute equivalent to 1/2 cup sugar
- 2 tablespoons sugar
- 1/2 cup mozzarella cheese, shredded

- 4 teaspoons baking powder
- 1/4 teaspoon salt

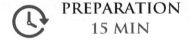 **PREPARATION**
15 MIN

 COOKING
20 MIN

 SERVES
20

DIRECTIONS

1. In a large bowl, beat egg substitute until frothy.

2. Stir in the milk, yogurt and vanilla.

3. Add mozzarella cheese and stir well.

4. Combine Carbquik, sugar substitute, baking powder and salt

5. Stir into almond milk mixture just until combined.

6. Bake in a preheated waffle iron according to manufacturer's directions until golden brown.

Nutrition: Calories 132, Total Fat 18 g, Cholesterol 2 mg, Sodium 273 mg, Total Carbohydrate 9 g, Protein 16 g, Fiber 2 g

96. ALMOND WAFFLE MIX

INGREDIENTS

- 4 cups almond flour
- 2 cups almond milk
- 1/4 cup toasted wheat germ
- 1/4 cup toasted oat bran
- 1 cup buttermilk blend powder
- 3 tablespoons baking powder
- 2 teaspoons baking soda
- 1 teaspoon salt
- 1/2 cup mozzarella cheese, shredded
- 2 eggs

- 1 cup water
- 2 tablespoons canola oil
- 1 tablespoons honey

 PREPARATION
10 MIN

 COOKING
10 MIN

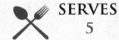 **SERVES**
5

DIRECTIONS

1. In a large bowl, combine the first nine ingredients.

2. Store in an airtight container in the refrigerator for up to 6 months.

3. Yield: 8-1/2 cups mix (about 4 batches).

To prepare chaffles:

4. Place 2 cups waffle mix in a bowl.

5. Combine the eggs, water, oil and honey.

6. Stir into waffle mix just until moistened.

7. Bake in a preheated waffle iron according to manufacturer's directions until golden brown.

Nutrition: Calories 284, Total Fat 19 g, Cholesterol 89 mg, Sodium 482 mg, Total Carbohydrate 11 g, Protein 15 g, Fiber 5 g

97. WHOLESOME KETO CHAFFLES

INGREDIENTS

- 1 cup almond flour
- 3 tablespoons ground flaxseed
- 3 teaspoons baking powder
- 1/2 teaspoon salt
- 2 eggs, separated
- 1/2 cup mozzarella cheese, shredded
- 2 cups almond milk
- 3 tablespoons canola oil
- 3 tablespoons unsweetened applesauce
- Mixed fresh berries, optional

 PREPARATION
15 MIN

 COOKING
5 MIN

 SERVES
12

DIRECTIONS

1. In a large bowl, combine the flour, flax, baking powder and salt.
2. Combine the egg yolks, almond milk, oil and applesauce.
3. Stir into dry ingredients until just moistened.
4. In a small bowl, beat egg whites until stiff peaks form; fold into batter.
5. Add mozzarella cheese and stir well.
6. Bake in a preheated waffle iron according to manufacturer's directions until golden brown.
7. Serve with berries if desired.

To freeze:

Arrange waffles in a single layer on sheet pans. Freeze overnight or until frozen.

Transfer to a resealable plastic freezer bag. Waffles may be frozen for up to 2 months.

To use frozen waffles: Reheat waffles in a toaster. Serve with berries and confectioners' sugar if desired.

Nutrition: Calories 278, Total Fat 19 g, Cholesterol 70 mg, Sodium 456 mg, Total Carbohydrate 11 g, Protein 18 g, Fiber 4 g

98. NUTTER BUTTER CHAFFLES

INGREDIENTS

For the chaffles:

- 2 tbsp sugar-free peanut butter powder
- 2 tbsp maple (sugar-free) syrup
- 1 egg, beaten
- ¼ cup finely grated mozzarella cheese
- ¼ tsp baking powder
- ¼ tsp almond butter
- ¼ tsp peanut butter extract
- 1 tbsp softened cream cheese

For the frosting:

- ½ cup almond flour
- 1 cup peanut butter
- 3 tbsp almond milk
- ½ tsp vanilla extract
- ½ cup maple (sugar-free) syrup

 PREPARATION
20 MIN

 COOKING
0 MIN

 SERVES
6

DIRECTIONS

1. Preheat the waffle iron.
2. Meanwhile, in a medium bowl, mix all the ingredients until smooth.
3. Open the iron and pour in half of the mixture. Close the iron and cook until crispy, 6 to 7 minutes.
4. Remove the chaffle onto a plate and set aside.
5. Make a second chaffle with the remaining batter.
6. While the chaffles cool, make the frosting.
7. Pour the almond flour in a medium saucepan and stir-fry over medium heat until golden.
8. Transfer the almond flour to a blender and top with the remaining frosting ingredients. Process until smooth.
9. Spread the frosting on the chaffles and serve afterward.

Nutrition: Calories 239, Fats 19.48 g, Net Carbs 7.92 g, Protein 9.52 g

99. WONDERFUL CHAFFLES

INGREDIENTS

- 2 ¼ cups almond flour
- 1 teaspoon baking soda
- 1 teaspoon baking powder
- ½ teaspoon salt
- ¼ cup butter
- ¼ cup Swerve
- ½ cup mozzarella cheese, shredded
- 3 egg yolks
- 2 cups buttermilk
- 3 egg whites

 PREPARATION
15 MIN

 COOKING
5 MIN

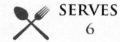 **SERVES**
6

DIRECTIONS

1. Preheat waffle iron. In a medium bowl, sift together almond flour, baking soda, baking powder and salt; set aside.

2. In a large bowl, cream butter and sweetener until light and fluffy. Add mozzarella cheese and stir well.

3. Beat in egg yolks. Blend in flour mixture alternately with buttermilk.

4. In a large glass or metal mixing bowl, beat egg whites until stiff peaks form.

5. Fold 1/3 of the whites into the batter, then quickly fold in remaining whites until no streaks remain.

6. Spray waffle iron with non-stick cooking spray, or lightly brush with oil. Ladle the batter onto preheated waffle iron. Cook the chaffles until golden and crisp. Serve immediately.

Nutrition: Calories 329, Total Fat 11.1 g, Cholesterol 126 mg, Sodium 638 mg, Total Carbohydrate 46.2 g, Protein 10.8 g

100. YEAST CHAFFLES

INGREDIENTS

- 2 cups almond milk
- 1 (0.25 ounce) package active dry yeast
- 1/2 cup warm water (110 degrees F/45 degrees C)
- 1/2 cup butter, melted
- 1 teaspoon salt
- 1 teaspoon sugar substitute
- 1/2 cup mozzarella cheese, shredded
- 3 cups almond flour
- 2 eggs, slightly beaten
- 1/2 teaspoon baking soda

 PREPARATION 30 MIN

 COOKING 10 MIN

 SERVES 6

DIRECTIONS

1. Warm the almond milk in a small saucepan until it bubbles, then remove from heat.

2. In a small bowl, dissolve yeast in warm water. Let stand until creamy, about 10 minutes.

3. In a large bowl, combine almond milk, yeast mixture, butter, salt, sugar substitute and flour. Add mozzarella cheese and stir well.

4. Mix thoroughly with rotary or electric mixer until batter is smooth.

5. Cover and let stand at room temperature overnight.

6. The next morning, stir beaten eggs and baking soda into the batter; beat well.

7. Spray preheated waffle iron with non-stick cooking spray. Pour mix onto hot waffle iron.

8. Cook until golden brown.

Nutrition: Calories 434, Total Fat 29.3 g, Cholesterol 109 mg, Sodium 661 mg, Total Carbohydrate 9.8 g, Protein 16.8 g

101. YOGURT CHAFFLES

INGREDIENTS

- 1 ¼ cups almond flour
- 1 ½ teaspoons baking powder
- 1 teaspoon baking soda
- ¼ teaspoon salt
- 2 cups (16 ounces) plain yogurt
- ¼ cup butter, melted
- 2 eggs
- 2 tablespoons honey
- ½ cup mozzarella cheese, shredded
- Raspberry, peach or strawberry low carbs yogurt
- Raspberries, blueberries

 PREPARATION
30 MIN

 COOKING
0 MIN

 SERVES
6

DIRECTIONS

1. In a bowl, combine the almond flour, baking powder, baking soda and salt.

2. Beat in plain yogurt, butter, eggs mozzarella cheese and honey until smooth.

3. Bake in a preheated waffle iron according to manufacturer's directions until golden brown.

4. Top with flavored yogurt and fruit.

Nutrition: Calories 516, Total Fat 24 g, Cholesterol 204 mg, Sodium 1089 mg, Total Carbohydrate 29 g, Protein 15 g, Fiber 1 g

CHAPTER 10: WHAT ARE THE ADVANTAGES OF KETOSIS?

Accomplishing a condition of ketosis can have numerous advantages from getting interminable ailments advancing execution. While the benefits are all around archived, the fundamental instrument of activity isn't altogether known. The eating regimen improves the capacity of mitochondria, the force plants of our cells, to convey our bodies' vitality needs in a way that diminishes aggravation and oxidative pressure. Through upgrading how our body utilizes vitality, we brace our bodies' capacity to battle a few illnesses just as take no the stressors of our cutting edge method for living.

The "Exemplary Keto" Approach

The reason behind going keto was straightforward: patients could be kept in a fasted state uncertainly on the off chance that they constrained their starch admission with the goal that their bodies consumed fat rather than glucose. Moving the dietary proportion for fat expelled sugar from the circulation system and set off the body to expend a corrosive known as ketone bodies. Effectively following the eating routine persuaded the authority to act metabolically as though it was starving.

Another Mayo Clinic doctor named Dr. Peterman gets acknowledgment for institutionalizing the eating routine into the "great keto" approach that is still followed today. Right now, specialists advocate for a 4:1 proportion of fat to protein and carbs, with 90 percent of calories originating from fat, six percent from protein, and only four percent from carbs. Although these proportions are as yet thought about the highest quality level, a 3:1 balance was likewise viewed as gainful.

Natural products (with some restraint): berries, avocado, rhubarb and coconut

In the beginning, emphases of the ketogenic diet, specialists underscored the significance of exact estimations for precise outcomes, implying that nourishment was frequently overloaded to the gram before utilization to keep members destined for success.

The outcome? An eating routine as viable as fasting for treating epilepsy that could be kept up for far longer. Presently in its subsequent century, the fundamentals of the eating methodology remain generally unaltered. Nutritionists recommended that members devour one gram of protein for every kilogram of body weight, 10-15 day by day grams of starches, and top off the rest of their eating regimen with fat.

Dietary Fat Delivers Results

How precisely does the ketogenic diet work? Researchers, despite everything, aren't sure. The essential hypothesis is that the regular structure of ketones makes them have an enemy of electrical impact on the mind. Great electric motivations trigger seizures, so getting these leveled out keeps seizures from happening.

Not long after the eating regimen formerly picked up prevalence for treating epilepsy, specialists began seeing advantages of ketosis that went outside seizure ability to control. Kids entertained with the eating routine were seen as being less crabby, progressively alarm, and simpler to train. These kids likewise rested better around evening time and had more vitality. (Further research in the mid-2000s approved these cases).

Coming back to Mainstream Attention

By the 1990s, the ketogenic diet was everything except overlooked, and the individuals who contemplated it consigned it to the domain of authentic interest, as opposed to medicinal truth.

So, what changed? The television program Dateline merits a significant part of the credit for reintroducing Americans to the ketogenic diet. An October 1994 scene wrote about the instance of Charlie, a two-year-old with extreme epilepsy whose seizures were wild until he began the keto diet. When Charlie looked for treatment at John Hopkins, less than ten kids were being controlled the ketogenic diet every year.

Watchers observed how the ketogenic diet lessened Charlie's seizures, and the show set off a blast of logical enthusiasm for it. The eating system pulled in so much consideration that the kid's dad coordinated the film "First Do No Harm" in 1997 about their involvement in the eating regimen, which featured Meryl Streep and disclosed on national TV.

The Modern Era of the Ketogenic Diet

After the resurgence of enthusiasm for following the ketogenic diet, it was before long offered in emergency clinics as a reasonable choice for treating epileptic patients. Today the ketogenic diet is accessible at practically all significant kids' emergency clinics, and it keeps on drawing in logical enthusiasm for its job in the neurological issue.

In any case, the narrative of the ketogenic diet doesn't end with epilepsy. If the eating plan's just favorable position was that it treated a generally uncommon ailment, far fewer individuals would be keen on it today. Instead, a great many people today are interested in the eating regimen for its capability to assist them with getting in shape. It's not so much clear when the keto diet initially stood out as a weight reduction arrangement, yet the early and late nineties were commanded by the Atkins diet and eating plan with a comparative point of view of carbs. This recharged enthusiasm for the eating routine's belongings made analysts investigate what it could offer in any case sound people, and the discoveries are noteworthy.

CONCLUSION

Keto diet can be a complicated affair, especially when you are starting out. This is especially the case when it comes to desserts, sugary food, and some diary stuff. If you are an ardent keto diet follower, I hope that my sweet and savory chaffle recipes cookbook will help you overcome the challenges you have been facing when preparing. Low-carb chaffles are super-easy to make, and the ingredients are readily available in your local supermarket or grocery store.

Regularly, keto dieters' lookout for ways to be accurate on the diet while searching for ways to make life easier at that. Chaffles are one of those foods that bring on a stimulating effect to the low-carb lifestyle. I find them to be an easy fix, and thankfully, they can be enjoyed different times of the day.

Meanwhile, while I found waffles to be addictive back then, I would say chaffles are waffles on steroids. They are moreish! Now, there isn't the need to deal with bulky, flour stuffed pastries when cheese and egg offer a better version. This blend, therefore, makes dieting simpler as chaffles are enriched with healthy fats and mostly with no carbs. Reaching ketosis just got easier!

Finally, they are convenient for prep-ahead meals. And we know how prepping meals aids with effective keto dieting. Chaffles can be frozen for later use, and they taste excellent when warmed and enjoyed later. Once you are hooked on chaffles, they will become a crucial part of your feeding because of the benefits that they bring. As soon as you quickly fall in love with chaffles, you will find that there are two major ways to enjoy them: sweet and savory. With that said, just like any other food, the key to making your chaffles tasty is by having the right tools and owning the ingredients.

Here are some of my tips that I have learned from my mistakes and successes. They will help you to make incredibly tasty chaffle recipes.

Many, if not all, chaffle recipes require you to use a teaspoon of baking powder or almond flour to give them a slightly more waffle-like texture and make them crispier.

Another tip for preparing really tasty chaffles is giving them ample time to cook. Always avoid opening the waffle prematurely as it may affect the doneness or crispness of your chaffles. If anything, the best chaffles tend to be those that are cooked for a slightly longer period.

I hope that my sweet and savory chaffle recipes cookbook will help you overcome the challenges you have been facing when preparing. Low-carb chaffles are super-easy to make, and the ingredients are readily available in your local supermarket or grocery store.